T0315090

SPORTS RESEARCH WITH ANALYTICAL SOLUTION USING SPSS®

SPORTS RESEARCH WITH ANALYTICAL SOLUTION USING SPSS®

J. P. VERMA
Centre for Advanced Studies
Lakshmibai National Institute of Physical Education

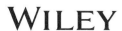

Library of Congress Cataloging-in-Publication Data has been applied for

Set in 10/12pt Times by SPi Global, Pondicherry, India

Printed in the United States of America

10   9   8   7   6   5   4   3   2   1

This book is dedicated to my father

Shri O P Verma

for his encouragement, support
and
continued confidence in me

CONTENTS

PREFACE

During the past three decades of my teaching statistics to the graduate students, I felt the need to produce a book that will help them in identifying research problems and solving them by means of a robust statistical software. The SPSS package has been chosen for this text. While organizing many workshops on research, statistics, and data analysis in many of the universities in India and abroad, I observed almost universally that the students at the graduate level find it difficult to identify research problems and analyze them by using appropriate statistical techniques. With this background in mind, I decided to produce this book as a self-learning material for the sports scientists and physical educationists. The USP of this book is the ease of understanding the contents even with little background knowledge of statistics. Each chapter is self-contained and starts with the need of the analysis, its details, application areas, and step-by-step solved examples with SPSS. Emphasis has been laid on the interpretation of results produced by SPSS.

Based on the contents of the book and its prospects of teaching computing skills using SPSS, the book is a go-to-text for every researcher from masters-level studies onward.

This book aims to provide a crisp, clear, and easy understanding of the methods, processes, and statistical techniques used in sports research, free from excessive unrelated material that comes in the way of the student's understanding. In each chapter, short-answer questions, multiple choice questions, and assignments have been provided as practice exercises for the reader. Case studies have been provided at the end of each chapter so that the users can appreciate the use of the technique discussed in that chapter and analyzing their research data by using SPSS.

Common mistakes like using two-tailed test for testing one-tailed hypothesis, using the phrase "level of confidence" for defining the "level of significance" or using the statement "accepting null hypothesis" instead of "not able to reject the null hypothesis" have been explained clearly in the text so that the readers may avoid them while organizing and conducting their research.

A teacher who uses this book as a text will be comfortable because it contains some illustrative studies with simulated realistic data at appropriate places to clarify and discuss the analytical technique covered in each chapter. Further, instructor's resources in the form of associated SPSS data file and PPT presentation for each chapter will make this book more useful for them. Some of the examples cited in the text are from my colleagues' and my own research studies.

The book consists of 12 chapters. Chapter 1 is an introductory chapter that deals with the data types, data cleaning, and procedure to start SPSS on your system. Chapter 2 deals with descriptive profile. Many students prepare descriptive profile in their dissertation. Besides computing procedure through SPSS, a new approach has been shown towards the end of the second chapter to develop the profile graph that can be used for comparing different domain of the populations.

Chapter 3 explains the procedure of computing correlation matrix and partial correlations using SPSS. Emphasis has been placed on how to interpret these correlations.

Chapter 4 deals with the application of t-test in the three situations namely one sample, two sample independent, and two sample dependent groups. The use of one- and two-tailed tests has been discussed thoroughly.

Chapter 5 explains the independent measures analysis of variance (ANOVA). Procedures have been explained by using SPSS to apply one-way ANOVA with equal and unequal samples as well as two-way ANOVA. A graphical approach has been discussed for post-hoc analysis of means besides using the p-value concept. Interaction analysis in two-way ANOVA has been discussed in detail by using SPSS software.

Chapter 6 discusses the repeated measures ANOVA's for solving research designs where same subjects undergo all the treatments. This design is very useful in sports research if it is difficult to get more subjects in the study. One-way and two-way repeated measures ANOVA have been discussed by means of solved examples with SPSS. This will help the researchers to identify their research problems where repeated measures ANOVA may be applied.

In Chapter 7, the application of ANCOVA has been discussed by means of a research example. Readers can find the procedure of analyzing their data much easier after going through this chapter.

Chapter 8 explains various nonparametric tests used by the researchers in their studies. A step-by-step procedure of computing all nonparametric tests, including chi-square, has been discussed by means of solved example with SPSS software.

In Chapter 9, multiple regression analysis has been discussed. Both the approaches of stepwise and backward regressions have been deliberated in detail.

Discriminant analysis technique, another widely used multivariate technique, has been discussed in Chapter 10. This technique can be used for developing a classifi-catory model in sports. This technique has tremendous application in sports and physical education research. Discussions of all its basics have been elaborated upon so that even a nonstatistician can appreciate it and use it in their research study.

Chapter 11 discusses the use of logistic regression for developing a logit model in a situation where the dependent variable is dichotomous and independent variable is either metric or nonmetric.

Chapter 12 explains the factor analysis, one of the most important multivariate analysis techniques used for talent identification in sports. Basics of this technique have been discussed for the beginners before showing the procedure of applying factor analysis using SPSS. Interpretation of each and every output has been very carefully explained for easy understanding of the readers.

At each and every step, care has been taken so that the readers can learn to apply SPSS and understand the minute details for each of the analysis which they will undertake.

The purpose of this book is to give a brief and straightforward description of how to conduct a range of statistical analysis using the SPSS software. We hope the book will encourage the students and researchers for adopting the self-learning approach in using SPSS for analyzing their data.

Students and other readers are welcome to e-mail me their query related to any part of this book.

J. P. Verma, PhD
Email: vermajp@bsnl.in

ABOUT THE COMPANION WEBSITE

This book is accompanied by a companion website:

www.wiley.com/go/Verma/Sportsresearch

The website includes:

- SPSS® data files
- Answers to multiple choice questions
- PowerPoint® slide presentations

ACKNOWLEDGMENTS

I am grateful to Professor S. R. Gangopadhyay for his excellent efforts in editing and also for his support in the preparation of this book. I extend my heartfelt thanks to Subhash Joshi, my colleagues, and my students of physical education, not only in my university, but also in other Indian and foreign universities, who constantly interacted with me for their research problems. They always encourage me by posing some challenging research problems for which the solutions have been provided in this text.

I would like to express my sincere gratitude to Susanne Steitz-Filler, Senior Editor, John Wiley & Sons and her team for providing me all the support and encouragement in presenting this book to the audience in its present form. I am thankful to Sari Friedman for providing me all the support and timely guidance in the publication of this text. She was very cooperative and supportive in dealing all my queries during the whole process of publication. At last I would like to thank Mary Rosechelle Ponce, Project officer, Kumudhavalli Narasiman, Deputy Manager and Dipak Durairaj, Production Editor in producing this book by copywriting, typesetting and editing the entire text.

I would like to place on record the contribution of my daughter Prachi and son Priyam for their valuable suggestions during preparation of this text. Finally, I must thank my wife Dr (Mrs) Haripriya Verma for not only providing a peaceful atmosphere during the long hours of working on this project but also contributing tremendously in checking the manuscript.

J. P. VERMA, PhD
Email: vermajp@bsnl.in

1

INTRODUCTION TO DATA TYPES AND SPSS OPERATIONS

LEARNING OBJECTIVES

After completing this chapter, you should be able to do the following:

- Understand different data types generated in research
- Learn the nature of variables
- Know various data cleaning methods
- Learn to install SPSS package in computer
- Prepare data file in SPSS

1.1 INTRODUCTION

Due to large stake involved in sports, research in this area is gaining momentum in different universities of the world. Even developing countries have started introducing sports sciences in different universities. The sole purpose is to create specific knowledge required for enhancing sports performance. Everyday, enormous data is being generated in the area of sports all over the world, which can be used to draw meaningful conclusions. Scientists have started organizing experiments by taking athletes as subjects. It is therefore required to support these scientists with analytical skill

---

Sports Research with Analytical Solution using SPSS®, First Edition. J. P. Verma.
© 2016 John Wiley & Sons, Inc. Published 2016 by John Wiley & Sons, Inc.
Companion website: www.wiley.com/go/Verma/Sportsresearch

set to carry out their business. Since they deal with the data, it is essential that they are aware of its nature. Depending upon the data types, one identifies the relevant analytical technique for addressing research issues. Sports research can broadly be classified into two categories: descriptive and analytical. In descriptive research, the nature of dataset is investigated from different perspectives. Several statistics like mean, standard deviation, coefficient of variation, skewness, kurtosis, and percentiles are used to describe the characteristics of the dataset. Many interesting facts about the population can be investigated by using these descriptive statistics. Analytical research broadly follows two approach: exploratory and confirmatory. In explorative research, focus is on discovering the hidden relationships. It is done by hypothesis testing, data modeling, and using multivariate analysis. On the other hand, in confirmatory studies, some of the facts are either confirmed or denied on the basis of hypothesis testing.

Numerous statistical techniques are available to the researchers for analyzing their research data. Selection of an appropriate technique depends upon the research questions being investigated in the study. Due to complexities of different analytical solutions in sports research, one needs to use some user-friendly software package. This chapter will acquaint you with different types of data that are generated in sports research and some of the widely used statistical techniques by the research scholars to solve them for answering different research questions by using the most popular IBM SPSS Statistics package.

1.2 TYPES OF DATA

It is essential to know the types of data generated in research studies because choosing statistical test for analyzing data depends upon its type. Data can be classified into two categories: metric and nonmetric. Metric data is analyzed by using parametric tests such as t, F, Z, correlation coefficient, etc., whereas nonparametric tests such as Wilcoxon signed-ranked, Chi-square, Mann–Whitney U, and Kruskal Wallis are used to analyze nonmetric data.

Parametric tests are more reliable than the nonparametric, but to use such tests certain assumptions must be satisfied. On the other hand, nonparametric tests are more flexible, easy to use, and not many assumptions are required to use them.

Nonmetric and metric data are also known as qualitative and quantitative data, respectively. Nonmetric data is further classified into nominal and ordinal. On the other hand, metric data is classified into interval and ratio. These classification is based on the level of measurements. The details of these four types of data have been discussed under two categories: qualitative data and quantitative data.

1.2.1 Qualitative Data

Qualitative data is a categorical measurement and is expressed not in terms of numbers, rather by means of a natural language description. It is often known as "categorical" data. For instance, smoking habit = "smoker" and gender = "male" are the examples of categorical data. These data can be measured on two different scales: nominal and ordinal.

1.2.1.1 Nominal Scale Variables measured on this scale are known as categorical variables. Categorical variables result from a selection of categories. Examples might be response (agree, disagree), sports specialization, race, religion, etc. If in a class 30 subjects are male and 20 are female, no gradation is possible. In other words, 30 do not indicate that the males are better than the female in some sense.

1.2.1.2 Ordinal Scale Variables that are assessed on the ordinal scale are also known as categorical variables, but here the categories are ordered. Such variables are also called "ordinal variables." Categorical variables that assess performance (good, average, poor, etc.) are ordinal variables. Similarly, the variables that measure attitude (strongly agree, agree, undecided, disagree, and strongly disagree) are also ordinal variables. On the basis of the order of these variables, we may not know the magnitude of the measured phenomenon of an individual, but we can always grade them. For instance, if A's playing ability in soccer is good and B's is average, we can always conclude that the A is better than B, but how much is not known. Moreover, the distance between the ordered categories is also not same and measurable.

1.2.2 Quantitative Data

Quantitative data is a numerical measurement expressed in terms of numbers. It is not necessary that all numbers are continuous and measurable. For instance, the roll number is a number, but not something that one can add or subtract. Quantitative data are always associated with a scale measure. These data can be measured on two different types of scales: interval and ratio.

1.2.2.1 Interval Scale The interval scale is a quantitative measure. It also has an equidistant measure. But the doubling principle breaks down in this scale. The 4 marks given to an individual for his creativity do not explain that his nature is twice as good as the person with 2 marks. This is so because on this scale zero cannot be exactly located. Thus, variables measured on an interval scale have values in which differences are uniform, but ratios are not.

1.2.2.2 Ratio Scale The data on ratio scale has a meaningful zero value and has an equidistant measure (i.e., the difference between 30 and 40 is the same as the difference between 60 and 70). For example, 60 marks obtained in a test is twice that of 30. This is so because zero exists in the ratio scale. Height is another ratio scale quantitative measure. Observations that are counted or measured are ratio data (e.g., number of goals, runs, height, and weight).

1.3   IMPORTANT DEFINITIONS

1.3.1   Variable

A variable is a phenomenon that changes from time to time, place to place, and individual to individual. It can be numeric or attribute. Numeric variable can further be classified into discrete and continuous. *Discrete variable* is a numeric variable that assumes value from a limited set of numbers and is always represented in whole number. Examples of such variables are number of goals, runs scored in cricket, scores in basketball match, etc. *Continuous variable* is also a numeric variable, but it can take any value within a range and is usually represented in fraction. Examples of such variables are height, weight, and timings.

On the other hand, an attribute is a qualitative variable that takes sub-values of a variable, such as "male" and "female," "student" and "teacher," etc. An attribute is said to be mutually exclusive if its sub-values do not occur at the same time. For instance, gender is a mutually exclusive variable because it can take value either "male" or "female" but not both. Similarly in a survey, a person can choose only one option from a list of alternatives (as opposed to selecting as many that might apply).

1.3.1.1   Independent Variable   An independent variable can be defined as the one that can be manipulated by a researcher. In planning a research experiment to see the effect of different intensities of exercise on the performance, exercise intensity is an independent variable because the researcher is free to manipulate it.

1.3.1.2   Dependent Variable   A variable is said to be dependent if it changes as a result of the change in the independent variable. In the previous example, performance is a dependent variable because it is affected by the change in exercise intensity. In fact dependent variable can be defined as the variable of interest. In creating the graph, the dependent variable is taken along the Y-axis, whereas the independent variable is plotted on the X-axis.

1.3.1.3   Extraneous Variable   Any additional variable that may provide alternative explanation or create some doubt on the conclusions in an experimental study is known as extraneous variable. If the effect of three different teaching methods on the performance is to be compared, IQ of the subjects may be considered as an extraneous variable as it might affect the final outcomes in the experiment, if IQ of all the groups are not equal initially.

1.4   DATA CLEANING

Data needs to be organized before preparing a data file. There are more chances that a dataset may contain unusual data due to wrong feeding or due to extreme cases. And if it is so, the analyzed results may lead to erroneous conclusions. Analysts tend to waste lots of time in drawing valid conclusions if the data is erroneous. Thus, it is utmost important that the data must be cleaned before analysis. In cleaned data, analysis becomes straightforward and valid conclusions can be drawn from it.

In data cleaning, first an unusual data is detected and then it is corrected. Some of the common sources of errors are as follows:

- Typing errors in data entry
- Not applicable option or blank options are coded as "0"
- Data for one variable column is entered under the adjacent column
- Coding errors
- Data collection errors

1.5 DETECTION OF ERRORS

The wrongly fed data can be detected by means of descriptive statistics. Some useful approaches in this regard are given in the text.

1.5.1 Using Frequencies

One of the methods of cleaning data is to use frequency of each score obtained in descriptive statistics. Since most of the behavioral parameters are normally distributed; therefore, if any anthropometric or physical variable shows large frequency for any values, it must be checked for any systematic error.

1.5.2 Using Mean and Standard Deviation

Normally, the value of standard deviation is less than the mean, except in case of the distribution like negative binomial. Thus, if the value of standard deviation for any of the variables like age, height, or cardio-respiratory index is more than its mean, then some of the values of these variables must be negative. However, the value of these variables cannot be negative, and thus one may identify the wrongly fed data.

1.5.3 Logic Checks

Data error may also be detected by observing whether responses are logical or not? For example, one would expect to see 100% of responses, not 110%. Another example would be if a question is asked to female respondents about their periods and the reply is marked "yes," but you notice that the respondent is coded "MALE." Logical approach is to be adopted with full justification, to avoid the embarrassing situation like in reporting that 10% of the men in the sample had periods during training.

1.5.4 Outlier Detection

The unusual data can also be identified by detecting the outliers. Any data that lies outside the two sigma limits can be considered to be outlier. In other words, data lying outside the range mean ± 2SD may be identified as an outlier and may be removed from the dataset. If a liberal view is adopted, then one can take mean ± 3SD limits to detect the unusual data. The outlier can be detected in a dataset by means of Boxplot discussed in Chapter 2.

1.6 HOW TO START SPSS?

This book has been written by using the IBM SPSS software. The SPSS package needs to be activated on the computer before entering the data. This can be done by clicking the left button of the mouse on SPSS icon in the SPSS directory in the **Start** and **All Programs** option (if the SPSS directory has been created in the programs file). Using the command sequence shown in Figure 1.1, SPSS can be activated. The last box is marked SPSS, but usually it will be followed by the version you are using.

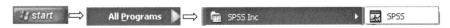

FIGURE 1.1   Sequence of commands for starting SPSS package.

By using the aforementioned command sequence and clicking **IBM SPSS Statistics 20** in the window shown in Figure 1.2, you will get the screen as shown in Figure 1.3 to prepare the data file or open the existing data file.

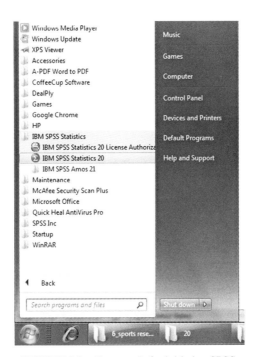

FIGURE 1.2   Commands for initiating SPSS.

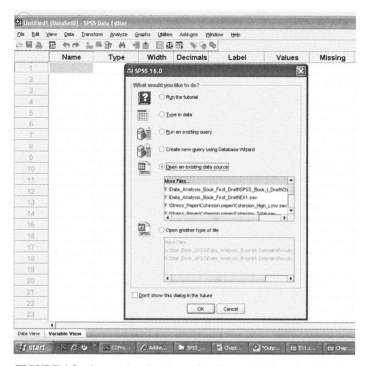

FIGURE 1.3 Screen showing the option for creating/opening data file.

If you are entering the data for a new problem and the file is to be created for the first time, check 'Type in data' option and if the existing file is to be opened or edited, then select the 'Open an existing data source' option in the window shown in Figure 1.3.

Click on **OK** to get the screen for defining variables in the **Variable View**.

1.6.1 Preparing Data File

The procedure of preparing data file shall be explained by means of the data shown in Table 1.1.

In SPSS, all variables need to be defined in the **Variable View** before feeding data. Once 'Type in data' option is selected in the screen shown in Figure 1.3, click on **Variable View**. This will allow you to define all variables in the SPSS. The blank screen shall look like as shown in Figure 1.4.

Now you are ready for defining variables row-wise.

1.6.1.1 Procedure for Defining Variables and Their Properties

Column 1: Under the column heading "Name," short names of the variables are defined. The variable name should essentially start with an alphabet only and may include underscore and numerals in between without any gap. If at all the variable needs to be defined in two words, then they must be joined by using the underscore such as Playing_Ability or Muscular_Strength.

TABLE 1.1 **Data on Anthropometric Parameters Obtained on College Badminton Players**

S.N.	Height (cm)	Weight (kg)	Arm Length (cm)	Leg Length (cm)	Trunk Length (cm)	Thigh Girth (cm)	Shoulder Width (cm)
1	177	66	82	89	91	50	36
2	172	75	74	90	85	52	41
3	180	68	85	87	91	51	44
4	189	49	81	96	91	54	48
5	180	55	75	95	86	47	37
6	175	74	82	89	88	51	43
7	187	73	86	93	92	52	42
8	181	69	73	96	84	50	44
9	171	68	75	87	86	54	43
10	180	62	78	92	91	48	39
11	177	66	72	91	85	53	44
12	163	68	71	88	77	52	45
13	162	65	73	87	76	54	46
14	168	67	74	89	78	53	48
15	165	69	75	91	79	51	47

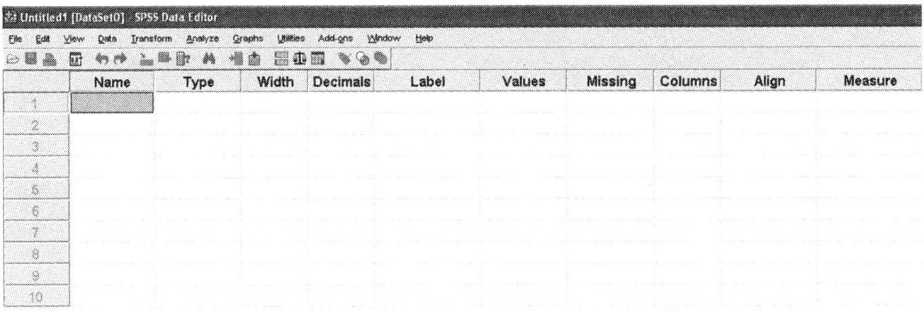

FIGURE 1.4   Blank format for defining variables.

Column 2: Under the column heading "Type," format of the variables (numeric or non-numeric) is defined. This can be done by double clicking the cell. The screen shall look like as shown in Figure 1.5.

Column 3: Under the column heading "Width," number of digits that a variable can have may be defined.

Column 4: In this column, the number of decimal a variable can have may be defined.

Column 5: Under the column heading "Label," full name of the variable can be written. User can take advantage of this facility to write expanded name of the variable.

Column 6: Under the column heading "Values," coding of the variable is defined by double clicking the cell if the variable is of classificatory in nature. For example, if there is a choice of choosing any one of the four sports—cricket, gymnastics, swimming, and athletics—then these sport categories can

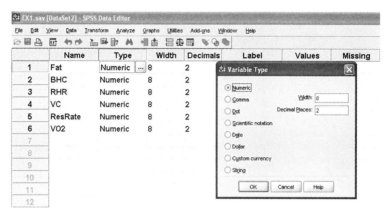

FIGURE 1.5 Defining variables and their characteristics.

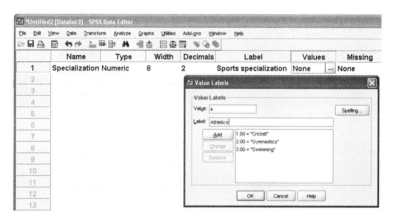

FIGURE 1.6 Defining code of nominal variable.

be coded as 1 = cricket, 2 = gymnastics, 3 = swimming, and 4 = athletics. While entering data into computer, these codes are entered as per the response of a particular subject. SPSS window showing the option for entering the code has been shown in Figure 1.6.

Column 7: In survey study, it is quite likely that a respondent may not reply certain questions. This creates the problem of missing value. Such missing value can be defined under column heading "Missing."

Column 8: Under the heading "Columns," the width of the column space where data is typed in **Data View** is defined (Figure 1.7).

Column 9: Under the column heading "Align," the alignment of data while feeding may be defined as left, right, or center.

Column 10: Under the column heading "Measure," the variable type may be defined as scale, ordinal, or nominal. Scale is used for interval and ratio data both.

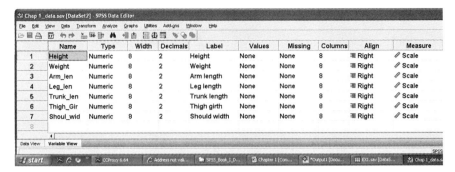

FIGURE 1.7   Variables along with their characteristics for the data shown in Table 1.1.

1.6.1.1.1   Defining Variables

1. Write short name of each of the seven variables as *Height, Weight, Arm_ len, Leg_len, Trunk_len, Thigh_Gir,* and *Shoul_wid* under the column heading "Name."
2. Under the column heading "Label," full names of these variables may be defined as *Height, Weight, Arm length, Leg length, Trunk length, Thigh girth,* and *Shoulder width.* One may define some other names as well.
3. Use default entries in rest of the columns.

After defining variables in **Variable View**, screen shall look like as shown in Figure 1.7.

1.6.1.1.2   Entering Data
After defining the variables, click the **Data View** option on the left corner in the bottom of the screen to open the format for entering data. For each variable, data can be entered column-wise. After entering data, the screen will look like as shown in Figure 1.8. Save the data file in the desired location before further processing.

After preparing the data file, one may use it for different types of statistical analysis available under the **Analyze** in SPSS. Various types of statistical analyses have been discussed along with their interpretations in different chapters of the book. Methods of data entry differ in different applications. Relevant details have been discussed in different chapters.

1.7   EXERCISE

1.7.1   Short Answer Questions

Note: Write answer to each of the questions in not more than 200 words.

Q.1   What do you mean by exploratory data analysis? Explain any one situation in research where such analysis can be applied.

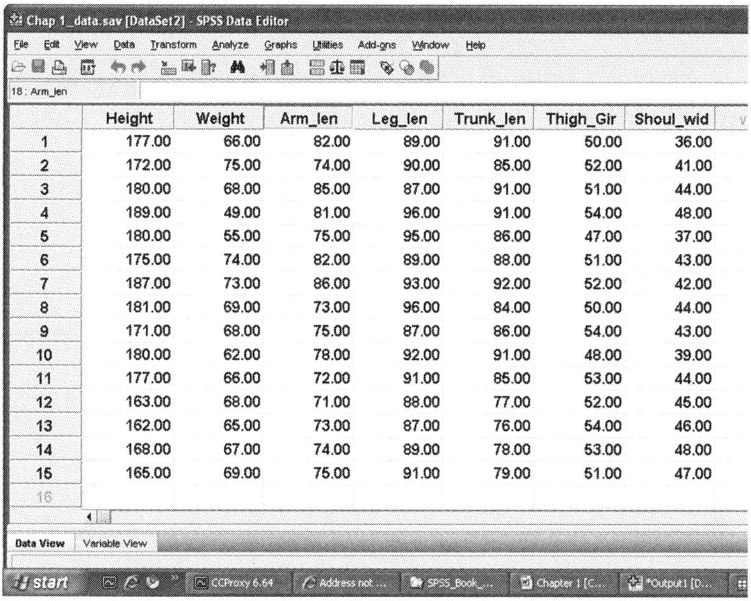

	Height	Weight	Arm_len	Leg_len	Trunk_len	Thigh_Gir	Shoul_wid
1	177.00	66.00	82.00	89.00	91.00	50.00	36.00
2	172.00	75.00	74.00	90.00	85.00	52.00	41.00
3	180.00	68.00	85.00	87.00	91.00	51.00	44.00
4	189.00	49.00	81.00	96.00	91.00	54.00	48.00
5	180.00	55.00	75.00	95.00	86.00	47.00	37.00
6	175.00	74.00	82.00	89.00	88.00	51.00	43.00
7	187.00	73.00	86.00	93.00	92.00	52.00	42.00
8	181.00	69.00	73.00	96.00	84.00	50.00	44.00
9	171.00	68.00	75.00	87.00	86.00	54.00	43.00
10	180.00	62.00	78.00	92.00	91.00	48.00	39.00
11	177.00	66.00	72.00	91.00	85.00	53.00	44.00
12	163.00	68.00	71.00	88.00	77.00	52.00	45.00
13	162.00	65.00	73.00	87.00	76.00	54.00	46.00
14	168.00	67.00	74.00	89.00	78.00	53.00	48.00
15	165.00	69.00	75.00	91.00	79.00	51.00	47.00

FIGURE 1.8 Format of data entry in most of the applications.

Q.2 What do you mean by ratio scale, and how is it different from interval scale?

Q.3 Under what situations should qualitative data be preferred? Explain its types with examples.

Q.4 Explain a situation in research where responses can be obtained on mutually exclusive attributes.

Q.5 What is an extraneous variable? How does it affect findings in an experiment? Suggest remedies for eliminating its effects.

Q.6 While feeding data in SPSS, what are the possible mistakes that a user may commit?

Q.7 Explain in brief as to how an error can be identified in data feeding.

1.7.2 Multiple Choice Questions

Note: Questions 1–10 have four alternative answers for each question. Tick mark the one that you consider the closest to the correct answer.

1 Read the following statements carefully:

(i) Parametric tests do not assume anything about the form of the distribution.

(ii) Nonparametric tests are simple to use.

(iii) Parametric tests are the most powerful, if their assumptions are satisfied.

(iv) Nonparametric tests are based upon the assumptions of normality.

Choose the correct statements.
(a) (i) and (ii)
(b) (i) and (iii)
(c) (ii) and (iii)
(d) (iii) and (iv)

2 If respondents were required to rate themselves on emotional strength on a 9-point scale, what type of data would be generated?
(a) Ratio
(b) Interval
(c) Nominal
(d) Ordinal

3 The term "categorical variables" are used for the data measured on
(a) Ratio and interval
(b) Interval and ordinal
(c) Interval and nominal
(d) Ordinal and nominal

4 In tossing an unbiased coin, one can get the following events E1: getting a head, E2: getting a tail. Choose the correct statement.
(a) E1 and E2 are independent.
(b) E1 and E2 are mutually exclusive.
(c) E1 and E2 are not equally likely.
(d) E1 and E2 are independent and mutually exclusive.

5 While creating a new data file in SPSS, which option should be used?
(a) Type in data
(b) Open an existing data source
(c) Open another type of file
(d) None

6 Identify valid name of a variable.
(a) CardioRes
(b) My Flexibility
(c) My Height
(d) Cardio-Res

7 While defining the types of the variable under the heading "Measure" in SPSS, what are the valid options out of the following:
 (i) Interval
 (ii) Scale
 (iii) Nominal
 (iv) Ordinal
(a) (i), (ii), and (iii)
(b) (i), (ii), and (iv)
(c) (i), (iii), and (iv)
(d) (ii), (iii), and (iv)

8   Choose the correct statement.
    (a) t-test and chi-square tests are parametric
    (b) t-test is parametric and chi-square test is nonparametric
    (c) t-test and chi-square tests are nonparametric
    (d) t-test is nonparametric and chi-square test is parametric

9   Runs scored in a cricket match is
    (a) Interval data
    (b) Ratio data
    (c) Nominal data
    (d) Ordinal data

10 In an experiment, the effect of different intensities of aerobic exercises on
    cardio-respiratory endurance has to be seen on the subjects. Choose the correct
    statement.
    (a) Aerobic intensity is a dependent variable and cardio-respiratory endurance
        is an independent variable.
    (b) Aerobic intensity is an independent variable and cardio-respiratory
        endurance is a dependent variable.
    (c) Aerobic intensities and cardio-respiratory endurance both are independent
        variables.
    (d) Aerobic intensities and cardio-respiratory endurance both are dependent
        variables.

2

DESCRIPTIVE PROFILE

LEARNING OBJECTIVES

After completing this chapter, you should be able to do the following:

- State circumstances in which a descriptive study can be undertaken
- Know about various statistics that can be used in profile study
- Understand the procedure for testing normality of data
- Learn to identify outliers in a dataset
- Learn to interpret various descriptive statistics
- Understand the application of descriptive statistics in sports research
- Explain the procedure of computing descriptive statistics using SPSS
- Discuss findings of the outputs generated by the SPSS in a descriptive study
- Describe methods used in preparing a profile chart in a descriptive study

2.1 INTRODUCTION

Most of the research studies are either descriptive or inferential in nature. In a descriptive study, basic characteristics of different parameters are studied; whereas in an inferential study, different kinds of inferences are drawn on various phenomena.

Sports Research with Analytical Solution using SPSS®, First Edition. J. P. Verma.
© 2016 John Wiley & Sons, Inc. Published 2016 by John Wiley & Sons, Inc.
Companion website: www.wiley.com/go/Verma/Sportsresearch

In both type of studies, generalized statements are made about the population on the basis of sample. In this section, we shall discuss about descriptive studies only.

In descriptive study, different statistics are computed to describe the nature of data. These statistics provide the summary of various measures in a dataset. Descriptive statistics are computed in almost all research studies.

The primary goal in a descriptive study is to describe a sample at one specific point in time without trying to make inferences or causal statements. Normally, there are three primary reasons to conduct such studies:

1. To provide knowledge about the system
2. To help in need assessment and planning resource allocation
3. To identify areas for further research

Descriptive studies are helpful in revealing patterns and relationships that might otherwise go unnoticed.

A descriptive study is undertaken in order to ascertain and describe the characteristics of the variables of interest in a given situation. For instance, a study of an institute in terms of the percentage of students who are in their postgraduate and undergraduate courses, gender composition, age grouping, and number of students belonging to different states can be considered as a descriptive study. Quite frequently, descriptive studies are undertaken in sports to understand the characteristics of a group of athletes such as age, participation level, fitness status, and skill performance.

Descriptive studies may also be undertaken to know the characteristics of institutes that offer similar programs. For example, one might want to know and describe the characteristics of the institutes that offer physical education programs. Thus, the goal of a descriptive study is to offer the researcher a profile or to describe the relevant aspects of the phenomena of interest of an individual institute, organization, industry, or a domain of population. In many cases, such information may be vital before considering certain corrective steps.

Descriptive statistics are used in conducting a profile study. In a typical profile study, we compute various descriptive statistics like mean, standard deviation (SD), coefficient of variation (CV), range, skewness, and kurtosis. These descriptive statistics explain different features of the data. For instance, mean explains an average value of the measurements, SD describes variation of scores around its mean value, CV provides relative variability of scores, range gives the maximum variation, skewness explains the symmetricity, and kurtosis describes the variation of a distribution.

In a descriptive study, one tries to obtain information concerning the current status of different phenomena. The purpose of such a study is to describe "what exists" with respect to situational variables. In such studies, the researcher first states an objective and then spells out various phenomena that are required to be investigated. Once the parameters required to be studied are identified, the method of data collection is planned to obtain a representative sample. It is important to define domain of the population clearly. The size of the sample should be decided on the basis of any of the two factors: cost or efficiency. For more information, readers are advised to refer to the book titled *Statistics for Exercise Science and Health with Microsoft Office Excel* (Verma, 2014) and *Repeated Measures Design for Empirical Researchers* (Verma, 2015).

Once the data is collected, it is compiled in a meaningful manner for drawing information. The nature of each variable can be studied by computing various descriptive statistics. If purpose of the study is analytical as well, then these data may further be analyzed for testing different formulated hypotheses.

On looking at the values of various descriptive statistics and graphical pictures, different kinds of generalizations and predictions can be made. While conducting descriptive studies, one gets an insight to identify the future scope of the related research studies.

2.2   EXPLANATION OF VARIOUS DESCRIPTIVE STATISTICS

In this section, different descriptive statistics that are used in descriptive studies shall be discussed in brief.

2.2.1   Mean

Each descriptive statistic reduces lots of data into a simpler summary. For instance, consider a simple number used to summarize how well a batsman is performing in cricket, the batting average. This single number is simply the number of runs scored in different matches divided by the number of matches played (assuming no not-out innings). A batsman whose average is 40 means every time he goes for bat, he scores 40. The single number describes a large number of discrete events. Similarly, consider the average height of basketball players in a team. This average number describes general height of a basketball player in the team. Thus, *mean* is an aggregate score that represents the whole sample.

2.2.2   Variance

Variance explains the variation of scores in dataset around its mean value. In other words, one can say that it measures the consistency. Higher variance indicates more heterogeneity in a group, whereas lower variance indicates more homogeneity of the scores. Square root of the variance is known as standard deviation.

Like variance, SD also explains the variability of scores around its mean value. By looking at the value of the SD, it is not possible to draw any conclusion about the variability of scores. It is because of the fact that the SD is an absolute variability. In order to know the extent of variability in the dataset, the SD has to be viewed in relation to the mean. Thus, SD cannot be used to compare the variability of two groups of scores having different means. To overcome this problem, another index of variability is defined which is known as CV. It is a relative variability and takes care of the mean value as well and is defined as follows:

$$CV = \frac{s}{\overline{X}} \times 100$$

where s is the standard deviation and $\overline{X}$ is the mean.

Since CV measures relative variability and is computed in percentage, it can be used to assess the variability of any variable with respect to its mean value. Further, it can also be used in comparing the variability of two groups in a situation when their mean values are not same. Since it is free from units, it can be used to compare the variability of two variables having different units.

Consider the data on sit-ups performance obtained on the students of class IX and XI on which the following statistics were obtained. Let us see what conclusion can be drawn from these information.

Class	IX	XI
Mean	35	25
SD	8	6
CV	$\frac{8}{35} \times 100 = 22.86\%$	$\frac{6}{25} \times 100 = 24\%$

The SD of the sit-ups data is larger in class IX in comparison to class XI, whereas CV is larger in class XI. Thus, it may be concluded that the variation among the student's performance in class XI on their sit-ups data is higher than that of the class IX students.

2.2.3 Standard Error of Mean

The standard error of the mean, SE $(\overline{X})$, is a measure of how much the mean varies from sample to sample drawn from the same population. The standard error of mean can be used to compare the observed mean to a hypothesized value. The two values may be different at 5% level if the ratio of the difference to the SE is less than -2 or greater than $+2$.

2.2.4 Skewness

Skewness gives an idea about the symmetricity of the data. It is measured by β_1.

$$\beta_1 = \frac{\mu_3^2}{\mu_2^3}$$

The value of β gives the magnitude of skewness only and does not provide the direction. Thus, another statistic γ_1 is used for skewness, which provides magnitude as well as direction both. The γ_1 is computed by the following formula:

$$\gamma_1 = \frac{\mu_3}{\left(\mu_2\right)^{3/2}}$$

For a symmetric distribution γ_1 is 0. A distribution having significant positive value of γ_1 has a long right tail, whereas a distribution having significant negative value of γ_1

(a)   (b)

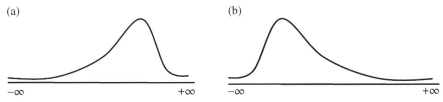

$-\infty$ $+\infty$ $-\infty$ $+\infty$

FIGURE 2.1   Distribution of IQ scores of the IIT and engineering students. (a) Negatively skewed curve and (b) positively skewed curve.

has a long left tail. In general, skewness value when more than twice its SE indicates a departure from symmetry. Thus, if the data is positively skewed, it simply means that the majority of the scores are less than its mean value; and in a negatively skewed curve, most of the scores are more than its mean value.

If the skewness of IQ scores for the IIT entrants is negative, then the distribution of the data would look like as shown in Figure 2.1a. Similarly, if the skewness of IQ scores for the students of engineering institute that does not have any ranking on the national list is positive, then the distribution of scores shall look like as shown in Figure 2.1b.

It can be concluded from Figure 2.1a that most of the IIT students have higher IQ scores in the group. Similarly, from Figure 2.1b, it may be interpreted that the majority of the engineering students have low IQ scores.

2.2.5   Kurtosis

Kurtosis is a statistical measure used for describing the distribution of the observed data around the mean. It measures the extent to which the observations cluster around the mean value.

It is measured by γ_2 and is computed as follows:

$$\gamma_2 = \beta_2 - 3 = \frac{\mu_4}{\mu_2^2} - 3$$

For a normal distribution, the value of kurtosis is zero. Positive value of kurtosis in a distribution indicates that the observations cluster more around its mean. In such situation, the curve is more peaked in comparison to that of normal distribution, whereas a distribution with negative kurtosis indicates that the observations cluster less around its mean and in that case the curve is more flat than that of the normal distribution. Depending upon the value of kurtosis, the distribution of scores can be classified into any one of the three categories: leptokurtic, mesokurtic, and platykurtic.

If for any variable the kurtosis is positive, the curve is known as leptokurtic, and it represents a low level of data fluctuation as the observations cluster around the mean. On the other hand, if the kurtosis is negative, the curve is known as platykurtic and that the data has more variability. Further, if the kurtosis is 0, the curve is classified as mesokurtic. The normal curve is a mesokurtic curve. These three types of curves are shown in Figure 2.2.

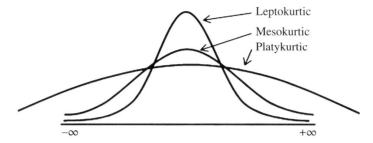

FIGURE 2.2   Distribution with different types of kurtosis.

2.2.6   Percentiles

Percentiles are used to develop norms on the basis of subject's performance. A given percentile indicates the percentage of scores below it and is denoted by P_x. For example, P_{40} is a score below which 40% scores lie. Median is also known as P_{50}, and it indicates that 50% scores lie below it.

Similarly, quartiles (the 25th, 50th, and 75th percentiles) divide the distribution into four quarters. If you want an equal number of groups other than four, select cut points for 'n' equal groups in SPSS. You can also specify any specific percentile value in SPSS for computation. Percentiles can be computed by choosing relevant option in SPSS, explained in the solved example.

2.3   APPLICATION OF DESCRIPTIVE STATISTICS

Descriptive statistics are used in studying the characteristics of a group of sub-jects. Such a study is often known as profile study. A profile study is undertaken in a situation where it is required to describe the nature of a particular population. For example, if a researcher is interested to know the basic traits of Indian wrestlers of interuniversity level, then all the wrestlers belonging to the univer-sities shall form the population in the study. One may typically investigate the following issues:

1. Testing normality of data
2. Identifying outliers in data
3. Understanding the nature of variables by investigating their SE, CV, skewness, and kurtosis
4. Developing percentile scale for each variable
5. Developing classification criteria
6. Comparison of performance on different parameters among the wrestlers in different weight categories

To cater to the aforementioned objectives, the following steps may be performed:

- Obtain data on physical, physiological, and psychological variables of the wrestlers.
- Test normality of data by using the Shapiro–Wilk test.
- Identify outliers by using boxplot.
- Compute largest and smallest scores, mean, SD, CV, SE, skewness, kurtosis, and quartile deviation for all parameters of the wrestlers.
- Compute percentile scores at decile points for all variables in order to develop a scale.
- Use properties of normal distribution for developing five-point classification criteria for all parameters so that an individual can be classified into any of the five categories: very good, good, average, poor, and very poor.
- Prepare profile charts of wrestlers in different age categories.

These computations can be done by using SPSS that shall be explained in the following sections.

2.3.1 Testing Normality of Data and Identifying Outliers

One of the assumptions in using all parametric tests is that the data should come from normal population. Normality of data can be checked by testing the significance of skewness and kurtosis. If these two statistics are not significant, then the data is normal. But what happens if the skewness is significant and kurtosis is not, or vice versa. To resolve this issue, the Shapiro–Wilk and Kolmogorov–Smirnov tests are used to test the normality of data. These tests can be applied by using SPSS.

The Shapiro–Wilk test is more suitable for testing normality in case of small sample (N ≤ 50), but it can be used for the sample size up to 2000. However, if the sample size is large, then the Kolmogorov–Smirnov test is used for checking normality of data. One of the limitations of these tests is that in case of large sample, you are more likely to get significant results. In other words, in large sample these tests become significant even for slight deviation from normality. While testing the normality with SPSS, one can also choose the option for identifying outliers using boxplot.

The procedure for testing normality of data and detecting outliers shall be explained by means of a solved example using SPSS. Let us consider the growth data obtained on school boys as shown in Table 2.1.

After preparing data file, follow the below mentioned sequence of commands as shown in the Fig. 2.3.

Analyze → Descriptive Statistics → Explore

After clicking on the **Explore** option, select variables for testing normality and identifying outliers as shown in Figure 2.4. Select all three variables from the left

TABLE 2.1   Growth Data Obtained on School Boys

S.N.	Age (years)	Height (cm)	Weight (lb)
1	9	150	105
2	11	152	99
3	10	154	108
4	13	158	106
5	12	162	103
6	12	149	100
7	11	165	99
8	10	156	110
9	9	158	103
10	10	160	105
11	12	162	110
12	11	163	115
13	9	160	120
14	12	185	123
15	11	165	135

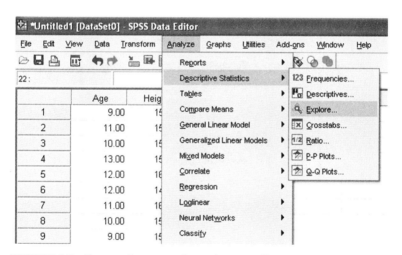

FIGURE 2.3   Command sequence for testing normality and identifying outliers.

panel and shift them to the "Dependent List" section of the screen. Click on **Statistics** command and select the 'Outliers' option. Let other options remain as it is selected by default.

After selecting option for outliers, click on **Continue.** Click on the **Plots** command in the same screen and then select the 'Normality plots with test' option as shown in Figure 2.5. This option will generate the output of the Shapiro–Wilk test and Q–Q plot. Let other options remain selected by default. Click on the **Continue** and **OK** options to get the outputs.

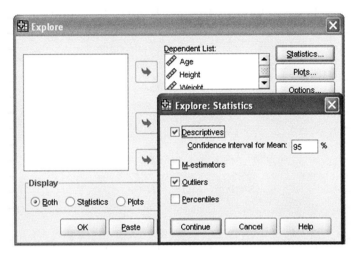

FIGURE 2.4   Option for selecting variables and detecting outliers.

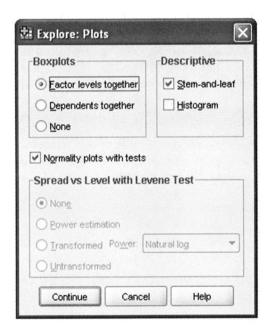

FIGURE 2.5   Option for computing the Shapiro–Wilk test and Q–Q plot.

Select the following outputs from the output window of SPSS:

1. Tests of normality
2. Q–Q plot
3. Boxplot for identifying outliers.

TABLE 2.2   Tests of Normality for the Data on Memory Recall

	Kolmogorov–Smirnov			Shapiro–Wilk		
	Statistics	df	Significance	Statistic	df	Significance
Age	0.163	15	0.200	0.918	15	0.179
Height	0.211	15	0.070	0.850	15	0.017*
Weight	0.210	15	0.075	0.872	15	0.036*

* Significance at 5% level.

2.3.1.1   *Test of Normality* Table 2.2 shows the Kolmogorov–Smirnov and Shapiro–Wilk test statistics. If these tests are significant, then the data is non-normal. Thus, for the data to be normal these tests should be nonsignificant. Since the Shapiro–Wilk test is significant for the height (p=0.017) and weight (0.036), it may be concluded that the data for height and weight are non-normal, whereas age is normally distributed.

2.3.1.2   *Q–Q Plot for Normality* Q–Q plot is a graphical way of checking the normality of data. It compares the two probability distributions by plotting their Quantiles against each other. If distribution of sample data are similar to that of standard normal distribution, all the points in the Q–Q plot will lie very close to the line. It can be seen from Figure 2.6 that the points are not on or close to the lines for the height and weight variables, whereas points are mostly near the line in case of age data.

2.3.1.3   *Test for Outliers* The outlier is an unusual data which a researcher tries to remove from the sample if the results drawn from the sample need to be generalized for the population of interest. If the researcher feels that the data is genuine, then he may decide to keep it in the study. Figure 2.7 shows the Boxplot for all three variables. It describes the distribution of data and identifies outliers if any. Usually, any data outside the mean $\pm 2SD$ is taken as outlier. The SPSS computes outlier on the basis of interquartile range. Any data less than $Q_1 - (Q_3 - Q_1)/2$ or more than $Q_3 + (Q_3 - Q_1)/2$ is identified as outlier by the SPSS. However, you may keep the data in your sample even if it lies outside this range provided you are convinced that such score is genuine and can be obtained by the subjects easily. It can be seen in Figure 2.7b that the 14th score is an outlier. Similarly, Figure 2.7c shows that the SPSS has detected 15th data as an outlier.

Example 2.1

Consider a study in which physiological profile of a university men's hockey player needs to be developed by using their data shown in Table 2.3. Let us see how various descriptive statistics can be computed using SPSS software.

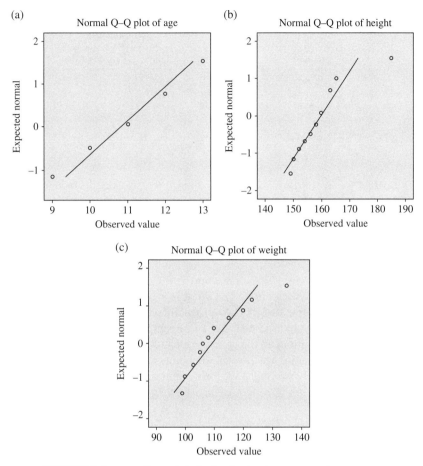

FIGURE 2.6 (a–c) Normal Q–Q plot for the data on growth parameter.

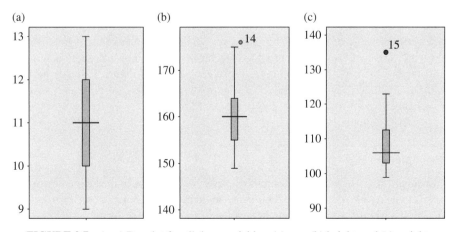

FIGURE 2.7 (a–c) Boxplot for all three variables: (a) age, (b) height, and (c) weight.

TABLE 2.3   Data on Physiological Parameters Obtained on University Hockey Players

S.N.	Fat%	BHC	RHR	VC	Resp. Rate	VO$_2$ max
1	9.90	38	68	3.5	21	57.05
2	11.5	40	73	3.0	24	57.15
3	15.9	44	78	2.6	23	53.46
4	15.3	27	73	2.5	25	49.86
5	5.90	60	67	4.0	19	46.36
6	13.4	55	71	2.5	22	49.86
7	9.00	34	70	3.5	25	46.26
8	15.4	56	69	3.0	17	46.26
9	5.50	54	66	3.7	21	42.66
10	15.40	60	67	2.7	23	46.26
11	9.00	37	77	3.1	20	53.46
12	13.4	60	72	5.0	20	46.27
13	9.8.0	60	68	3.6	24	42.66
14	15.4	36	72	3.0	20	46.26
15	9.00	60	70	3.5	21	53.46
16	5.80	31	75	3.0	21	42.66
17	13.40	45	67	3.0	23	42.66
18	13.60	50	72	3.5	23	53.46
19	13.70	53	70	3.5	22	57.05
20	13.70	37	71	3.0	21	43.66

Fat%, fat percentage; BHC, breath-holding capacity in sec; RHR, respiratory heart rate in beat/min; VC, vital capacity in liters; Resp. rate, respiratory rate in no. of inhale/min; VO$_2$ max, VO$_2$ max in mL/g/min.

2.4   COMPUTATION OF DESCRIPTIVE STATISTICS USING SPSS

2.4.1   Preparation of Data File

Data file in SPSS needs to be prepared before SPSS commands are used for computing descriptive statistics. It is advised to go through Chapter 1 for starting the SPSS package for preparing the data file.

After starting the SPSS and selecting the option 'Type in data,' you will be taken to the SPSS data editor. The sequence of SPSS commands is as follows:

Start

    All Programs

        SPSS Inc

            SPSS 22.0

                Type in data

Now you are ready for defining variables row-wise.

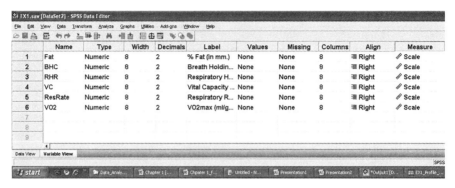

FIGURE 2.8   Defining variables along with their characteristics.

2.4.2   Defining Variables

In this example, there are six variables that need to be defined along with their properties. The procedure is as follows:

1. Click on **Variable View** to define variables and their properties.
2. Write short names of all six variables as *Fat*, *BHC*, *RHR*, *VC*, *ResRate*, and VO$_2$ under the column heading "Name."
3. Under the column heading "Label," full name of these variables may be defined as *% Fat*, *Breath-Holding Capacity*, *Respiratory Heart Rate*, *Vital Capacity*, *Respiratory Rate*, and VO$_2$ *max*.
4. Use default entries in rest of the columns.

After defining the variables in **Variable View**, the screen shall look like as shown in Figure 2.8.

2.4.3   Entering Data

Once all six variables have been defined in the **Variable View**, click on the **Data View** option on the left corner in the bottom of the screen to open the format for entering the data. For each variable, data can be entered column-wise. After entering data, screen will look like as shown in Figure 2.9. Save the data file in the desired location before further processing.

2.4.4   SPSS Commands

After entering all data in the **Data View**, do the following steps for computing descriptive statistics.

1. *Initiating SPSS commands*: In **Data View**, click on the following commands in sequence:

Analyze → Descriptive Statistics → Frequencies

The screen shall look like as shown in Figure 2.10.

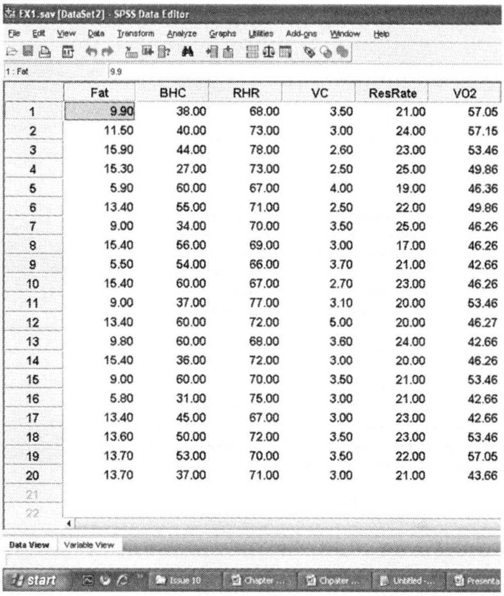

FIGURE 2.9 Method of data entry in **Data View**.

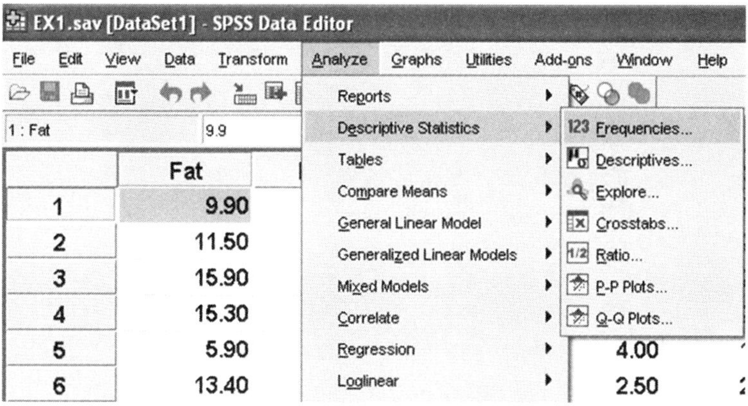

FIGURE 2.10 Command sequence for computing descriptive statistics.

2. *Selecting variables*: After clicking on "Frequencies", you will be taken to the next screen for selecting variables for which descriptive statistics need to be computed. The screen shall look like as shown in Figure 2.11. Do the following:

(a) Select all six variables *Fat*, *BHC*, *RHR*, *VC*, *ResRate*, and VO$_2$ in the left panel and bring them into the "Variable(s)" section in the right panel.

The variables can be selected one by one or all at once. The screen will look like as shown in Figure 2.11.

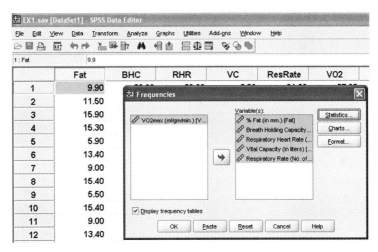

FIGURE 2.11   Selection of variables for descriptive analysis.

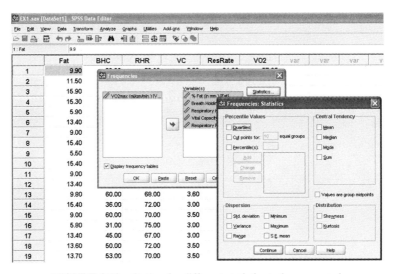

FIGURE 2.12   Option for different statistics to be computed.

3. *Selecting option for computation*: After selecting variables, options need to be selected for the computation of various statistics. Do the followings:

   (a) Click on the **Statistics** command to get the screen as shown in Figure 2.12 for selecting the following options:

      (i) Check 'Quartiles' and 'Cut points for *10* equal groups' options in "Percentile Values" section.

      (ii) Check 'Mean,' 'Median,' and 'Mode' options in "Central Tendency" section.

(iii) Check 'Std. deviation,' 'Variance,' 'Range,' 'Minimum,' 'Maximum,' 'Range,' and 'S.E. mean' in "Dispersion" section.

(iv) Check 'Skewness' and 'Kurtosis' in "Distribution" section.

Remarks

(a) Here, you have four different classes of statistics like "Percentile Value," "Central Tendency," "Dispersion," and "Distribution" that can be computed. Any or all the options may be selected under the categories "Central Tendency," "Dispersion," and "Distribution." Under the category "Percentile Values," quartiles can be checked for computing Q_1 and Q_3. For computing percentiles at decile points, cut points can be selected as 10. Similarly, if the percentiles are required to be computed in the interval of 5, cut points may be selected as 5.

(b) In using the option "Cut points" for the percentiles, output contains some additional information on frequency in different segments. If the researcher is interested, the same may be incorporated in findings; otherwise it may be ignored.

(c) *Percentile* option is selected, if percentile values at different intervals are required to be computed. For example, if we are interested in computing P_4, P_{16}, P_{27}, P_{39}, etc., then these numbers are added in the Percentile options.

(d) Under the heading "Percentile Values," 'Quartiles' option has been checked and the value of 'Cut points for' has been taken as 10; whereas under the heading "Central Tendency," "Dispersion," and "Distribution," all options have been checked.

4. *Option for graph*: The option of **Chart** command can be used if graph is required to be constructed. Any one of the options under this section like Bar Charts, Pie Charts, or Histograms may be selected. If no chart is required, then option "None" may be selected. Click on **Continue** and **OK** for outputs.

5. *Getting outputs*: All the results would be generated into output window. The output panel shall have lots of results. It is up to the researcher to select the relevant outputs in their results. In the output window of SPSS, the relevant outputs may be selected by pressing the right click of the mouse and copying them into the word file. In this example, the output generated will look like as shown in Table 2.4.

2.5   INTERPRETATIONS OF THE RESULTS

Different interpretations can be made from the results in Table 2.4. However, some of the important findings that can be drawn are as follows:

1. Mean and median for all the variables are nearly equal.
2. SE of mean is least for the vital capacity, whereas it is the maximum for the breath-holding capacity.

TABLE 2.4 Output Showing Values of Different Statistics of Physiological Parameters

	Fat%	Breath-Holding Capacity (sec)	Respiratory Heart Rate (beat/min)	Vital Capacity (L)	Respiratory Rate (No. of Inhalation/min)	VO$_2$ max (mL/g/min)
N Valid	20	20	20	20	20	20
Missing	0	0	0	0	0	0
Mean	11.7000	46.8500	70.8000	3.2600	21.7500	48.8390
Std. error of mean	0.77392	2.49871	0.74197	0.13087	0.45811	1.15884
Median	13.4000	47.5000	70.5000	3.0500	21.5000	46.3150
Mode	9.00[a]	60.00	67.00[a]	3.00	21.00	42.66[a]
Std. deviation	3.46106	11.17457	3.31821	0.58526	2.04875	5.18249
Variance	11.979	124.871	11.011	0.343	4.197	26.858
Skewness	−0.565	−0.203	0.617	1.288	−0.319	0.376
Std. error of skewness	0.512	0.512	0.512	0.512	0.512	0.512
Kurtosis	−0.964	−1.446	−0.071	2.936	0.070	−1.286
Std. error of kurtosis	0.992	0.992	0.992	0.992	0.992	0.992
Range	10.40	33.00	12.00	2.50	8.00	14.49
Minimum	5.50	27.00	66.00	2.50	17.00	42.66
Maximum	15.90	60.00	78.00	5.00	25.00	57.15
Sum	234.00	937.00	1416.00	65.20	435.00	976.78
Percentiles 10	5.8100	31.3000	67.0000	2.5100	19.1000	42.6600
20	9.0000	36.2000	67.2000	2.7600	20.0000	42.8600
25	9.0000	37.0000	68.0000	3.0000	20.2500	44.3100
30	9.2400	37.3000	68.3000	3.0000	21.0000	46.2600
40	10.5400	41.6000	70.0000	3.0000	21.0000	46.2600
50	13.4000	47.5000	70.5000	3.0500	21.5000	46.3150
60	13.5200	53.6000	71.6000	3.5000	22.6000	49.8600
70	13.7000	55.7000	72.0000	3.5000	23.0000	53.4600
75	14.9000	59.0000	72.7500	3.5000	23.0000	53.4600
80	15.3800	60.0000	73.0000	3.5800	23.8000	53.4600
90	15.4000	60.0000	76.8000	3.9700	24.9000	57.0500

[a] Multiple modes exist. The smallest value is shown.

3. As a guideline, a skewness value more than twice its SE indicates a departure from symmetry. Owing to this principle, only vital capacity is positively skewed as its value is 1.288 that is more than twice its SE (2×0.512). Thus, it can be interpreted that most of the subject's performance on vital capacity is less than the mean value.

4. SPSS uses $\gamma_2 (= \beta_2 - 3)$ statistic for kurtosis. If kurtosis value is greater than two times of its SE, it may be considered significant. For a normal distribution, kurtosis value is 0. If for any variable the value of kurtosis is positive, then its distribution is leptokurtic, which indicates low level of data fluctuation around its mean, whereas negative kurtosis indicates large degree of variation among data and in that case the distribution is known as platykurtic. In this example, kurtosis for the vital capacity is 2.936, which is significant. Since kurtosis is positive, the shape of the curve is leptokurtic indicating less variation among subject's vital capacity performance around their mean value.

5. Minimum and maximum values of the parameter can give some interesting facts and provide range of variation. For instance, fat% of the university hockey players is in the range of 5.5–15.9%. Since for an adult male, fat% should be in the range of 10–20%; therefore, it can be interpreted that hockey players had less fat in their body. This is rightly so as the hockey players need to have an athletic body due to the very nature of the game.

6. Similarly, respiratory heart rate is in the range of 66 and 78. This indicates that some of the players had better conditioning of heart whereas others need to improve upon on this parameter.

7. Percentile scales can be used to draw various conclusions about different parameters. For instance, P_{40} for the fat% is 10.54, which indicates that around 40% of the hockey players had fat below the 10.54% which may be categorized as lean. Similarly, P_{30} for the respiratory heart rate is 68. This indicates that 30% of the hockey players were very fit and 70% needs to improve their fitness as lower pulse rate is the sign of better fitness.

2.6 DEVELOPING PROFILE CHART

A researcher who undertakes a profile study generally computes various statistics that are described in Table 2.4. The significant findings can be explained while writing interpretation of the results as shown earlier. However, it would be more interesting to prepare a graphical profile as well by using minimum score, maximum score, mean, and SD of all the parameters shown in Table 2.4.

After manipulating the data as per the following steps, functionality of EXCEL can be used to prepare a graphical profile of the hockey players.

Step 1: Segregate the descriptive statistics like minimum score, maximum score, mean, and SD of all the parameters from Table 2.4. The same has been shown in Table 2.5.

TABLE 2.5   Selected Statistics of the Physiological
Parameters of University Hockey Players

	Min	Max	Mean	SD
Fat	5.5	15.9	11.7	3.46
BHC	27	60	46.85	11.17
RHR	66	78	70.8	3.32
VitCap	2.5	5	3.26	0.59
ResRate	17	25	21.75	2.05
VO$_2$ max	42.66	57.15	48.84	5.18

TABLE 2.6   Standard Scores of the Physiological
Parameters

	Min (Z)	Mean (Z)	Max (Z)
Fat	−1.79	0	1.21
BHC	−1.78	0	1.18
RHR	−1.45	0	2.17
VitCap	−1.29	0	2.95
ResRate	−2.32	0	1.59
VO$_2$ max	−1.19	0	1.6

TABLE 2.7   Transformed Standard Scores of the
Physiological Parameters

	Min	Mean	Max
Fat	32.1	50	62.1
BHC	32.2	50	61.8
RHR	35.5	50	71.7
VitCap	37.1	50	79.5
ResRate	26.8	50	65.9
VO$_2$ max	38.1	50	66.0

Step 2: Convert minimum score, maximum score, and mean of each variable into
their standard scores by using the following transformation:

$$Z = \frac{X - \bar{X}}{S}$$

Thus, mean of all the variables will become zero. The values so obtained are shown
in Table 2.6.

Step 3: Convert these Z values into their linear transformed scores by using the
transformation $Z_1 = 50 + 10 \times Z$. This way negative value of Z can be converted
into positive. Descriptive statistics shown in the form of linearly transformed
scores are shown in Table 2.7.

Step 4: Use EXCEL graphic functionality for developing line diagram to show the
profile of university hockey players. The profile chart so prepared is shown in
Figure 2.13.

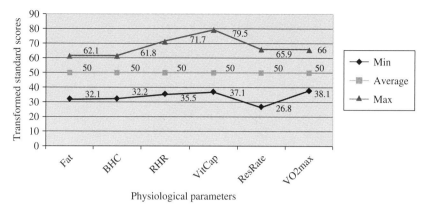

FIGURE 2.13   Physiological profiles of university hockey players.

2.7   SUMMARY OF SPSS COMMANDS

1. Start SPSS by using the following commands:

   Start → All Programs → SPSS Inc → SPSS 20.0 → Type in Data

2. Click on **Variable View** and define the variables *Fat*, *BHC*, *RHR*, *VC*, *ResRate*, and *VO$_2$* as a 'Scale' variable.

3. Once the variables are defined, type data for these variables by clicking on **Data View**.

4. In the **Data View**, follow the below mentioned command sequence for generating descriptive statistics.

   Analyze → Descriptive Statistics → Frequencies

5. Select all variables from left panel and bring them into the right panel for computing various descriptive statistics.

6. Click on the **Statistics** command and select 'Percentile Values,' 'Central Tendency,' 'Dispersion,' and 'Distribution' options. Click on **Continue.**

7. Click on the **Charts** command and select the required chart, if graph is required.

8. Click on **OK** to get the output.

2.8   EXERCISE

2.8.1   Short Answer Questions

Note: Write the answer to each question in not more than 200 words.

Q.1   If mean performance of two groups is same, can it be said that both groups are equally good?

Q.2   What do you mean by absolute and relative variability? Explain them by means of examples.

Q.3   What is coefficient of variation? In what situation should it be computed? With the help of the following data on weight can it be concluded that group A is more variable than group B.

	Group A (lb)	Group B (lb)
Mean	110	170
SD	10	14

Q.4   Is there any difference between SE of mean and error in computing the mean? Explain by means of an example.

Q.5   If skewness of a set of data is zero, can it be said that it is normally distributed? If yes, how? And if no, how it can be checked for its normality?

Q.6   If performance of a student is 95th percentile in a particular subject, can it be concluded that he is very intelligent in that subject? Explain your answer.

Q.7   What does quartile measures? In what situation should it be used?

2.8.2   Multiple Choice Questions

Note: Questions 1–10 have four alternative answers for each question. Tick mark the one that you consider the closest to the correct answer.

1   If an investigator is interested to know as to how many students in a college have come from different regions of the country and how many of them have opted for science studies. The study may be categorized as follows:
    (a) Descriptive
    (b) Inferential
    (c) Philosophical
    (d) Descriptive and Inferential both

2   Choose the correct sequence of commands to compute descriptive statistics.
    (a) Analyze → Descriptive Statistics → Frequencies
    (b) Analyze → Frequencies → Descriptive Statistics
    (c) Analyze → Frequencies
    (d) Analyze → Descriptive Statistics

3   Choose nonparametric statistics.
    (a) Mean and Median
    (b) Mean and SD
    (c) Median and SD
    (d) Median and QD

4   SE of mean can be defined as follows:
    (a) Error in computing mean
    (b) Difference in sample and population mean
    (c) Variation in the mean values among the samples drawn from the same population
    (d) Error in measuring the data on which mean is computed

5   The value of skewness for a given set of data shall be significant if
    (a) Skewness is more than twice its SE
    (b) Skewness is more than its SE
    (c) Skewness and SE are equal
    (d) Skewness is less than its SE

6   Kurtosis in SPSS is assessed by
    (a) β_2
    (b) $\beta_2 + 3$
    (c) $\beta_2 - 3$
    (d) $2\beta_2$

7   In order to prepare a profile chart, minimum score for each variable is converted into
    (a) Percentage
    (b) Standard score
    (c) Percentile score
    (d) Rank

8   While selecting option for percentile in SPSS, cut points are used for
    (a) Computing Q_1 and Q_3
    (b) Generating percentiles at decile points only
    (c) Cutting Q_1 and Q_3
    (d) Generating percentiles at fixed interval points

9   If IQ for a group of students is positively skewed, what conclusions could be drawn?
    (a) Most of the students are less intelligent.
    (b) Most of the students are more intelligent.
    (c) There are equal number of high- and low-intelligent students.
    (d) Nothing can be said about the intelligence of the students.

10 If distribution of a dataset is platykurtic, what can be said about its variability?
    (a) More variability exists.
    (b) Less variability exists.
    (c) Variability is equivalent to normal distribution.
    (d) Nothing can be said about the variability.

2.9   CASE STUDY ON DESCRIPTIVE ANALYSIS

Objective

A researcher wanted to study physiological characteristics of the college basketball players. A pilot study was conducted by him on a randomly selected sample of 20 basketballers on which the data was obtained on eight selected variables. The data so obtained are shown in Table 2.8.

Research Questions

The following research questions were investigated:

1. Whether all the data were normally distributed?
2. Whether the data contained any outlier?
3. How was the nature of variables?

Data Format

The format used for preparing data file in SPSS is shown in Table 2.8.

Analyzing Data

By using the commands **Analyze**, **Descriptive Statistics**, and **Explore** in sequence and by selecting the option 'Normality plots with tests,' the output for the Shapiro–Wilk test was obtained for all the variables for testing normality. The results so obtained are shown in Table 2.9. Further by selecting the option 'Outliers,' the box-plots were developed for identifying the outliers, if any, in all the variables. Boxplot for only those variables in which outliers were detected have been shown in Figures 2.14 and 2.15.

Further, for understanding the nature of data various descriptive statistics were computed by using the commands **Analyze, Descriptive Statistics,** and **Frequencies** in sequence and selecting options for different statistics in SPSS. The statistics so computed are shown in Table 2.10.

Testing Normality

It can be seen from Table 2.9 that the Shapiro–Wilk test is nonsignificant for all the variables, except weight and 9 min run/walk tests. Since the Shapiro test is significant for weight and 9 min run/walk test, the data for these two variables are non-normal although other variables are normally distributed.

Checking Outliers

Boxplot for weight and fat indicates that in each of these two variables, one outlier exists. Figure 2.14 shows that the 20th data for the weight, which is 87, is an outlier. Similarly, Figure 2.15 indicates that the second data of fat, that is, 23.35 is an outlier.

TABLE 2.8 Data on Physiological Parameters of College Basketballers

S.N.	Height (cm)	Weight (kg)	Grip Strength (kg)	Pulse Rate (beat/min)	Explosive Power (kt)	9 min Run/ Walk (mt.)	Body Density (g/cc)	Fat%
1	175	64	29	68	991.49	3000	1.07	13.34
2	171	54	29	84	1066.9	3000	1.08	23.35
3	159	50	26	88	698.36	2000	1.05	20.21
4	167	50	27	80	741.46	2400	1.06	15.5
5	158	49	25	80	502.49	2200	1.08	7.89
6	174	65	29	60	824.55	2600	1.06	17.81
7	165	58	22	84	403.1	2000	1.08	8.45
8	159	44	16	86	558.16	2800	1.08	10.44
9	157	55	30	88	719.58	1800	1.05	11.91
10	161	51	33	84	484.43	2500	1.08	8.72
11	162	54	20	75	1033.48	3000	1.07	11.57
12	161	50	18	63	994.68	2800	1.06	8.74
13	165	51	30	71	836.31	2600	1.07	11.89
14	161	57	21	84	928.6	3000	1.07	11.98
15	164	51	24	83	712.32	2800	1.07	13.13
16	165	54	24	76	716.04	2700	1.07	13.35
17	170	57	20	67	775.98	3000	1.07	15.75
18	159	51	24	79	612.92	3000	1.07	11.79
19	170	48	27	70	1204.47	3200	1.09	15.04
20	181	87	29	79	857.45	2000	1.04	10.12

TABLE 2.9 Tests of normality

	Kolmogorov–Smirnov[a]			Shapiro–Wilk		
	Statistic	df	Significance	Statistic	df	Significance
Height	0.162	20	0.177	0.923	20	0.112
Weight	0.221	20	0.012	0.746	20	0.000
Grip_Strength	0.151	20	0.200*	0.962	20	0.592
Pulse_Rate	0.173	20	0.117	0.922	20	0.108
Explosive	0.095	20	0.200*	0.982	20	0.960
Nine_Min_R/W	0.166	20	0.148	0.896	20	0.035
Body_Density	0.249	20	0.002	0.918	20	0.092
Fat	0.170	20	0.132	0.919	20	0.093

[a] Lilliefors significance correction.
* This is a lower bound of the true significance.

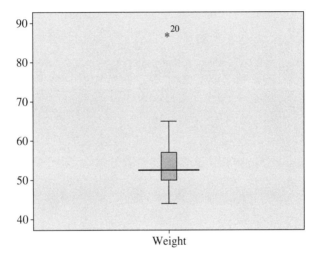

FIGURE 2.14 Boxplot showing outlier in weight data.

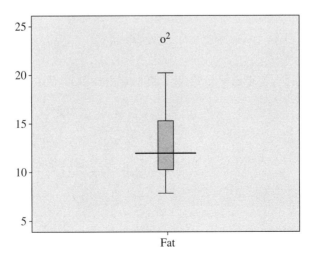

FIGURE 2.15 Boxplot showing outlier in fat data.

TABLE 2.10 Descriptive statistics

		Height	Weight	Grip_Strength	Pulse_Rate	Explosive	Nine_Min_RW	Body_Density	Fat
N	Valid	20	20	20	20	20	20	20	20
	Missing	0	0	0	0	0	0	0	0
Mean		1.6520E2	55.0000	25.1500	77.4500	783.1385	2620.000	1.0685	13.0490
Std. error of mean		1.45566	2.03263	1.01896	1.87290	47.42410	94.20023	0.00274	0.89666
Median		1.6450E2	52.5000	25.5000	79.5000	758.7200	2750.000	1.0700	11.9450
Mode		159.00[a]	51.00	29.00	84.00	403.10[a]	3000.00	1.07	7.89[a]
Std. deviation		6.50991	9.09019	4.55695	8.37587	2.12087E2	421.2762	0.01226	4.01000
Variance		42.379	82.632	20.766	70.155	4.498E4	177473.68	0.000	16.080
Skewness		0.868	2.493	−0.345	−0.667	0.086	−0.634	−0.638	1.054
Std. error of skewness		0.512	0.512	0.512	0.512	0.512	0.512	0.512	0.512
Kurtosis		0.178	7.956	−0.652	−0.610	−0.510	−0.855	0.335	1.068
Std. error of kurtosis		0.992	0.992	0.992	0.992	0.992	0.992	0.992	0.992
Range		24.00	43.00	17.00	28.00	801.37	1400.00	0.05	15.46
Minimum		157.00	44.00	16.00	60.00	403.10	1800.00	1.04	7.89
Maximum		181.00	87.00	33.00	88.00	1204.47	3200.00	1.09	23.35
Percentiles	10	1.5810E2	48.1000	18.2000	63.4000	486.2360	2000.0000	1.0500	8.4770
	20	1.5900E2	50.0000	20.2000	68.4000	569.1120	2040.0000	1.0600	9.0160
	25	1.5950E2	50.0000	21.2500	70.2500	634.2800	2250.0000	1.0600	10.2000
	30	1.6100E2	50.3000	22.6000	72.2000	702.5480	2430.0000	1.0630	10.7790
	40	1.6140E2	51.0000	24.0000	77.2000	717.4560	2600.0000	1.0700	11.8300
	50	1.6450E2	52.5000	25.5000	79.5000	758.7200	2750.0000	1.0700	11.9450
	60	1.6500E2	54.0000	27.0000	81.8000	831.6060	2800.0000	1.0700	13.2560
	70	1.6910E2	56.4000	29.0000	84.0000	907.2550	3000.0000	1.0770	14.5330
	75	1.7000E2	57.0000	29.0000	84.0000	975.7675	3000.0000	1.0800	15.3850
	80	1.7080E2	57.8000	29.0000	84.0000	994.0420	3000.0000	1.0800	15.7000
	90	1.7490E2	64.9000	30.0000	87.8000	1.0636E3	3000.0000	1.0800	19.9700

[a] Multiple modes exist. The smallest value is shown.

Understanding Nature of Data

It is evident from Table 2.9 that the data on weight and fat are skewed because their skewness is greater than two times of their SE. For instance, skewness of the weight is 2.493, which is greater than 2×0.512. Since skewness is positive for these two variables, the data is positively skewed for both these variables. It can be interpreted that most of the weight and fat scores of the basketballers were less than their respective mean values.

Since kurtosis for the weight (7.956) is more than two times of its SE (2×0.992), it is significant and the curve is leptokurtic. In other words, curve is more peak which indicated that there was less variation among the weights of basketballers.

Reporting

- Since the Shapiro–Wilk test was significant for weight and 9 min run/walk test, these two variables were non-normal although all other variables were normally distributed.
- One outlier in each of the dataset of weight and fat was identified.
- Data for weight and fat were positively skewed, indicating most of the data lying below the mean.
- Data for weight was also leptokurtic, indicating less variation around the mean value.

3

CORRELATION COEFFICIENT AND PARTIAL CORRELATION

LEARNING OBJECTIVES

After completing this chapter, you should be able to do the following:

- State the circumstances in which correlation and regression analysis can be used
- Learn to interpret the significance of correlation coefficient and partial correlation
- Construct hypothesis to test the significance of correlation coefficient
- Formulate research problems where correlation matrix and partial correlation can be used to draw conclusions
- Know the procedure of using SPSS in computing correlation matrix and partial correlation
- Interpret the output of SPSS in computing the correlation matrix and partial correlation

---

3.1 INTRODUCTION

Researchers in the area of sports science are always engaged in finding ways and means to improve the capability of athletes to enhance their performance. It is therefore important to know the parameters that affect the performance in different sports. Once the parameters responsible for performance are identified, an effective training

Sports Research with Analytical Solution using SPSS®, First Edition. J. P. Verma.
© 2016 John Wiley & Sons, Inc. Published 2016 by John Wiley & Sons, Inc.
Companion website: www.wiley.com/go/Verma/Sportsresearch

schedule can be developed to improve the performance. For instance, if a coach trains his budding athletes for the middle distance events, his first priority would be to develop their endurance and then try to improve their other parameters like strength, skills, and related techniques and tactics. This is so because endurance is highly associated with the performance of the middle distance event. Thus, it is important to identify the parameter that is highly related to the performance. This can be achieved by knowing the strength of relationship between a parameter and the performance. This strength of relationship between the two variables can be computed by a measure known as product moment correlation coefficient. In short, it is referred as correlation coefficient and is denoted by "r."

The correlation coefficient gives a fair estimate of the extent of relationship between the two variables, if the subjects are chosen randomly. But in most of the situations samples are purposive; and therefore, correlation coefficient in general may not give the correct picture of the real relationship. If a study is to be conducted on university students for developing a regression equation for estimating shot put performance, on the basis of some predictors, a sample may be drawn from all the university students who have participated in the interuniversity tournaments. The next job is to first identify the most contributing parameter to the shot put performance. And if the correlation coefficient between the performance and height comes out to be 0.8, it cannot be interpreted that height is highly related with the performance. It may be due to the fact that the subjects might have very good as well. Further, higher correlation might also be due to their higher coordinative ability, and leg strength. Thus, in this situation product moment correlation may not be considered as a good indicator of the real relationship between the height and shot put performance because the sample was purposive in nature. The sample is called "purposive" because it is not randomly chosen from the population of interest, rather has been obtained from a specific domain and for a specific purpose.

Since correlation does not explain the cause and effect relationship, another measure is computed to overcome this problem, which is known as partial correlation. This provides a real relationship between the two variables after partialling out the effect of other independent variables. Partial correlation is a statistical technique of eliminating the effects of independent variables after the data is collected. Another method of eliminating the effect of independent variables is to make them constant while collecting the data, but this is not feasible all the time. Let us understand this fact through this example. Consider a situation where the height and weight of 20 children with age ranging from 12 to 18 years are selected, and the correlation between the height and weight is computed as 0.75. Although this correlation is quite high, it cannot be considered as an indicator of a real relationship between height and weight. This higher correlation has been observed because all the children belong to the developmental age; and during this age, in general, if the height increases weight also increases. Thus, in order to find the real relationship between the height and weight, the age needs to be constant. Age can be made constant by taking all the subjects from the same age category. But it is not possible in the experimental situation once the data collection is over. Even if an experimenter tries to control the effect of one or more variable manually, it may not be possible to control the effect of other variables; otherwise, one might end up with getting one or two sample only for the study.

Although the correlation coefficient may not give a clear picture of the real relationship between the two variables, yet it provides inputs for computing partial and multiple correlations. And, therefore, in most of the analysis it is important to compute a correlation matrix for the set of variables in the study. This chapter discusses the procedure for computing correlation matrix and partial correlations, and their application in research.

3.2 CORRELATION MATRIX AND PARTIAL CORRELATION

Matrix is an arrangement of scores in rows and columns. If elements in a matrix are correlation coefficients, it is known as correlation matrix. Usually in correlation matrix upper diagonal values of the matrix are written. For instance, correlation matrix with the variables X_1, X_2, X_3, and X_4 may look like as follows:

	X_1	X_2	X_3	X_4
X_1	1	0.5	0.3	0.6
X_2		1	0.7	0.8
X_3			1	0.4
X_4				1

The lower diagonal values in the matrix are not written because of the fact that the correlation between X_2 and X_3 is the same as the correlation between X_3 and X_2.
    Some authors prefer to write this correlation matrix in the following form:

	X_1	X_2	X_3	X_4
X_1		0.5	0.3	0.6
X_2			0.7	0.8
X_3				0.4
X_4				

In this correlation matrix, diagonal values are not written as it is obvious that these values are 1 because correlation between the two same variables is always 1.
    In this section, we shall discuss product moment correlation and partial correlation along with testing of their significance.

3.2.1 Product Moment Correlation Coefficient

Product moment correlation coefficient is the measure of relationship between any two variables. When we refer to correlation matrix, it is a matrix of product moment correlation coefficients. It is represented by "r" and is given by the following formula:

$$r = \frac{N\Sigma XY - (\Sigma X)(\Sigma Y)}{\sqrt{\left[N\Sigma X^2 - (\Sigma X)^2\right]\left[N\Sigma Y^2 - (\Sigma Y)^2\right]}}$$

where, N is the number of paired scores. This coefficient r was developed by British mathematician Karl Pearson, hence it is also known as Pearson r. The limits of r are −1 to +1. In general, positive relationship means higher score on one variable tends to be paired with higher score on the other or lower score on one variable tends to be paired with lower score on the other. On the other hand, negative relationship means higher score on one variable tends to be paired with lower score on the other, and vice-versa.

One of the main limitations of the correlation coefficient is that it measures only linear relationship between the two variables. Further, it can be computed only when the data is measured either on an interval or ratio scale. The other limitation of the correlation coefficient is that it does not explain cause and effect relationship. To overcome this problem, partial correlation may be computed, which explains somewhat real relationship between the two variables with certain limitations.

3.2.1.1 Testing the Significance of Correlation Coefficient

After computing correlation coefficient, the next task is to check whether it actually explains some relationship or not. In other words, it is required to test the significance of r.

The following mutually exclusive hypotheses are used for testing the significance of correlation coefficient:

H_0: $\rho = 0$ (There is no correlation between the two variables.)

H_1: $\rho \neq 0$ (There is a significant correlation between the two variables.)

Here, ρ indicates population correlation coefficient whose significance is tested on the basis of the sample correlation. To test the null hypothesis H_0 any of the following three approaches may be used.

First Approach: The easiest way to test the null hypothesis is to compare the computed value of r with that of the critical value of r obtained from Table A.6 in the Appendix at $n-2$ degrees of freedom and some desired level of significance. If the calculated r is greater than critical r, null hypothesis is rejected; otherwise we fail to reject it. For instance, if the correlation between the height and self-esteem scores obtained on 25 individuals is 0.45, then the critical value of r required at 0.05 level of significance and $n-2$ (=23) df from Table A.6 in the Appendix can be seen as 0.396. Since calculated r, that is, 0.45 is greater than the critical value of r (=0.396), the null hypothesis is rejected at the significance level 0.05, and we may conclude that there is a significant correlation between the height and self-esteem.

Second Approach: Null hypothesis for testing the significance of correlation coefficient may be tested by using t-test. In this case, t-statistic is given by the following formula:

$$t = \frac{r}{\sqrt{1-r^2}}\sqrt{n-2}$$

Here "r" is the observed correlation and "n" is the number of paired data.

The calculated value of t is compared with that of the tabulated value of t (obtained from Table A.2 in the Appendix) at 0.05 level and $n - 2$ df.

Thus, if calculated $t > t_{0.05}(n - 2)$, H_0 is rejected at the significance level 0.05. and if calculated $t \leq t_{0.05}(n - 2)$, we fail to reject H_0.

Third Approach: In this approach, significance of correlation coefficient is tested on the basis of p value associated with t statistic. The p value can be defined as the smallest level of significance at which the null hypothesis would be rejected. The smaller the p value, the stronger is the evidence in favor of the research hypothesis. If the p value associated with t is 0.04 for a given correlation coefficient, it indicates that the chances of wrongly rejecting the null hypothesis are less than 5%. Thus, as long as p value is less than 0.05, correlation coefficient is significant and the null hypothesis is rejected at 5% level. On the other hand, if the p value is more than or equal to 0.05, the correlation coefficient is not significant and the null hypothesis is not rejected.

Note: The SPSS output follows third approach and provides p value for each of the correlation coefficient in the correlation matrix.

3.2.2 Partial Correlation

Partial correlation is a measure of relationship between two variables after controlling the effect of one or more independent variables. For example, one may compute partial correlation if it is required to see the relationship of leg strength with 100-meter performance after adjusting the effect of reaction time.

The partial correlation of X_1 and X_2 adjusted for X_3 is given by

$$r_{12.3} = \frac{r_{12} - r_{13}r_{23}}{\sqrt{\left(1 - r_{13}^2\right)\left(1 - r_{23}^2\right)}}$$

Like correlation coefficient, the limits of partial correlation are also -1 to $+1$.

Number of independent variable whose effects are controlled determines the order of a partial correlation. For example, first-order partial correlation is the one in which the effect of only one variable is controlled.

The generalized formula for $(n - 2)$th order partial correlation is given by

$$r_{12.34\ldots n} = \frac{r_{12.345\ldots(n-1)} - r_{1n.345\ldots(n-1)}r_{2n.345\ldots(n-1)}}{\sqrt{1 - r_{1n.345\ldots(n-1)}^2}\sqrt{1 - r_{2n.345\ldots(n-1)}^2}}$$

3.2.2.1 Assumptions Partial correlation is useful when the effect of one or more variables needs to be controlled. Following are the assumptions in partial correlation:

1. Partial correlation assumes that the data are measured either on interval or ratio scale.
2. In computing partial correlation, data should be linearly related with each other and no outlier should be present. Further data need to be normally distributed.

3.2.2.2 Testing the Significance of Partial Correlation   The significance of partial correlation is tested in a similar way as is done in case of product moment correlation.

In SPSS, testing the significance of partial correlation is done on the basis of p value. Partial correlation becomes significant if p value associated with r is less than 0.05 and nonsignificant otherwise.

3.3   APPLICATION OF CORRELATION MATRIX AND PARTIAL CORRELATION

If a researcher is interested to study the relationship between the performance in any sport and several independent variables, he may compute the correlation matrix, which might facilitate him to understand the extent of multicollinearity among independent variables besides understanding the pattern of relationship between performance and independent variables. While investigating the relationships using correlation matrix, it is relevant to know as to which variable is highly associated with the performance variable. With certain limitations, these highly associated variables with the performance may be identified by a coach to develop his training model for their athletes. Further, partial correlation may be used to identify the priority variables useful in developing a training model.

3.4   CORRELATION MATRIX WITH SPSS

Example 3.1

A study was conducted on college boys to investigate the relationship between 100-meter performance and physical variables. The data so obtained is shown in Table 3.1. Let us see how correlation matrix and partial correlation can be computed.

Solution: The first step is to compute the correlation matrix. Using the correlation matrix independent variables that have significant correlations with 100-meter performace shall be identified. Partial correlation shall be computed between 100-meter and the identified variables in order to know the most contributing physical variable to the 100-meter performance.

The correlation coefficients and partial correlations so obtained in the output from the SPSS shall be tested for their significance using p values.

3.4.1   Computation in Correlation Matrix

3.4.1.1 Preparation of Data File   Before using SPSS commands for the computation of correlation matrix, a data file needs to be prepared. After starting SPSS and selecting the option 'Type in data,' you will be taken to **Variable View** option where all the variables need to be defined. The sequence of SPSS commands is as follows:

Start

  All Programs

TABLE 3.1   Data on Physical Performance

S.N.	100-Mt.	Leg Str.	Back Str.	Sit-Ups	SBJ	Vert. Jump	30-Mt. Race
1	13.20	80	71	23	2.24	0.70	4.20
2	13.20	72	80	26	1.91	0.31	4.50
3	14.13	76	62	25	2.05	0.61	5.00
4	13.01	46	72	26	1.85	0.28	4.40
5	14.09	65	60	20	1.81	0.12	5.12
6	15.49	80	80	30	1.80	0.19	5.60
7	14.82	76	92	27	2.00	0.14	5.00
8	14.45	95	86	32	2.20	0.42	4.6
9	14.90	74	91	25	2.12	0.09	5.10
10	17.72	70	59	26	2.05	0.29	5.21
11	14.57	70	59	28	2.19	0.30	4.80
12	15.54	110	85	25	1.70	0.34	5.22
13	16.65	70	60	33	1.45	0.33	5.26
14	14.56	85	80	30	1.96	0.31	4.60
15	15.16	85	83	30	2.25	0.49	4.61
16	15.15	67	65	29	1.90	0.67	4.99
17	14.39	90	76	23	1.95	0.33	4.66
18	13.01	65	62	29	2.20	0.65	4.33
19	15.51	100	90	35	1.35	0.26	5.01
20	14.36	120	105	31	1.90	0.37	4.75

100-Mt., 100-meter timings in sec; Leg Stre., Leg strength in kg; Back Stre., Back strength in kg; Sit-ups, Sit-ups in nos.; SBJ, Standing broad jump in mt.; Vert. Jump, Vertical jump in mt.; 30-Mt. Race, 30-meter run timing in sec.

> IBM SPSS Statistics
> > IBM SPSS Statistics 20
> > > Type in Data

Now you are ready for defining variables row-wise.

3.4.1.2   Defining Variables   Here seven variables need to be defined. Since all the variables are quantitative in nature, they are treated as scale in SPSS. The procedure of defining the variables is as follows:

1. Click on **Variable View** button to define variables and their properties.
2. Write short name of the variables as *HundredMt*, *LegStr*, *BackStr*, *SitUps*, *SBJ*, *VertJump*, and *ThirtyMt* under the column heading "Name."
3. Under the column heading "Label," define full name of these variables as 100-meter timing in sec, Leg strength in kg, Back strength in kg, Sit-ups in numbers,

standing broad jump in cm, vertical jump in cm, and 30-meter timing in sec. There is no restriction in defining the full name of each variable. One can take liberty to write any relevant name of the variable without any restrictions.

4. Under the column heading "Measure," select the option 'Scale' for all the variables, as all these variables are quantitative in nature.

5. Use default entries in rest of the columns.

After defining variables in the **Variable View**, the screen will look like as shown in Figure 3.1.

3.4.1.3 Entering Data   Once all the seven variables are defined, click the **Data View** option on the left corner in the bottom of the screen to open the format for entering data. For each variable enter the data column-wise. After entering the data, the screen will look like as shown in Figure 3.2. Save the data file in the desired location before further processing.

3.4.1.4 SPSS Commands   After entering all the data in the **Data View**, the following steps should be followed for computing correlation matrix:

1. *Initiating SPSS Commands for Correlation Matrix*: In the **Data View**, click the following commands in sequence:

Analyze → Correlate → Bivariate

The screen shall look like as shown in Figure 3.3.

2. *Selecting Variables*: After clicking the "Bivariate" option, you will be taken to the next screen for selecting variables for generating correlation matrix. Select all the variables from left panel and bring them to the right panel by using the arrow key. The variable selection may be made one by one or all at once. After selecting the variables, the screen will look like as shown in Figure 3.4.

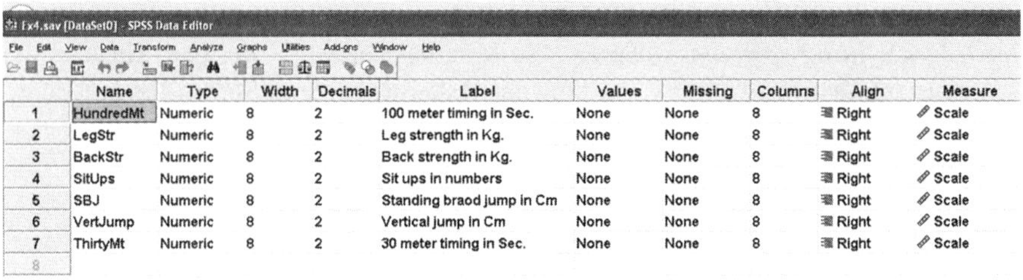

	Name	Type	Width	Decimals	Label	Values	Missing	Columns	Align	Measure
1	HundredMt	Numeric	8	2	100 meter timing in Sec.	None	None	8	Right	Scale
2	LegStr	Numeric	8	2	Leg strength in Kg.	None	None	8	Right	Scale
3	BackStr	Numeric	8	2	Back strength in Kg.	None	None	8	Right	Scale
4	SitUps	Numeric	8	2	Sit ups in numbers	None	None	8	Right	Scale
5	SBJ	Numeric	8	2	Standing braod jump in Cm	None	None	8	Right	Scale
6	VertJump	Numeric	8	2	Vertical jump in Cm	None	None	8	Right	Scale
7	ThirtyMt	Numeric	8	2	30 meter timing in Sec.	None	None	8	Right	Scale
8										

FIGURE 3.1   Defining variables along with their characteristics.

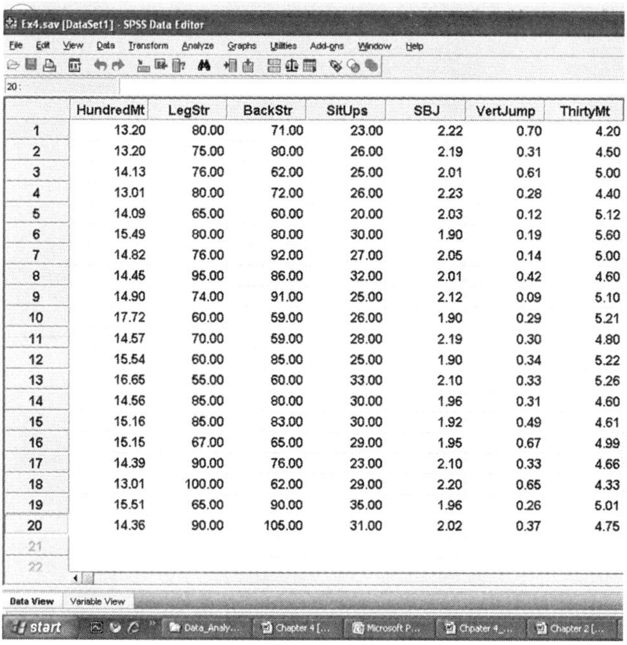

	HundredMt	LegStr	BackStr	SitUps	SBJ	VertJump	ThirtyMt
1	13.20	80.00	71.00	23.00	2.22	0.70	4.20
2	13.20	75.00	80.00	26.00	2.19	0.31	4.50
3	14.13	76.00	62.00	25.00	2.01	0.61	5.00
4	13.01	80.00	72.00	26.00	2.23	0.28	4.40
5	14.09	65.00	60.00	20.00	2.03	0.12	5.12
6	15.49	80.00	80.00	30.00	1.90	0.19	5.60
7	14.82	76.00	92.00	27.00	2.05	0.14	5.00
8	14.45	95.00	86.00	32.00	2.01	0.42	4.60
9	14.90	74.00	91.00	25.00	2.12	0.09	5.10
10	17.72	60.00	59.00	26.00	1.90	0.29	5.21
11	14.57	70.00	59.00	28.00	2.19	0.30	4.80
12	15.54	60.00	85.00	25.00	1.90	0.34	5.22
13	16.65	55.00	60.00	33.00	2.10	0.33	5.26
14	14.56	85.00	80.00	30.00	1.96	0.31	4.60
15	15.16	85.00	83.00	30.00	1.92	0.49	4.61
16	15.15	67.00	65.00	29.00	1.95	0.67	4.99
17	14.39	90.00	76.00	23.00	2.10	0.33	4.66
18	13.01	100.00	62.00	29.00	2.20	0.65	4.33
19	15.51	65.00	90.00	35.00	1.96	0.26	5.01
20	14.36	90.00	105.00	31.00	2.02	0.37	4.75

FIGURE 3.2 Data file for the correlation matrix.

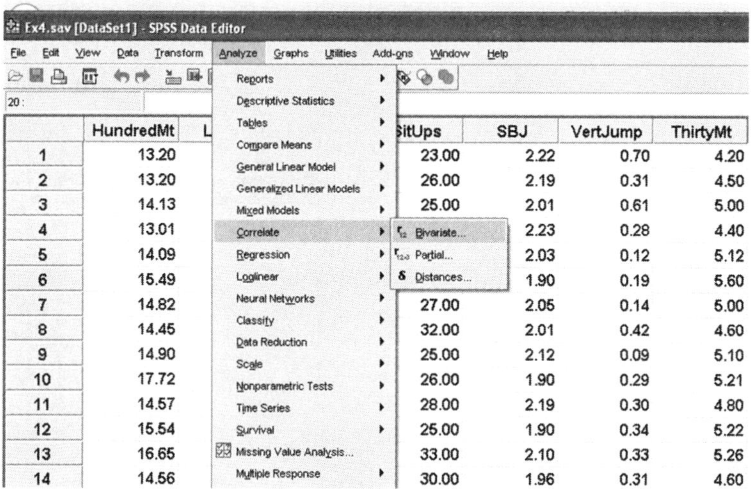

FIGURE 3.3 Commands sequence for computing correlation matrix.

3. *Selecting Options for Computation*: After selecting variables, option needs to be defined. Do the following:
   (a) In the screen shown in Figure 3.4, ensure that the options ‘Pearson’, ‘Two-tailed,’ and ‘Flag significant correlations’ are checked. By default, they are checked.

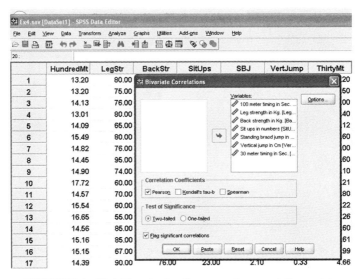

FIGURE 3.4   Variable selection for computing correlation matrix.

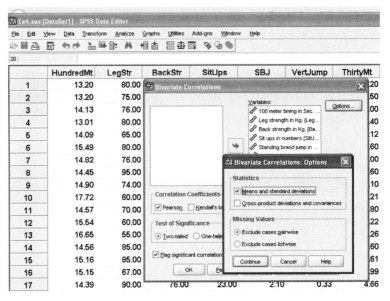

FIGURE 3.5   Option for computing correlation matrix and other statistics.

(b) Clicking **Options** command will take you to the screen as shown in Figure 3.5. Check 'Means and standard deviations' option. Click on **Continue**.

(c) Use default entries in other options. Readers are advised to try other options, and see what changes they get in their output.

TABLE 3.2   Descriptive Statistics

Variables	Mean	SD	N
100-Meter timing (sec)	14.6955	1.18314	20
Leg strength (kg)	89.8000	16.98482	20
Back strength (kg)	75.9000	13.45519	20
Sit-ups (numbers)	27.6500	3.73145	20
Standing broad jump (mt.)	1.9440	0.24481	20
Vertical jump (mt.)	0.3600	0.18047	20
30-Meter timing (sec)	4.8480	0.36068	20

4. *Getting the Output*: After clicking on **OK**, the output shall be generated in the output window. The two outputs, one for descriptive statistics and the other for correlation matrix, so generated are shown in Tables 3.2 and 3.3, respectively.

3.4.2   Interpretations of Findings

Values of mean and standard deviation for all the variables are shown in Table 3.2. These values may be used for further analysis in the study.

Further, actual output shows the full correlation matrix, but only upper diagonal values of correlation coefficients are shown in Table 3.3. This table shows the correlation coefficients along with their associated p values and sample size. One asterisk (*) indicates significance of correlation at 5% level, whereas two asterisks (**) indicate significance at 1% level. In this example, the research hypothesis is a two-tailed, which states "There is a significant correlation between the two variables." The following conclusions may be drawn from the results obtained in Table 3.3:

1. The 100-meter performance is significantly correlated with 30-meter performance at 1% level.
2. The correlation between leg strength and back strength is highly significant at 1% level. Whereas 30 meter timing is significantly correlated with standing broad jump as well as with vertical jump performance at 5% level.
3. All those correlation coefficients having p values less than 0.05 are significant at 5% level and are marked with an asterisk (*), whereas correlations significant at 1% level have been marked with two asterisks (**).

3.5   PARTIAL CORRELATION WITH SPSS

While computing partial correlation in SPSS, user needs to specify variables between which the partial correlation is computed along with the variables whose effects need to be controlled. In partial correlation, one of the variables is usually performance variable or criterion variable, and the other is the independent variable having the highest correlation with it. Depending upon the situation, a researcher may choose any variable other than the highest correlated variable with dependent variable for computing partial correlation. In this example, partial correlation shall be computed between 100-meter performance (X_1) and that of 30-meter performance (X_7) after eliminating the effect of Leg strength (X_2) and Standing broad jump (X_5). This is because the X_7 is highly correlated with the performance variable X_1. The decision of eliminating the effect of variables X_2 and X_5 has been taken because these are the only two significantly correlated variables with X_1 besides X_7. However, one may investigate the relationship between X_1 and X_2 after eliminating the effect of the variables X_5 and X_7. Similarly, partial correlation between X_1 and X_5 may also be investigated after eliminating the effects of the variables X_2 and X_7. The procedure of computing these partial correlations with SPSS has been discussed in the subsequent sections.

3.5.1 Computation of Partial Correlations

3.5.1.1 Preparation of Data File   The same data file that was prepared for computing correlation matrix shall be used for computing the partial correlations. Thus, the procedure for defining the variables and entering the data for all the variables is exactly the same as was done in the case of computing correlation matrix.

3.5.1.2 SPSS Commands   After entering all the data in the **Data View**, do the following steps for computing partial correlations.

1. *Initiating SPSS Commands for Partial Correlation*: In **Data View**, click the following commands in sequence:

   Analyze → Correlate → Partial

   The screen shall look like as shown in Figure 3.6.
2. *Selecting Variables for Partial Correlation*: After clicking on the "Partial" option, you will be directed to the next screen for selecting variables for computing partial correlations.
   (a) Select the two variables *100-meter timing* (X_1) and *30-meter timing* (X_7) from the left panel, and bring them into the "Variables" section in the right panel. X_1 and X_7 are the two variables between which we are interested to know the real relationship after controlling the effect of Leg strength (X_2) and Standing broad jump (X_5). Thus, Select the variables, Leg strength (X_2) and Standing broad jump (X_5), from the left panel and bring them into the "Controlling for" section in the right panel. X_2 and X_5 are the two variables whose effects are to be eliminated.

      Here, selection of variable is made either one by one or all at once. After specifying variables, the screen shall look like as shown in Figure 3.7.
3. *Selecting Options for Computation*: After selecting the two variables for partial correlation and identifying the controlling variables, option needs to be defined for the computation of partial correlation. In Figure 3.7, ensure that the options

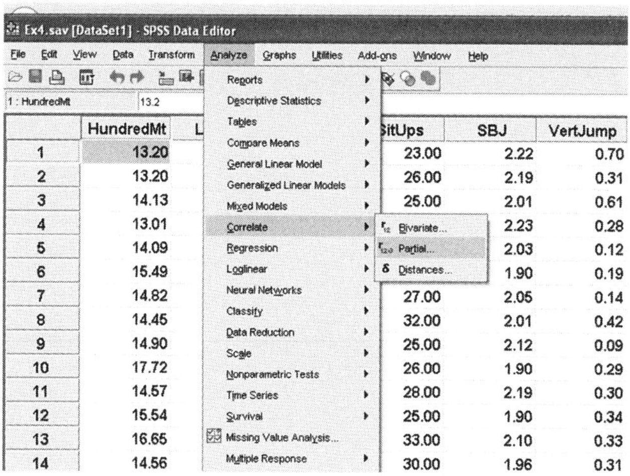

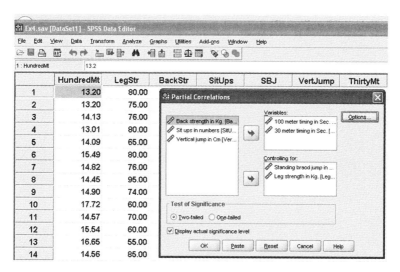

FIGURE 3.6 Command sequence for computing partial correlation.

FIGURE 3.7 Variable selections in partial correlation.

'Two-tailed' and 'Display actual significance level' are checked. In fact, they are checked by default. Do the following:

(a) Click **Options** command, you will get the screen as shown in Figure 3.8. Then check 'Means and standard deviations' option. Click on **Continue**.

(b) Use default entries in other options. Readers are advised to try other options and see what changes they get in their outputs.

(c) Click on **OK** to get the results.

TABLE 3.3 Correlation Matrix

	100 Mt. (X₁)	Leg Str. (X₂)	Back Str. (X₃)	Sit-Ups (X₄)	SBJ (X₅)	VJ (X₆)	30 Mt. (X₇)
100 Mt. (X_1) Pearson correlation	1	0.191	−0.061	0.323	−0.365	−0.287	0.743**
Sig. (two-tailed)		0.420	0.799	0.165	0.113	0.220	0.000
N	20	20	20	20	20	20	20
Leg Str. (X_2) Pearson correlation		1	0.694**	0.314	−0.171	0.004	0.106
Sig. (two-tailed)			0.001	0.177	0.471	0.986	0.657
N		20	20	20	20	20	20
Back Str. (X_3) Pearson correlation			1	0.304	−0.093	−0.309	−0.024
Sig. (two-tailed)				0.192	0.696	0.185	0.920
N			20	20	20	20	20
Sit-Ups (X_4) Pearson correlation				1	−0.330	0.074	0.096
Sig. (two-tailed)					0.155	0.756	0.687
N				20	20	20	20
SBJ (X_5) Pearson correlation					1	0.363	−0.509*
Sig. (two-tailed)						−0.116	0.022
N					20	20	20
VJ (X_6) Pearson correlation						1	−0.499*
Sig. (two-tailed)							0.025
N						20	20
30 Mt. (X_7) Pearson correlation							1
Sig. (two-tailed)							
N							20

* Correlation is significant at 0.05 level (two-tailed).
** Correlation is significant at 0.01 level (two-tailed).

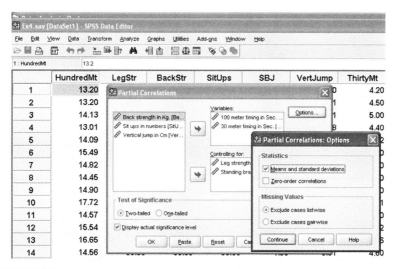

FIGURE 3.8   Option selection in computing partial correlation and other statistics.

TABLE 3.4   Descriptive Statistics

Variables	Mean	SD	N
100-meter timing (sec)	14.6955	1.18314	20
30-meter timing (sec)	4.8480	0.36068	20
Leg strength (kg)	76.4000	12.25346	20
Standing broad jump (mt.)	2.0480	0.11423	20

4. *Getting the Output*: The results are generated in the output panel. It will have two tables: one for descriptive statistics and the other for correlation matrix. These outputs can be selected using the right click of the mouse and may be pasted in the word file. In this example, the output so generated by the SPSS will look like as shown in Tables 3.4 and 3.5.

3.5.2   Interpretation of Partial Correlation

Table 3.4 shows descriptive statistics for the variables chosen for computing the partial correlation. Values of mean and standard deviations may be utilized for further analysis.

In Table 3.5, partial correlation between 100-meter performance (X_1) and 30-meter performance (X_7) after controlling the effect of Leg strength (X_2) and Standing broad Jump (X_5) is shown as 0.265. Since p value associated with this partial correlation is 0.289 in the table which is more than 0.05, it is not significant. It may be noted that correlation coefficient between 100-meter performance and 30-meter performance

TABLE 3.5   Partial Correlation Between 100-meter (X_1) and 30-meter (X_7) Performance After Controlling the Effect of Leg Strength (X_2) and Standing Broad Jump (X_5)

Control Variables			100-meter timing (sec) (X_1)	30-meter timing (sec) (X_7)
Leg strength (kg) (X_2) and *Standing broad jump* (mt.) (X_5)	100-meter timing (sec) (X_1)	Correlation	1.000	0.265
		Significance (two-tailed)	—	0.289
		df	0	16
	30-meter timing (sec) (X_7)	Correlation	0.265	1.000
		Significance (two-tailed)	0.289	—
		df	16	0

Remark: Readers are advised to compute partial correlations of different orders with the same data.

in Table 3.3 is 0.743, which is highly significant; but when the effects of Leg strength and Standing broad jump are eliminated, the actual correlation drops drastically. Thus, it may be concluded that there is no real relationship between 100-meter performance and 30-meter performance as far as this sample is concerned.

3.6   SUMMARY OF THE SPSS COMMANDS

3.6.1   For Computing Correlation Matrix

1. Start SPSS by using the following commands:

   Start → All Programs → SPSS Inc → SPSS 20.0

2. Click **Variable View** and define the variables *HundredMt*, *LegStr*, *BackStr*, *SitUps*, *SBJ*, *VertJump*, and *ThirtyMt* as scale variables.
3. Once variables are defined, type the data column-wise for these variables by clicking **Data View**.
4. In **Data View**, click on the following commands in sequence for generating correlation matrix.

   Analyze → Correlate → Partial

5. Select all the variables from left panel and bring them to the "Variables" section in the right panel.
6. Ensure that the 'Pearson,' 'Two-tailed,' and 'Flag significant correlations' are checked by default.
7. Click on **Options** command and check 'Means and standard deviations' option. Click on **Continue** and **OK** to get the outputs.

3.6.2　For Computing Partial Correlations

1. Follow steps 1–3 as discussed earlier.
2. Using the same data file, apply the following commands sequence for computing partial correlation:

Analyze → Correlate → Partial

3. Select the two variables between which the partial correlation needs to be computed. Select those variables whose effects are to be controlled in the "Controlling for" section.
4. After selecting the variables, click on the **Options** command. Check 'Means and standard deviation' option. Click on **Continue** and **OK** for outputs.

3.7　EXERCISE

3.7.1　Short Answer Questions

Note: Write answer to each of the questions in not more than 200 words.

Q.1　"Product moment correlation coefficient is a useless measure of relationship as it does not explain cause and effect relation between two variables." Comment on this statement.

Q.2　Describe a research situation where partial correlation can be used.

Q.3　Compute correlation coefficient between X and Y and interpret your findings, considering that Y and X are perfectly related by the equation $Y = X^2$

X:	−2	−1	0	1	2
Y:	4	1	0	1	4

Q.4　How will you test the significance of partial correlation using t-test?

Q.5　What does p value refers to? How is it used in testing the significance of product moment correlation coefficient?

3.7.2　Multiple Choice Questions

Note: Questions 1–10 have four alternative answers for each question. Tick mark the one that you consider the closest to the correct answer.

1　In testing the significance of product moment correlation, degrees of freedom for t-test is
  (a) $N-1$
  (b) N
  (c) $N+1$
  (d) $N-2$

2   If sample size increases, the value of correlation coefficient required for its significance
    (a) Increases
    (b) Decreases
    (c) Remains constant
    (d) May increase or decrease

3   Product moment correlation coefficient measures the relationship which is
    (a) Real
    (b) Linear
    (c) Curvilinear
    (d) None of the above

4   Given that $r_{12} = 0.8$ and $r_{12.3} = 0.15$ where X_1 is Performance, X_2 is Height, and X_3 is Leg strength. What interpretation can be drawn?
    (a) Height is an important contributory variable to the performance.
    (b) Leg strength affects the relationship between performance and height in a negative fashion.
    (c) Leg strength has got nothing to do with the performance.
    (d) It seems there is no real relationship between performance and height.

5   If p value for a partial correlation is 0.03, what conclusion can be drawn?
    (a) Partial correlation is not significant at 5% level.
    (b) Partial correlation is significant at 1% level.
    (c) Partial correlation is significant at 5% level.
    (d) Partial correlation is not significant at 10% level.

6   Partial correlation is computed with the data that are measured on
    (a) Interval scale
    (b) Nominal scale
    (c) Ordinal scale
    (d) Any scale

7   In computing correlation matrix with SPSS all variables are defined as
    (a) Nominal
    (b) Ordinal
    (c) Scale
    (d) Any of the nominal, ordinal, or scale option depending upon the nature of variable.

8   In computing correlation matrix in SPSS, which of the following command sequence is used?
    (a) Analyze → Bivariate → Correlate
    (b) Analyze → Correlate → Bivariate
    (c) Analyze → Correlate → Partial
    (d) Analyze → Partial → Bivariate

TABLE 3.6 Data on Self-Concept and Physical Parameters of Swimmers

S.N.	Self-Concept (X_1)	Strength (X_2)	Flexibility (X_3)	Static Balance (X_4)	Speed of Movement (X_5)	Agility (X_6)	Endurance (X_7)
1	169	8	21	33	33	14	980
2	151	21	18	35	36	13	1199
3	190	19	13	41	41	11	1471
4	170	26	19	48	38	12	1316
5	179	30	15	60	31	13	1306
6	188	16	9	32	36	12	1517
7	177	25	17	56	46	12	1555
8	153	21	13	49	34	11	1297
9	162	19	19	38	35	11	1706
10	149	9	20	30	27	13	1640
11	170	12	18	21	35	14	1143
12	146	19	19	36	27	12	1170
13	162	9	16	39	42	13	1146
14	157	28	14	34	37	11	1602
15	154	17	12	38	38	12	1369

9 While computing partial correlation in SPSS the variables selected, in "Controlling for" section are
   (a) All independent variables except the two between which partial correlation is computed.
   (b) Any of the independent variables as it does not affect partial correlation.
   (c) Only those variables whose effects need to be eliminated.
   (d) None of the above is correct.

10 The limits of partial correlation are
   (a) -1 to 0
   (b) 0 to 1
   (c) Sometimes more than 1
   (d) -1 to $+1$

3.7.3 Assignment

A study was conducted on swimmers to know the relationships of self-concept with that of physical parameters. The data so obtained are shown in Table 3.6. Compute the following:

1. Correlation matrix with all seven variables.
2. Partial correlations: $r_{12.7}$, $r_{12.76}$, and $r_{12.763}$

3.8 CASE STUDY ON CORRELATION

Objective

A researcher was interested to investigate as to how fat% of college students relates with different profile parameters. A sample of 15 college students was randomly drawn on which the data on the selected variables was obtained, which are shown in Table 3.7.

Research Questions

The following research questions were investigated:

1. Whether different profile variables have different level of relationship with fat%?
2. Can some of the variables be identified, which are exclusively related with the fat% after eliminating the effect of other variables?

Data Format

The format used for preparing data file in SPSS is shown in Table 3.7.

TABLE 3.7 Data Format Used in SPSS

S.N.	Fat_X_1	Weight_X_2	Pulse Rate_X_3	Expl_Power_X_4	Nine_Min_R/W_X_5	Body_Density_X_6	Height_X_7	LBW_X_8
1	21.23	50	80	698.36	2800	1.05	161	47.26
2	13.06	60	80	937.83	3000	1.07	174	48.69
3	21.76	56	92	678.20	2000	1.05	167	43.81
4	19.30	55	96	697.70	2200	1.05	165	44.39
5	11.66	49	80	750.45	2400	1.07	169	43.28
6	18.08	48	88	754.61	2400	1.05	154	40.15
7	19.30	59	84	824.05	2400	1.06	170	49.65
8	19.35	49	80	726.50	1800	1.05	163	39.50
9	12.58	48	81	887.50	2400	1.06	160	41.95
10	12.71	50	84	924.85	2800	1.06	158	43.63
11	11.92	43	60	786.00	2000	1.07	160	37.84
12	27.81	57	100	678.00	3000	1.05	157	40.44
13	17.46	51	84	637.50	2600	1.06	151	42.60
14	19.23	57	92	744.45	2400	1.06	161	46.65
15	22.70	66	92	1220.85	2000	1.05	163	56.96

Fat, in %; Weight, in kg; Pulse Rate, in b/m; Explosive Power, in kg.cm; 9 Min R/W, in mt.; Body Density, in g/cc; Height, in cm; LBW, in kg.

Analyzing Data

In order to address the research issues, a correlation matrix was computed. By using significant correlations with the Fat% different partial correlations were computed in order to find the independent contribution of the independent variables with fat%.

Describing Relationship

The correlation matrix was obtained by using the commands **Analyze**, **Correlate**, and **Bivariate Correlation** in sequence and by checking the 'Pearson' option. The matrix so obtained is shown in Table 3.8. It can be seen from this table that the fat% is significantly correlated with weight (p=0.044), pulse rate (p=0.003), and body density (p=0.000).

Partial Correlations

On this basis of the sampled data, only three variables weight (X_2), pulse rate (X_3), and body density (X_6) are significantly correlated with the fat%. It was interesting to investigate their independent contribution to the fat% by eliminating the effect of the other two variables. This was done by computing three partial correlations: $r_{12.36}$, $r_{13.26}$, and $r_{16.23}$. These partial correlations were obtained by using the commands **Analyze**, **Correlate**, and **Partial** in sequence and by selecting the variables whose effect was to be eliminated. Table 3.9 shows the partial correlation between the fat% and weight after eliminating the effect of pulse rate and body density. This correlation 0.439 is not significant. It is worth noting that although the correlation between the fat% and weight (0.527) in Table 3.8 was found to be significant, after eliminating the effect of pulse rate and body density, this correlation (0.439) has become nonsignificant. It may thus be concluded that there is no significant correlation between fat% and weight. Similarly, Table 3.10 indicates that the partial correlation between fat% and pulse rate (0.084) after eliminating the effect of weight and body density is insignificant.

On the other hand, Table 3.11 reveals that the partial correlation between fat% and body density after eliminating the effect of weight and pulse rate is −0.712, which is significant (p=0.006). It is worth noting that the correlation between fat% and body density before eliminating the effect of these variables was −0.801 in Table 3.8. It may thus be concluded on the basis of the sampled data that a real relationship exists between fat% and body density.

Reporting

- Fat% seems to be significantly correlated with weight, pulse rate, and body density.

TABLE 3.8 Correlation Matrix

		Fat_X_1	Weight_X_2	Pulse Rate_X_3	Expl_Power_X_4	9 Min R/W_X_5	Body_Density_X_6	Height_X_7	LBW_X_8
Fat_X_1	Pearson correlation	1	0.527*	0.711**	−0.165	0.000	−0.801**	−0.169	0.232
	sig. (two-tailed)		0.044	0.003	0.557	0.999	0.000	0.547	0.405
Weight_X_2	Pearson correlation	0.527*	1	0.627*	0.480	0.107	−0.242	0.420	0.828**
	sig. (two-tailed)	0.044		0.012	0.070	0.704	0.385	0.119	0.000
PulseRate_X_3	Pearson correlation	0.711**	0.627*	1	−0.048	0.175	−0.650**	−0.075	0.301
	sig. (two-tailed)	0.003	0.012		0.865	0.533	0.009	0.791	0.275
Expl_power_X_4	Pearson correlation	−0.165	0.480	−0.048	1	−0.080	0.124	0.251	0.676**
	sig. (two-tailed)	0.557	0.070	0.865		0.776	0.660	0.367	0.006
Nine_MinRW_X_5	Pearson correlation	0.000	0.107	0.175	−0.080	1	0.204	−0.088	0.057
	sig. (two-tailed)	0.999	0.704	0.533	0.776		0.466	0.754	0.841
Body_Density_X_6	Pearson correlation	−0.801**	−0.242	−0.650**	0.124	0.204	1	0.317	−0.090
	sig. (two-tailed)	0.000	0.385	0.009	0.660	0.466		0.249	0.749
Height_X_7	Pearson correlation	−0.169	0.420	−0.075	0.251	−0.088	0.317	1	0.431
	sig. (two-tailed)	0.547	0.119	0.791	0.367	0.754	0.249		0.109
LBW_X_8	Pearson correlation	0.232	0.828**	0.301	0.676**	0.057	−0.090	0.431	1
	sig. (two-tailed)	0.405	0.000	0.275	0.006	0.841	0.749	0.109	

* Correlation is significant at the 0.05 level (two-tailed).
** Correlation is significant at the 0.01 level (two-tailed).

TABLE 3.9   Correlations $r_{12.36}$

Control Variables			Fat_X_1	Weight_X_2
Pulse rate_X_3 and Body_ density_X_6	Fat_X_1	Correlation	1.000	0.439
		Significance (two-tailed)	—	0.134
		df	0	11
	Weight_X_2	Correlation	0.439	1.000
		Significance (two-tailed)	0.134	—
		df	11	0

TABLE 3.10   Correlations $r_{13.26}$

Control Variables			Fat_X_1	Pulse Rate_X_3
Weight_X_2 and Body_density_X_6	Fat_X_1	Correlation	1.000	0.084
		Significance (two-tailed)	—	0.784
		df	0	11
	PulseRate_X_3	Correlation	0.084	1.000
		Significance (two-tailed)	0.784	—
		df	11	0

TABLE 3.11   Correlations $r_{16.23}$

Control Variables			Fat_X_1	Body_Density_X_6
Weight_X_2 and Pulse rate_X_3	Fat_X_1	Correlation	1.000	−0.712
		Significance (two-tailed)	—	0.006
		df	0	11
	Body_ density_X_6	Correlation	−0.712	1.000
		Significance (two-tailed)	0.006	—
		df	11	0

- Partial correlation indicated that there was no real correlation between fat and weight as well as between fat% and pulse rate once the effect of other independent variables was removed.
- On the basis of the sampled data, significant partial correlation between fat% and body density suggested that there was a real relationship between them.

4

COMPARING MEANS

LEARNING OBJECTIVES

After completing this chapter, you should be able to do the following:

- Understand different forms of t-statistic
- Identify t-test appropriate in different research situations
- Know the assumptions in using t-test
- Understand the difference between one-tailed and two-tailed hypotheses
- Describe the situations in which one-tailed and two-tailed tests should be used
- Compute different t-statistics by using SPSS package
- Interpret the results of t-tests obtained in SPSS.

4.1 INTRODUCTION

This chapter describes the procedure for comparing means of two populations in hypothesis testing experiments. In comparative studies, we intend to compare the means of two groups and our focus is to test whether the difference between the two group means is significant. By comparing the sample means, we intend to find whether these samples come from the same population. In other words, we try to infer whether their population means are equal or not. We may come across many research

Sports Research with Analytical Solution using SPSS®, First Edition. J. P. Verma.
© 2016 John Wiley & Sons, Inc. Published 2016 by John Wiley & Sons, Inc.
Companion website: www.wiley.com/go/Verma/Sportsresearch

situations where it is desired to compare the performance of two groups. For instance one may wish, to compare IQ of boys and girls, effect of two aerobic programs on endurance or effect of two relaxation techniques on improving functional efficiency. In all such situations, samples are used to test the equality of population means.

For comparing two group means, two statistical tests "t" and "z" are used in a situation where data are measured on metric scale. In case of small sample where population variance is unknown, t-test is used, whereas z-test is used in large sample (N $\geq$30). For all practical purposes, a sample is said to be small, if it is less than 30 and large if it is equal to or more than 30. Since t-distribution approaches to z-distribution as sample size approaches to infinity, the t-test can be considered as a specific case of the z-test. Thus, t-test can be used for large sample, but the z-test cannot be used for small sample if population variance is unknown.

Once the value of "t" is calculated from the sample of size n, a critical value of t at a desired level of significance and $n-1$ degrees of freedom (df) can be obtained from Table A.2. Comparing the calculated value of t with this tabulated t facilitates us to know whether the difference between the groups is likely to have been a chance finding. The level of significance, also called the alpha level, is usually set at 0.05 or 0.01. The 0.05 level of significance means that the null hypothesis may be wrongly rejected five times in hundred similar experiments conducted on the same population.

In this chapter, we shall discuss three different statistical tests: one-sample t-test, two-sample t-test for independent groups, and paired t-test for related groups.

4.2 ONE-SAMPLE t-TEST

A t-test can be defined as a statistical test in which the test statistic follows a Student's t-distribution under the assumption of null hypothesis. A one-sample t-test is used for comparing the mean value of a sample to a predefined population mean. It is assumed that the population mean is known (or defined) in advance. An example of a one-sample t-test would be a comparison of the mean heart rate of a population to a given reference value.

In one-tailed test, an experimenter is interested to verify whether the population mean is larger than or smaller than a given value, whereas in a two-tailed test, it is required to know whether the population mean differs from the given value. Here, it is not of much interest to know the direction of difference.

In using one-sample t-test, it is assumed that the distribution of the population from which the sample has been drawn is normal. The t-distribution depends on the sample size. Its parameter is called the df, which is equal to $n-1$, where n is the sample size.

In one-sample test, t-statistic is computed by the formula

$$t = \frac{\overline{X} - \mu}{s/\sqrt{n}}, \quad S = \sqrt{\frac{1}{n-1}\Sigma\left(X - \overline{X}\right)^2}$$

After calculating t, its significance value (p value) is obtained. This p value is provided by the SPSS output. If p value is below the threshold level of significance (usually 0.05 or 0.01), then the null hypothesis is rejected in favor of the alternative hypothesis, otherwise it is not.

4.2.1 Application of One-Sample t-Test

The following situation will explain the application of one-sample t-test. A specific protocol of exercise used in a physical therapy center brings relief to the spondylitis patients within a 20-day session. When introducing a new set of exercise, it is administered to 25 patients, and the days until the exercise shows an effect are recorded. The mean days of getting the relief is 16 days with a standard deviation (SD) of 4 days. Can it be concluded that the new exercise reduces the time until a patient receives relief from spondylitis pain?

In this example, sample mean (the mean relief days for spondylitis patients) requires to be compared with a predefined limit. Here, the limit is fixed and well known in advance. Had the limit not been predefined but obtained from another sample (i.e., another group of spondylitis patients receiving the old exercise), one would have to apply a two-sample t-test for independent samples.

4.3 TWO-SAMPLE t-TEST FOR UNRELATED GROUPS

A two-sample t-test is used to test whether the difference between two population means is significant. All t-tests are usually called Student's t-tests. But strictly speaking, this name should be used only if the variances of the two populations are also assumed to be equal. In case the assumption of equality of variances is violated, then the Welch's t-test is used. Readers are advised to read some other text for this test.

We often want to compare the means of two populations, such as, comparing the effect of two training programs, skills of two groups, speed in two different sports etc. In all these situations, two-sample t-test is used. This two sample t-test is used if the samples are independent and identically distributed. Consider an experiment in which the effect of two conditioning programs on fitness level needs to be compared. Two randomly selected group of subjects may be taken in the study. These two groups may be exposed to two different conditioning programs. Assuming that initial fitness level of both the groups is same, the null hypothesis of no difference in their final fitness scores may be tested by applying the two-sample t-test. In this case, both the samples are independent because the subjects in both the groups are different.

4.3.1 Assumptions While Using t-Test

While using the two-sample t-test the following assumptions are made:

- Population from which the samples have been drawn is normally distributed.
- Variances of both the populations are equal.
- Samples are independent to each other.

Since it is assumed that σ_1^2 and σ_2^2 are equal, we can compute the estimate of pooled variance by computing S^2 after combining the two samples. The purpose of pooling the data is to obtain a better estimate of the population variance. The estimate of pooled variance is a weighted sum of mean square variances. Thus, if the sample sizes n_1 and n_2 are equal, then S^2 is just an average of the individual mean square variances of the two samples. The overall df is the sum of the individual df for the two-samples, that is,

$$df = df_1 + df_2 = (n_1 - 1) + (n_2 - 1) = n_1 + n_2 - 2.$$

Computation of t-statistic is same irrespective of testing a two-tailed or one-tailed hypothesis. The only difference in testing these hypotheses is in their testing criteria and the critical values of "t." These cases shall be discussed in the following sections.

4.3.2 Case I: Two-Tailed Test

In two-tailed test if the null hypothesis is rejected, it may be concluded that the group means differ significantly and one cannot interpret as to which group mean is higher. The testing procedure is as follows:

1. Hypotheses to be tested

$$H_0 : \mu_1 = \mu_2$$
$$H_1 : \mu_1 \neq \mu_2$$

2. Test statistic

$$t = \frac{\overline{x}_1 - \overline{x}_2}{S\sqrt{\left(\dfrac{1}{n_1} + \dfrac{1}{n_2}\right)}}$$

where

$$S = \sqrt{\frac{(n_1 - 1)S_1^2 + (n_2 - 1)S_2^2}{n_1 + n_2 - 2}}$$

3. Degrees of freedom $n_1 + n_2 - 2$
4. Decision criteria

If calculated $|t| > t_{\alpha/2}$, H_0 is rejected at α significance level and if calculated $|t| \leq t_{\alpha/2}$, we fail to reject H_0.

4.3.3 Case II: Right Tailed Test

Here, it is desired to test whether the mean of the first group is more than that of the second group. If null hypothesis is rejected, it may be concluded that the first group mean is significantly larger than that of the second group mean. The testing procedure shall be as follows:

1. Hypotheses to be tested

$$H_0 : \mu_1 = \mu_2$$
$$H_1 : \mu_1 > \mu_2$$

2. Test statistic

$$t = \frac{\overline{x}_1 - \overline{x}_2}{S\sqrt{\left(\dfrac{1}{n_1} + \dfrac{1}{n_2}\right)}}$$

where

$$S = \sqrt{\frac{(n_1 - 1)S_1^2 + (n_2 - 1)S_2^2}{n_1 + n_2 - 2}}$$

3. Degrees of freedom $n_1 + n_2 - 2$
4. Decision criteria
   If calculated $t > t_\alpha$, H_0 is rejected at α significance level.
   and if calculated $t \le t_\alpha$, we fail to reject H_0.

4.3.4 Case III: Left Tailed Test

Here it is desired to test whether mean of the first group is less than that of the second group. In other words, the researcher is interested in a particular group. In this testing if the null hypothesis is rejected, it can be concluded that the mean of the first group is significantly less than that of the second group. The testing procedure is as follows:

1. Hypotheses to be tested

$$H_0 : \mu_1 = \mu_2$$
$$H_1 : \mu_1 < \mu_2$$

2. Test statistic

$$t = \frac{\overline{x}_1 - \overline{x}_2}{S\sqrt{\left(\dfrac{1}{n_1} + \dfrac{1}{n_2}\right)}}$$

where

$$S = \sqrt{\frac{(n_1 - 1)S_1^2 + (n_2 - 1)S_2^2}{n_1 + n_2 - 2}}$$

3. Degrees of freedom $n_1 + n_2 - 2$
4. Decision criteria

   If calculated $t < -t_\alpha$, H_0 is rejected at α significance level.

   and if calculated $t \geq -t_\alpha$, we fail to reject H_0.

4.3.5 Application of Two-Sample t-Test

Two-sample t-test is used to compare means of the two independent groups. Consider a situation where a coach has developed two circuit training programs for his athletes and wish to know whether they differ in their effectiveness. Since he does not have an idea as to which program may be more effective, he would prefer to organize a two-tailed test as mentioned in Case I. Let us consider another situation where a conditioning program is going on in a university for the last many years. A newly appointed fitness consultant claims that his proposed program is better in comparison to the existing one in improving fitness status of the subjects. The authority may decide to conduct a study on two independent samples where t-test discussed in Case II may be used. The sole contention in testing the hypothesis in this study is to check whether the proposed progarm is better than the existing one or not. If the same experiment is conducted to test whether the proposed conditioning program improves the timing of athletes in a 400-meter event, then the t-test discussed in Case III may be used. Here it is of interest to see whether average timing of athletes on the 400-meter event reduces in the proposed conditioning group in comparison to that of existing conditioning group.

4.4 PAIRED t-TEST FOR RELATED GROUPS

Paired t-test is used to test a null hypothesis that the difference between two responses measured on the same subjects has a mean value of zero. Let us suppose we measure shooting accuracy of basketballers before and after a training program. If the training program is effective, we expect the shooting accuracy to improve for most of the basketballers after the training. Thus, to know the effectiveness of the program, a paired t-test is used. This paired t-test is also known as "repeated measures" t-test.

In using the paired t-test, sample must be paired data obtained on the same unit or sets of data obtained on the same subjects before and after the experiment. A typical example of the paired t-test may be a situation where subjects are tested on cardiorespiratory endurance before and after a 4-week aerobic program. Thus, paired t-test is used in a situation where the subjects are same in pre- and post-testing.

While applying paired t-test for two related groups, a pair-wise difference, D_i, is computed for all n-paired scores. This D_i, a new variable, follows the t-distribution. The $\bar{D}$ and S_D are the mean and root mean squares of the D_i's respectively. Thus, paired t-statistic is computed as follows:

$$t = \frac{\bar{D}}{S_D / \sqrt{n}}$$

While applying paired t-test, it is assumed that the distribution of scores obtained by pair-wise difference is normal and the differences are a random sample. An experiment where the paired difference is computed is often more powerful, since it can eliminate differences in the samples that increase the total variance σ^2. When the comparison is made between groups (of similar experimental units), it is called blocking. The paired difference experiment is an example of a randomized block experiment.

If normality assumption is violated, Wilcoxon signed-rank test may be used as a nonparametric test for paired difference designs. Whether two-tailed or one-tailed test is used, the test statistic remains the same and only decision-making strategy and the critical values of the t changes. All these situations have been discussed later.

4.4.1 Case I: Two-Tailed Test

Using this test, difference between means of the post- and pre experiment data is compared; and if the null hypothesis is rejected, one can only say that the post experiment mean differs from the pre experiment mean and no conclusion can be drawn as to which group mean is higher. The testing procedure shall be as follows:

1. Hypotheses to be tested

$$H_0 : \mu_1 - \mu_2 = 0 \qquad \text{[Post experiment is group 1}$$
$$\text{and pre experiment is group 2]}$$
$$H_1 : \mu_1 \neq \mu_2$$

2. Test statistic

$$t = \frac{\bar{D}}{S_D / \sqrt{n}}$$

where

$$\bar{D} = \bar{X}_1 - \bar{X}_2, \quad S_D = \sqrt{\frac{1}{n-1} \Sigma \left(D - \bar{D} \right)^2}$$

3. Degrees of freedom $n - 1$
4. Decision criteria
   If calculated $|t| > t_{\alpha/2}$, H_0 is rejected at α significance level.
   and if calculated $|t| \leq t_{\alpha/2}$, we fail to reject H_0.

4.4.2 Case II: Right Tailed Test

In most of the situations, we are interested to know as to whether there is an improvement after the treatment effect. Thus, in all such situations it is desired to test whether the difference between post- and pre experiment means is greater than zero. In such testing if null hypothesis is rejected, it may be concluded that the post experiment group mean is significantly higher than that of the pre experiment group. The testing procedure shall be as follows:

1. Hypotheses to be tested

$$H_0 : \mu_1 - \mu_2 = 0 \quad \text{[Post experiment is group 1}$$
$$\text{and pre experiment is group 2]}$$
$$H_1 : \mu_1 - \mu_2 > 0$$

2. Test statistic

$$t = \frac{\bar{D}}{S_D / \sqrt{n}}$$

Here

$$\bar{D} = \bar{X}_1 - \bar{X}_2, \quad S_D = \sqrt{\frac{1}{n-1}\Sigma(D-\bar{D})^2}$$

3. Degrees of freedom $n-1$
4. Decision criteria
   If calculated $t > t_\alpha$, H_0 is rejected at α significance level.
   and if calculated $t \le t_\alpha$, we fail to reject H_0.

4.4.3   Case III: Left Tailed Test

In case of timing events, it is required to test whether mean timing of the post experiment group is less than that of the pre experiment group. In such cases, left tailed testing is done. In other words, the researcher is interested to know whether there is a significant improvement in the timing event. In such testing if the null hypothesis is rejected, it can be concluded that the first group mean is significantly lower than that of the second group. The testing procedure shall be as follows:

1. Hypotheses to be tested

$$H_0 : \mu_1 - \mu_2 = 0 \quad \text{[Post experiment is group 1}$$
$$\text{and pre experiment is group 2]}$$
$$H_1 : \mu_1 - \mu_2 < 0$$

2. Test statistic

$$t = \frac{\bar{D}}{S_D / \sqrt{n}}, \quad S_D = \sqrt{\frac{1}{n-1}\Sigma(D-\bar{D})^2}$$

Here

$$\bar{D} = \bar{X}_1 - \bar{X}_2$$

3. Degrees of freedom $n-1$
4. Decision criteria

If calculated $t < -t_\alpha$, H_0 is rejected at α significance level.
and if calculated $t \geq -t_\alpha$, we fail to reject H_0.

4.4.4 Application of Paired t-Test

Application of the paired t-test can be understood by considering the following situation. In an institution, it has been observed that the research students are becoming lethargic due to lot of academic load and no compulsive physical activity. It is therefore, decided to launch a 40-min workout for them so that their muscular strength can be improved. Before launching the program it is decided to test the effectiveness of the programme hence the workout may be given to 20 randomly chosen research students for 6 weeks. These subjects may be tested for their muscular strength by means of strength index before and after the 6-week workout program. In order to know the effectiveness of the workout, the paired t-test may be used. Since in this situation we are interested in the improvement of post experiment mean, we may use the testing protocol discussed earlier in Case II.

Now consider another situation where an exercise scientist wishes to see the effectiveness of an aerobic program on agility by means of a 4×10-meter shuttle run. Here she would compare the mean agility score before and after the aerobic program. In this situation she would choose one-tailed test as discussed in Case III because the aerobic program will always reduce the timing on the 4×10-meter shuttle run but will never increase it. Here the intention is to test whether improvement in agility is significant or not. Even if the performance on agility is deteriorated due to noncooperation of the subjects or due to other lifestyle habits during experimentation, it will not affect the experiment because the whole contention of testing is to know whether the aerobic program is effective or not.

4.5 ONE-SAMPLE t-TEST WITH SPSS

Example 4.1

Fat% of 15 college football players is shown in Table 4.1. Do these data support the assumption that the mean fat% of college footballers is equal to 10.5? Let us test this hypothesis at 5% level and interpret the findings.

Solution: The hypotheses that need to be tested are as follows:

$$H_0 : \mu = 10.5$$
$$H_1 : \mu \neq 10.5$$

Once the value of t-statistic is computed by the SPSS, it shall be tested for its significance. SPSS output also gives the significance level (p value) along with calculated t. If p value is less than 0.05, the null hypothesis is rejected at 5% level, otherwise not.

TABLE 4.1   Fat% of Football Players

S.N.	Fat%
1	9.90
2	11.50
3	15.90
4	15.30
5	12.50
6	13.40
7	9.00
8	15.40
9	10.20
10	15.40
11	9.00
12	13.40
13	9.80
14	15.40
15	10.20

4.5.1   Computation in t-Test for Single Group

4.5.1.1   Preparations of Data File   After starting the SPSS as discussed in Chapter 1, select 'Type in data' option for preparing data file.

4.5.1.2   Defining Variables   There is only one variable in this example that needs to be defined along with its properties. Since the variable is quantitative in nature, it shall be treated as scale. The procedure of defining the variable and its characteristics in SPSS is as follows:

1. Click on **Variable View** to define variable and its properties.
2. Write short name of the variable as *Fat* under the column heading "Name."
3. Under the column heading "Label," the full name of the variable may be defined as *Fat%*. One can choose some other name of this variable as well.
4. Under the column heading "Measure," select the option 'Scale' for the variable *Fat* as this is a quantitative variable.
5. Use default entries in rest of the columns.

After defining the variable in **Variable View**, the screen shall look like as shown in Figure 4.1.

Note: More than one variable can be defined in the **Variable View** for computing t statistic for each variable.

4.5.1.3 *Entering Data* Once the variable is defined in the **Variable View**, click on **Data View** as shown in Figure 4.1 to open the format for entering the data column-wise. After entering the data, the screen will look like as shown in Figure 4.2. Save the data file in the desired location before further processing.

4.5.1.4 *SPSS Commands* After entering all the data in **Data View**, the following steps should be followed for computing t-statistic:

1. *Initiating SPSS commands:* In the **Data View**, click on the following commands in sequence:

$$\text{Analyze} \rightarrow \text{Compare Means} \rightarrow \text{One} - \text{Sample T Test}$$

The screen shall look like as shown in Figure 4.3.

2. *Selecting variables:* After clicking the "One-Sample T Test" option, you will be directed to the next screen for selecting variable for computing t-statistic. Select *Fat%* variable from left panel and bring it to the right panel by clicking the arrow sign. In case of more number of variables, you may select them as

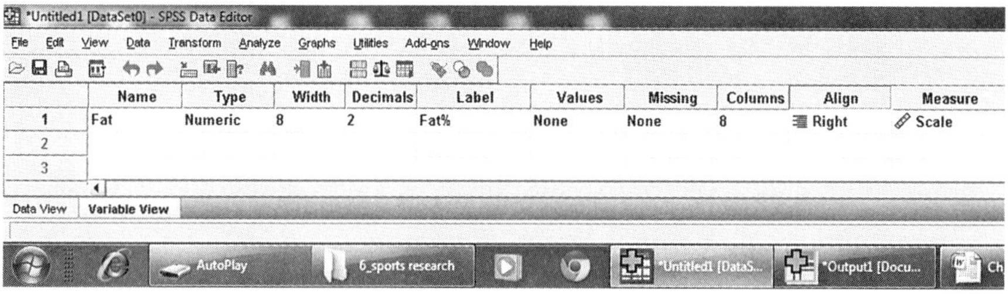

FIGURE 4.1 Variable along with its characteristics for the data shown in Table 4.1.

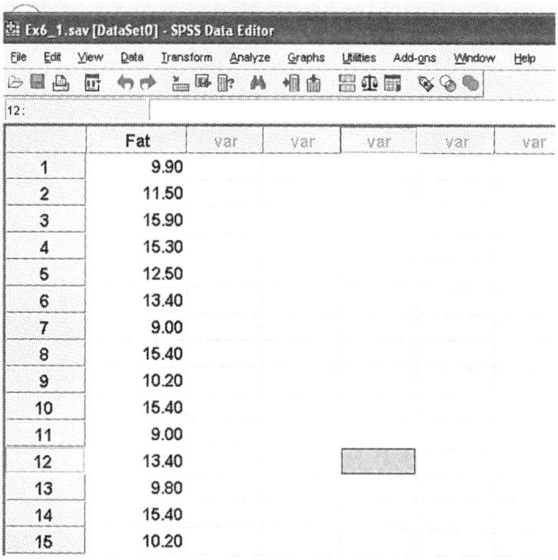

FIGURE 4.2 Screen showing entered data for the fat% in **Data View**.

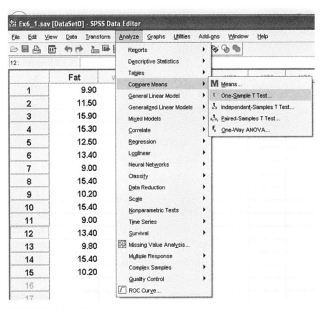

FIGURE 4.3   Command sequence in computing one-sample t-test.

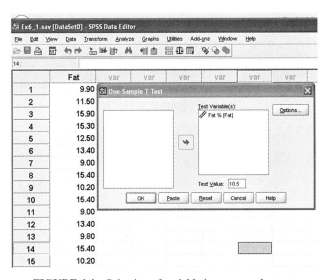

FIGURE 4.4   Selection of variable in one-sample t-test.

well for computing t value for each variable. The screen shall look like as shown in Figure 4.4.

3. *Selecting options for computation:* After selecting the variable, option needs to be defined for the one-sample t-test. Do the following:

   (a) In the screen shown in Figure 4.4, enter the "test value" as 10.5. This is the population mean for fat% that we need to verify in the hypothesis.

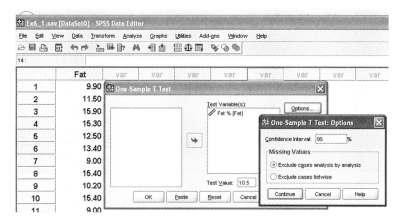

FIGURE 4.5   Selecting options for computing one-sample t-test.

(b) Click the **Options** command, you will get the screen as shown in Figure 4.5. Enter the confidence interval as 95% and click on **Continue** to get back the screen shown in Figure 4.4.

The confidence interval is chosen to get the confidence limits of mean based on sample data. Since in this example hypothesis needs to be tested at 5% level, the confidence interval has been chosen as 95%.

(c) Click on **OK**.

4. *Getting the output:* After clicking on **OK** in the screen as shown in Figure 4.4, you will get the output window. The relevant outputs may be selected by using right click of the mouse and may be copied in the word file. The following results shall be picked up:

(a) Sample statistics showing mean, SD, and standard error

(b) t-table showing the value of t and its significance level.

In this example, all the outputs so generated by the SPSS will look like as shown in Tables 4.2 and 4.3. The model way of writing the results of one-sample t-test has been shown in Table 4.4.

4.5.2 Interpretation of Findings

The values of mean, SD, and standard error of mean are given in Table 4.2. The average fat% of the footballers is 12.42. For an average adult, the fat% is in the range of 10–20% of their body weight; and therefore, it can be interpreted that an average footballer had an athletic body because their fat% was close to the ideal fat%.

From Table 4.4 it can be seen that the t value is equal to 2.836, and its associated p value is 0.013. Since p value is less than 0.05, it may be concluded that the null hypothesis is rejected at 5% level. Hence, it may be inferred that the average fat% of footballers is not equal to 10.5.

TABLE 4.2   One-Sample Statistics

	N	Mean	SD	SE Mean
Fat%	15	12.4200	2.62249	0.67712

TABLE 4.3   One-Sample t Test

Test Value = 10.5						
					95% Confidence Interval of the Difference	
	t	df	Sig. (2-Tailed)	Mean Difference	Lower	Upper
Fat%	2.836	14	0.013	1.92000	0.4677	3.3723

TABLE 4.4   t-Table for the Data on Fat%

Mean	SD	Mean Difference	t Value	p Value
12.42	2.62	1.92	2.836	0.013

4.6   TWO-SAMPLE t-TEST FOR INDEPENDENT GROUPS WITH SPSS

Example 4.2

In a study, flexibility of 15 gymnasts and 16 athletes was measured by sit and reach test. Can it be concluded from the data shown in Table 4.5 that the flexibility of gymnasts and athletes was different at 0.05 significance level?

Solution: The hypotheses that need to be tested are as follows:

$$H_0 : \mu_{Gym} = \mu_{Ath}$$

$$H_1 : \mu_{Gym} \neq \mu_{Ath}$$

Once the value of t-statistic is computed by the SPSS, it shall be tested for its significance. One of the conditions for using the two-sample t-test for independent groups is that the variance of the two groups must be equal. To do so, Levene's F-test shall be used to test the null hypothesis of equality of variances. If p value associated with the F-test is more than 0.05, the null hypothesis may be retained and this will ensure the homogeneity assumption required for using t-test.

Another important feature for this test is the method of data feeding in SPSS. Readers should note the procedure of defining variables and feeding data carefully. In this example, there are two variables *Sport* and *Flexibility*. *Sport* is a nominal variable whereas *Flexibility* is a scale variable.

TABLE 4.5   Data on Flexibility in Inches

S.N.	Gymnasts	Athletes
1	11.5	9.0
2	12.5	8.5
3	13.0	10.5
4	11.5	11.0
5	12.5	10.5
6	10.5	8.5
7	11.0	7.5
8	12.5	8.0
9	11.5	7.5
10	9.5	7.0
11	10.5	7.5
12	11.5	8.0
13	10.0	7.0
14	11.5	7.5
15	12.0	8.5
16		7.5

4.6.1   Computation in Two-Sample t-Test

4.6.1.1   Preparations of Data File   After starting the SPSS as discussed in Chapter 1, variables need to be defined by selecting 'Type in data' option.

4.6.1.2   Defining Variables   There are two variables *Sport* and *Flexibility* in this example that need to be defined along with their properties. Do the following:

1. Click on **Variable View** button to define variables and their properties.
2. Write short name of the variables as *Sport* and *Flexibility* under the column heading "Name."
3. Under the column heading "Label," full name of these variables may be defined as *Sport group* and *Flexibility of the subject*, respectively. Readers may choose some other names of these variables as well.
4. For the *Sport* variable double click the cell under the column heading "Values" and add the following values to different levels:

Value	Label
1	Gymnasts
2	Athletes

The screen for defining the values shall look like as shown in Figure 4.6.
5. Under the column heading "Measure," select option "Nominal" for the *Sport* and 'Scale' for the *Flexibility*.
6. Use default entries in rest of the columns.

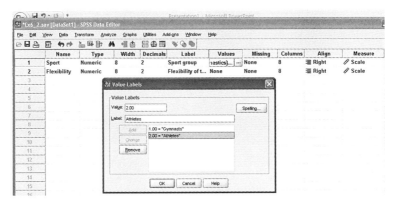

FIGURE 4.6   Defining code of nominal variable.

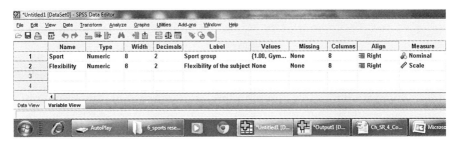

FIGURE 4.7   Defining variables along with their characteristics.

After defining variables in **Variable View**, the screen shall look like as shown in Figure 4.7.

4.6.1.3   Entering Data   Once both the variables are defined in the **Variable View**, click on **Data View** on the left corner in the bottom of the screen shown in Figure 4.7 to open the data entry format. For the *Sport* variable, type the first 15 scores as '1' and the next 16 scores as '2' in the column. This is because the value '1' denotes gymnasts, and there are 15 flexibility scores for them as shown in Table 4.5. Similarly, the value '2' denotes athletes, and there are 16 flexibility scores for them. After entering data, the screen will look like as shown in Figure 4.8.

4.6.1.4   SPSS Commands   After entering all the data in **Data View**, do the following steps:

1. *Initiating SPSS commands:* In **Data View**, go to the following commands in sequence:

   Analyze → Compare Means → Independent – SamplesT Test

   The screen shall look like as shown in Figure 4.9.

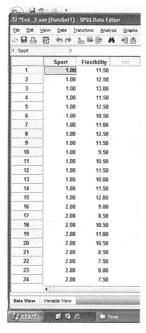

FIGURE 4.8   Format of data entry in **Data View**.

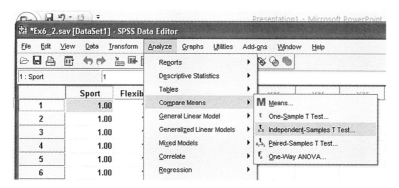

FIGURE 4.9   Command sequence in two-sample t-test.

2. *Selecting variables:* After clicking the 'Independent-Samples T Test' option, you will be directed to the next screen for selecting variables for the two-sample t-test. Select *Flexibility* variable from left panel and bring it to the "Test Variable" section in the right panel. Similarly, select the *Sport* variable from the left panel and bring it to the "Grouping Variable" section in the right panel.

   (a) Once both these variables are selected enter 1 and 2 in Groups 1 and 2, respectively, by clicking on "Define Groups."

   (b) Click on **Continue** after selecting both variables, the screen shall look like as shown in Figure 4.10.

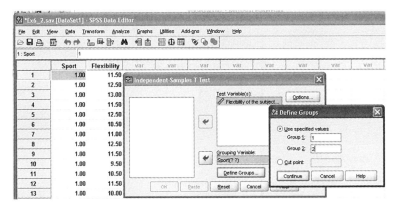

FIGURE 4.10   Selection of variables in two-sample t-test.

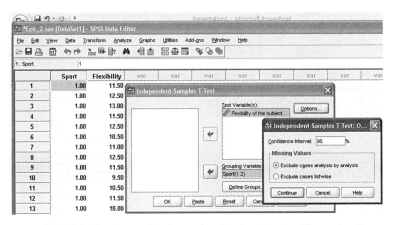

FIGURE 4.11   Screen showing option for choosing significance level.

Note: Many variables can be defined in the **Variable View** in the same data file for computing several t values for different independent groups.

3. *Selecting options for computation:* After selecting variables, option need to be defined for the two-sample t-test. Do the following:

(a) Click on the **Options** command to get the screen as shown in Figure 4.11.

(b) Enter the Confidence Interval as 95% and click on **Continue** to get back to the screen shown in Figure 4.10.

By default the confidence interval is 95%. However, if desired, it may be changed to some other level. The confidence level is the one at which hypothesis needs to be tested. In this problem, the hypothesis is required to be tested at a significance level of 0.05, and, therefore, the confidence level here shall be 95%. One may choose the confidence level as 90 or 99%, if the level of significance for testing the hypothesis is 0.10 or 0.01, respectively.

(c) Click on **OK** in the screen shown in Figure 4.10.

4. *Getting the output:* Click on **OK** to generate results. In the output window of SPSS, the relevant outputs can be selected by using right click of the mouse and may be copied into the word file. The following outputs have been selected in the analysis:

(a) Descriptive statistics of the groups.

(b) "F" and "t" values for testing the equality of variances and equality of means, respectively.

In this example, all outputs so generated by the SPSS will look like as shown in Tables 4.6 and 4.7. The model way of writing the results of two-sample t-test for independent samples has been shown in Table 4.8.

4.6.2 Interpretation of Findings

The following interpretations can be made on the basis of the results shown in the outputs:

1. The values of mean, SD, and standard error of mean for gymnasts and athletes are given in Table 4.6. The mean flexibility of gymnasts is larger than that of athletes. However, whether this difference is significant or not has to be tested by using the two-sample t-test for unrelated groups.

2. One of the conditions for using the two-sample t-test for independent groups is that the variance of the two groups must be equal. To test the equality of variances, Levene's test has been used. In Table 4.7, F value is 0.833, which is nonsignificant, as the p value is 0.369, which is more than 0.05. Thus, the null hypothesis of equality of variances may be retained, and it is concluded that the variances of the two groups are equal.

3. It can be seen from Table 4.7 that the value of t-statistic is 7.42. This t value is significant as the p value associated with it is 0.000, which is less than 0.05. Thus, the null hypothesis of equality of population means of two groups is rejected, and it may be concluded that the flexibility of gymnasts and athletes is different.

4. If it is desired to test the hypothesis as to whether the flexibility of gymnasts is higher than that of athletes or not, one tailed test should be used. In that case, the hypotheses would be as follows:

$$H_o : \mu_{Gym} = \mu_{Ath}$$

$$H_1 : \mu_{Gym} > \mu_{Ath}$$

TABLE 4.6 Descriptive Statistics of the Groups

	Sport Group	N	Mean	SD	SE (Mean)
Flexibility in inch	Gymnasts	15	11.43	0.9976	0.25758
	Athletes	16	8.375	1.27148	0.31787

TABLE 4.7 F and t Table for Testing the Equality of Variances and Equality of Means of Two Independent Groups

	Levene's Test for Equality of Variance		t-Test for Equality of Means						95% Confidence Interval of the Difference	
	F	Sig.	t	df	Sig. (2-Tailed)	Mean Difference	SE Difference		Lower	Upper
Flexibility										
Equal variances assumed	0.833	0.369	7.42	29.00	0.000	3.06	0.412		2.21	3.901
Equal variances not assumed			7.48	28.16	0.000	3.06	0.409		2.22	3.896

TABLE 4.8   t-Table for the Data on Flexibility Along with F Value

Groups	Mean	SD	Mean Difference	SE of Mean Difference	t Value	p Value	F Value	p Value
Gymnasts	11.43	0.998	3.06	0.412	7.42	0.000	0.833	0.369
Athletes	8.38	1.271						

In using one-tailed test, the value of t (=7.42) should be compared with tabulated $t_{0.05}(n_1 + n_2 - 2)$. Here $n_1 = 15$ and $n_2 = 16$ and, therefore, from Table A.2, for one-tailed hypothesis the value of $t_{0.05}(29) = 1.699$. Since calculated value of t (=7.42) is greater than tabulated t (=1.699), H_0 may be rejected, and it may be concluded that flexibility of the gymnasts is significantly higher than that of the athletes.

4.7   PAIRED t-TEST FOR RELATED GROUPS WITH SPSS

Example 4.3

Fifteen women participated in an 8-week management program. Their weights were measured before and after the program, which are shown in Table 4.9. Let us apply paired t-test to find whether the weight management program was effective at 0.05 significance level.

Solution: The hypotheses that need to be tested are as follows:

$$H_0 : \mu_{Post} = \mu_{Pre}$$

$$H_1 : \mu_{Post} \neq \mu_{Pre}$$

TABLE 4.9   Weights of Women in lb

Postprogram	Preprogram
155	160
158	170
159	160
165	175
145	150
150	158
146	145
158	169
168	172
162	167
152	155
128	132
136	135
138	142
139	147

Once the value of t-statistic for the paired sample is computed by the SPSS, it needs to be tested for its significance.

In this problem there are two variables *Pre-Testing weight* and *Post-Testing weight*. For both these variables, data shall be entered in two different columns unlike the way it was feeded in two-sample t-test for unrelated groups.

4.7.1 Computation in Paired t-Test

4.7.1.1 Preparations of Data File Start SPSS the way it was done in the Example 4.2 and select 'Type in data' option for defining variables.

4.7.1.2 Defining Variables Here the two variables preprogram weight and postprogram weight need to be defined along with their properties. Both these variables are scale variables as they are quantitative in nature.

1. Click on **Variable View** to define variables and their properties.
2. Write short name of the variables as *Post_Wt* and *Pre_Wt* under the column heading "Name."
3. Under the column heading "Label," full name of these variables may be defined as *Postprogram Weight* and *Preprogram Weight*, respectively. Readers may choose some other names of these variables if so desired.
4. Under the column heading "Measure," select the option 'Scale' for both variables.
5. Use default entries in rest of the columns.

After defining variables in the **Variable View**, the screen shall look like as shown in Figure 4.12.

4.7.1.3 Entering Data Once both the variables are defined in **Variable View**, click on **Data View** on the left corner in the bottom of the screen shown in Figure 4.12 to open the format for entering the data column-wise. After entering data, the screen will look like as shown in Figure 4.13.

4.7.1.4 SPSS Commands After entering data in the **Data View**, perform the following steps:

1. *Initiating SPSS commands:* In **Data View**, click the following commands in sequence:

   Analyze → Compare Means → Paired – Samples T Test

   The screen shall look like as shown in Figure 4.14.
2. *Selecting variables:* After clicking **Paired-Samples T Test**, the next screen will appear for variable selection. Select the variable *Postprogram Weight* and

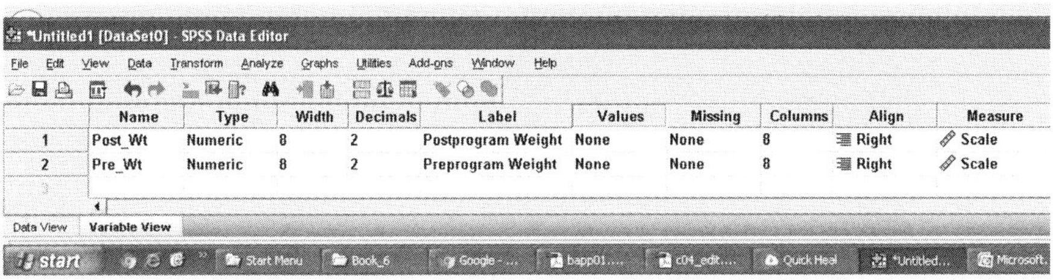

	Name	Type	Width	Decimals	Label	Values	Missing	Columns	Align	Measure
1	Post_Wt	Numeric	8	2	Postprogram Weight	None	None	8	Right	Scale
2	Pre_Wt	Numeric	8	2	Preprogram Weight	None	None	8	Right	Scale

FIGURE 4.12 Defining variables along with their characteristics.

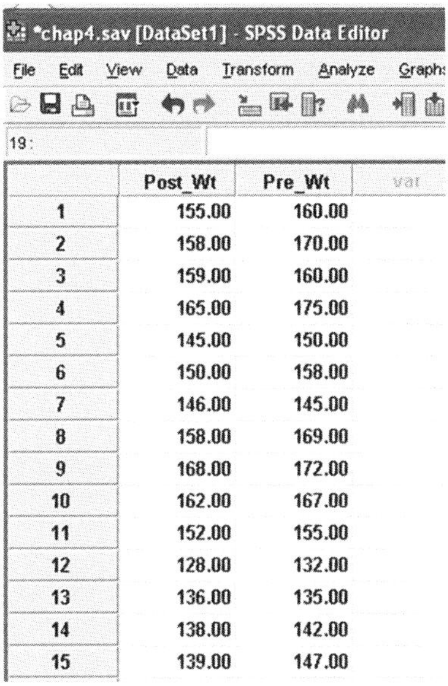

	Post_Wt	Pre_Wt
1	155.00	160.00
2	158.00	170.00
3	159.00	160.00
4	165.00	175.00
5	145.00	150.00
6	150.00	158.00
7	146.00	145.00
8	158.00	169.00
9	168.00	172.00
10	162.00	167.00
11	152.00	155.00
12	128.00	132.00
13	136.00	135.00
14	138.00	142.00
15	139.00	147.00

FIGURE 4.13 Data Entry format in paired t-test.

Preprogram Weight from left panel, and bring them to the right panel as variable 1 and variable 2 of pair 1. After selecting both the variables, the screen shall look like as shown in Figure 4.15.

Note: Many pairs of variables can be defined in the **Variable View** in the same data file for computing several paired t-tests. These pairs of variables can be selected together in the screen shown in Figure 4.15.

3. *Selecting options for computation:* After selecting variables, option needs to be defined for computing paired t-test. Do the following:
   (a) On the screen shown in Figure 4.15 click on **Options** command, you will get the screen where confidence level is selected as 95% by default. Click on **Continue**. One can define the confidence level as 90 or 99% if the level of significance for testing the hypothesis is 0.10 or 0.01, respectively.

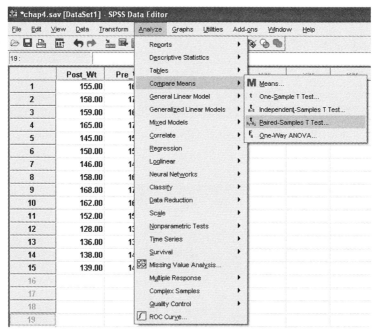

FIGURE 4.14 Command sequence in paired t-test.

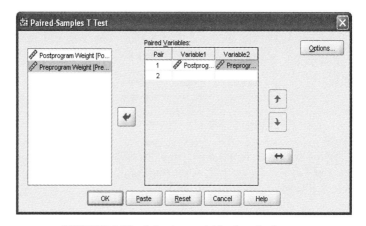

FIGURE 4.15 Selecting variables in paired t-test.

4. Click on **OK** to generate the different outputs. The following outputs shall be selected for discussion:

   (a) Paired samples statistics

   (b) Paired t-test table

5. In this example, selected outputs generated by the SPSS will look like as shown in Tables 4.10 and 4.11.

TABLE 4.10 Paired Sample Statistics

	Mean	N	SD	SE (Mean)
Pair 1				
Postprogram Weight	150.60	15	11.69	3.02
Preprogram Weight	155.80	15	13.60	3.51

TABLE 4.11 Paired t-Test Table

	Paired Differences							
				95% Confidence Interval of the Difference				
	Mean	SD	SE (Mean)	Lower	Upper	t	df	Sig. (2-Tailed)
Pair 1 Postprogram Weight – Preprogram Weight	−5.20	3.99	1.03	−7.41	−2.99	−5.053	14	0.000

4.7.2 Interpretation of Findings

The following interpretations can be made on the basis of the results shown in the earlier output:

1. The values of the mean, SD, and standard error of the mean for the data on weight in the post- and preprogram are shown in Table 4.10. These values can be used for further analysis.
2. It can be seen from Table 4.11 that the value of t-statistic is 5.053. This t-statistic is significant as its corresponding p value is 0.000, which is less than 0.05. Thus, the null hypothesis of equality of mean weights in post- and preprogram groups is rejected, and it may be concluded that the average weight of the women in post- and preprogram groups in the weight management program is not same. However, in order to conclude whether the weight reduction program is effective or not, one tailed test should be used. The hypotheses that need to be tested in that shall be

$$H_o : \mu_{Post} = \mu_{Pre}$$
$$H_1 : \mu_{Post} < \mu_{Pre}$$

For left tailed test, the value of tabulated t at 0.05 level of significance and 14 (N−1=14) df can be seen from Table A.2, which is equal to 1.761. Since calculated value of t (−5.053) is less than tabulated $t_{0.05}(14)$ (−1.761), H_0 may be rejected, and it may be concluded that the weight management program is effective.

4.8 SUMMARY OF SPSS COMMANDS FOR t-TESTS

4.8.1 One-Sample t-Test

1. Start SPSS by using the following sequence of commands:

    Start → All Programs → SPSS Inc → SPSS 20.0

2. Click on **Variable View** and define the variable *Fat*.
3. Type the data by clicking on **Data View**.
4. In **Data View**, follow the below mentioned sequence of commands:

    Analyze → Compare Means → One − Sample t Test

5. Select *Fat%* from left panel, and bring it to the right panel by using the arrow command.
6. Enter the test value as 10.5. This is the population mean of Fat%, which we need to verify in the hypothesis.
7. By clicking on the **Options** command, ensure that the confidence interval is selected as 95%, and then click on **Continue**. Confidence level can be entered as 90 or 99% if the level of significance for testing the hypothesis is 0.10 or 0.01, respectively.
8. Click on **OK** for outputs.

4.8.2 Two-Sample t-Test for Independent Groups

1. Start SPSS the way it is done in case of one-sample t-test.
2. In the **Variable View** define *Sport* as a 'Nominal' and *Flexibility* as 'Scale' variable.
3. In the **Variable View** under column heading "Values" define '1' for gymnast and '2' for athlete for *Sport* variable.
4. In **Data View** feed the first 15 entries as 1 and next 16 entries as 2 for the *Sport* variable. Under the column *Flexibility*, enter the first group of flexibility data and then in the same column enter the second group of flexibility data.
5. In **Data View**, the following sequence of commands must be followed for computing the value of t:

    Analyze → Compare Means → Independent-Samples T Test

6. Select *Flexibility* and *Sport* variables from left panel, and bring them to the "Test Variable" and "Grouping Variable" sections in the right panel, respectively.
7. Define values 1 and 2 as two groups for the grouping variable *Sport*.
8. By clicking on the **Options** command, ensure that the confidence interval is selected as 95%, and then click on **Continue**.
9. Click on **OK** for generating outputs.

4.8.3   Paired t-Test

1. Start SPSS the way it is done in case of one-sample t-test.
2. In the **Variable View** define *Post_Wt* and *Pre_Wt* as 'Scale' variables.
3. In the **Data View** the following sequence of commands must be followed for computing the value of t after entering the data for both the variables:

$$\text{Analyze} \rightarrow \text{Compare Means} \rightarrow \text{Paired-Samples T Test}$$

4. Select variables *Pre_Wt* and *Post_Wt* from left panel, and bring them into the right panel as variable 1 and variable 2 of pair 1.
5. By clicking on the **Options** command, ensure that the confidence interval is selected as 95%, and click on **Continue** and **OK** for generating the outputs.

4.9   EXERCISE

4.9.1   Short Answer Questions

Note: Write answer to each of the following questions in not more than 200 words.

Q.1   Discuss a situation where one-sample t-test can be used. Explain the formula and procedure of testing the hypothesis.

Q.2   In comparing two group means, write down steps used in testing the hypothesis.

Q.3   Under what situation paired t-test should be used? Can it be used if sample size differs?

Q.4   What do you mean by pooled SD? How will you compute it?

Q.5   In testing the hypothesis concerning the equality of two group means (independent groups), what is the difference in testing two-tailed and one-tailed hypotheses?

Q.6   Write steps in using paired t-test for testing the effectiveness of a training program.

4.9.2   Multiple Choice Questions

Note: Questions 1–10 have four alternative answers for each question. Tick mark the one that you consider the closest to the correct answer.

1   Choose the most appropriate statement
   (a) t-test cannot be used for large sample
   (b) z-test cannot be used for large sample
   (c) t-test can be used for large sample test
   (d) Both t-test and z-test can be used for small sample

2   Sample is said to be small, if it is
    (a) 39
    (b) 31
    (c) 29
    (d) 30

3   In two-tailed hypothesis, the critical region is
    (a) divided in both the tails in $1:4$ proportion
    (b) lying in right tail only
    (c) lying in left tail only
    (d) divided in both the tails

4   If an investigator is interested to test the effectiveness of a training program in enhancing the muscular strength and the hypotheses are developed as follows:

$$H_0 : \mu_{Post} = \mu_{Pre}$$

$$H_1 : \mu_{Post} > \mu_{Pre}$$

    The critical region lies
    (a) in right tail only
    (b) in left tail only
    (c) in both the tails
    (d) None of the above is correct.

5   In using two-sample t-test, certain assumptions are made. Choose the most appropriate one
    (a) Variances of both the populations are equal.
    (b) Variances of both the populations are not necessarily equal.
    (c) No assumption is made on the population variance.
    (d) Variance of one population is larger than other.

6   If Cal $t < t_\alpha$, choose the most appropriate statement
    (a) H_0 may be accepted
    (b) H_0 is rejected
    (c) H_0 is not rejected
    (d) H_1 may be accepted

7   If it is desired to compare cardio-respiratory endurance of undergraduate and postgraduate students, which is the most appropriate set of hypotheses?
    (a) $H_0: \mu_{UG} = \mu_{PG}; H_1: \mu_{UG} \neq \mu_{PG}$
    (b) $H_0: \mu_{UG} = \mu_{PG}; H_1: \mu_{UG} > \mu_{PG}$
    (c) $H_0: \mu_{UG} = \mu_{PG}; H_1: \mu_{UG} < \mu_{PG}$
    (d) $H_0: \mu_{UG} \neq \mu_{PG}; H_1: \mu_{UG} = \mu_{PG}$

8   In testing the following set of hypotheses

$$H_0: \mu_1 = \mu_2$$

$$H_1: \mu_1 < \mu_2$$

Choose the most appropriate statement
(a) If calculated $t \leq t_\alpha$, H_0 may not be rejected
(b) If calculated $t < -t_\alpha$, H_0 may be rejected
(c) If calculated $t > -t_\alpha$, H_0 may be rejected
(d) None of the above is correct

9 If there are N pairs of score and paired t-test is used for comparing means of both the groups, what will be the df for t-statistic?
(a) N
(b) $2N - 2$
(c) $N + 1$
(d) $N - 1$

10 If reaction time of 14 sprinters and 16 gymnasts is to be compared using t-test, what would be its df?
(a) 28
(b) 30
(c) 2
(d) 29

11 To see the effectiveness of a circuit training program on the shooting accuracy, which of the SPSS command shall be used?
(a) One-sample t-test
(b) Independent samples t-test
(c) Paired t-test
(d) None of the above

4.9.3 Assignment

1. A random sample of 20 college athletes was tested for their performance on sit-ups. Their scores were as follows:

23, 26, 25, 26, 20, 29, 27, 27, 25, 26, 28, 25, 29, 29, 29, 29, 23, 28, 35, 31

Can it be concluded that all the college athletes have mean sit-ups equal to 30?

4.10   CASE STUDY

1   Case Study on Comparing two Independent Group Means

Objective

In a sports medicine unit of a university, a researcher wanted to investigate whether breath-holding capacity of hockey and swimming players differs due to the very nature of their events. He conducted a study in which 20 hockey and 20 swimming players who represented the university in the competition were selected for the study. The breath-holding capacity was tested on them before the competition, which is shown in Table 4.12.

Research Question

The main issue of investigation was whether due to the nature of the sports the breath-holding capacity of the players of hockey and swimming differs.

Data Format

The format used for preparing data file in SPSS is shown in Table 4.13.

TABLE 4.12   Breath-Holding Capacity (in sec) of players

Hockey	Swimming
38	45
40	44
44	41
27	39
60	80
55	65
34	45
56	50
54	65
60	65
37	45
60	72
60	65
36	42
60	58
31	45
45	42
50	55
53	48
37	42

TABLE 4.13   Data Format Used in SPSS

Breath-Holding Capacity	Group	
38	1	
40	1	
44	1	
27	1	
60	1	
55	1	
34	1	
56	1	
54	1	
60	1	$n_1 = 20$ (Hockey)
37	1	
60	1	
60	1	
36	1	
60	1	
31	1	
45	1	
50	1	
53	1	
37	1	
45	2	
44	2	
41	2	
39	2	
80	2	
65	2	
45	2	
50	2	
65	2	
65	2	$N_2 = 20$ (Swimming)
45	2	
72	2	
65	2	
42	2	
58	2	
45	2	
42	2	
55	2	
48	2	
42	2	

Group coding: 1, hockey; 2, swimming.

TABLE 4.14 Independent Samples Test

		Levene's Test for Equality of Variances		t-Test for Equality of Means						95% Confidence Interval of the Difference	
		F	Sig.	t	df	Sig. (2-Tailed)	Mean Difference	SE Difference		Lower	Upper
Breath-Holding Capacity	Equal variances assumed	0.070	0.793	−1.577	38	0.123	−5.80000	3.67749		−13.24469	1.64469
	Equal variances not assumed			−1.577	37.778	0.123	−5.80000	3.67749		−13.24613	1.64613

Analyzing Data

To investigate research issue a two-sample t-test was applied for testing the null hypothesis that the difference between hockey and swimming group means of breath-holding capacity is zero against the alternative hypothesis that it is not. The obtained value of t in the output was tested for its significance. The two-sample t-test was used because the data in both the groups were not related. A two-sample t-test was applied in SPSS by using the commands: **Analyze**, **Compare Means**, and **Independent Samples t-Test** in sequence. The output was obtained by selecting the test variable and grouping variable in the SPSS dialog box. The results so obtained are shown in Table 4.14. One of the assumptions in using the two-sample t-test for independent groups is that the population variance of these two groups is same. This was tested by using the Levene's test in SPSS. Since in Table 4.14 the F value is 0.070, which is not significant, it may be concluded that the variance of the two groups does not differ significantly. Hence assumption of equality of variance is satisfied for using the t-test. Since absolute value of t (1.577) is not significant ($p=0.123$), the null hypothesis may not be rejected. It may thus be concluded that the breath-holding capacity of hockey and swimming does not differ.

Reporting

- Since the absolute value of t ($=1.577$) is not significant ($p=0.123$), it may be concluded that the breath-holding capacity does not differ among hockey and gymnastics players.

2   Case Study on Paired t-Test

Objective

An exercise scientist developed a circuit training program for improving anaerobic capacity of tennis players. In order to test its effectiveness he conducted a study in which 20 national-level tennis players were randomly selected. They were tested for their anaerobic capacity before and after implementing the circuit training program for 6 weeks. The data so obtained are shown in Table 4.15.

Research Question

The researcher wanted to test whether the circuit training program improves the anaerobic capacity?

Data Format

The format used for preparing data file in SPSS is shown in Table 4.15.

**TABLE 4.15 Data Format Used in
SPSS for Anaerobic Capacity (in sec)**

Post_test	Pre_Test
16.45	13.05
20.47	13.03
14.87	10.48
13.96	11.73
13.48	16.00
12.80	10.14
13.96	12.21
13.84	12.13
15.36	14.12
15.46	12.73
16.84	10.08
17.60	13.16
18.19	17.32
16.97	11.93
15.54	16.13
14.08	13.96
28.05	17.90
22.18	16.34
27.47	16.45
17.93	17.78

TABLE 4.16 Paired Samples Test

	Paired Differences							
				95% Confidence Interval of the Difference				Sig.
	Mean	SD	SE Mean	Lower	Upper	t	df	(2-Tailed)
Pair 1 Post testing data – pre testing data	3.44150	3.50343	0.78339	1.80184	5.08116	4.393	19	0.000

Analyzing Data

In order to address the research issue a paired t-test was applied for testing the null hypothesis that the difference of post- and pre-training means is zero against the alternative hypothesis that it is not. The obtained value of t in the output was tested for its significance. The paired t-test was used because the data in both the groups were related to each other. The paired t-test was applied in SPSS by using the commands: **Analyze**, **Compare Means**, and **Paired Samples t-Test** in sequence.

The output was obtained by selecting both variables in the dialog box. The results so obtained are shown in Table 4.16. Since the value of t is significant (p=0.000), the null hypothesis may be rejected and alternative hypothesis is accepted. It may thus be concluded that the circuit training program is effective in increasing the anaerobic capacity among the tennis players.

Reporting

- Since the paired t-test is significant (p < 0.01) at 1% significance level, it may be concluded that the circuit training program is effective in improving the anaerobic capacity of the tennis players.

5

INDEPENDENT MEASURES ANOVA

LEARNING OBJECTIVES

After completing this chapter, you should be able to do the following:

- Learn to interpret the model involved in analysis of variance
- Describe the situations in which one-way and two-way analysis of variance should be used
- Explain the assumptions used in two-way analysis of variance
- Construct hypotheses to be tested in a research study
- Interpret various terms involved in analysis of variance
- Understand the steps involved in solving one-way and two-way analysis of variance
- Interpret the significance of F-statistic using p value
- Know the procedure of making data file for analysis of variance in SPSS
- Learn the steps involved in using SPSS for solving problems with one-way and two-way analysis of variance and
- Explain the outputs obtained in analysis of variance.

Sports Research with Analytical Solution using SPSS®, First Edition. J. P. Verma.
© 2016 John Wiley & Sons, Inc. Published 2016 by John Wiley & Sons, Inc.
Companion website: www.wiley.com/go/Verma/Sportsresearch

5.1   INTRODUCTION

Analysis of variance (ANOVA) is a group of statistical techniques that can be used to compare means of three or more groups. In this analysis, the null hypothesis of no difference among the group means is tested against the alternative hypothesis that at least one group mean differs. In ANOVA, variability in a dependent variable is studied as a function of independent variables. The total variability is split into different components and then the significance of these components is tested. In ANOVA if the effect of only one factor on some dependent variable is investigated, then the technique is known as one-way ANOVA. If the effect of two factors is investigated simultaneously, then the technique is referred as two-way ANOVA. Whatever statistical design is used in a research study, it is always analyzed by the ANOVA technique. Depending upon the way treatments (independent variable) are allocated to the subjects, the ANOVA is classified into three different categories: independent measures ANOVA, repeated measures ANOVA, and mixed ANOVA. If each subject receives only one treatment, then such studies are investigated by using one-way independent measures ANOVA; whereas if each subject in the sample receives all the treatments, then repeated measures ANOVA is used to test the hypothesis. Independent measures ANOVA is also known as between-groups design, whereas repeated measures ANOVA is referred to as within-subjects design. However, if one of the factors is between-groups and another is a within subjects, then the design is known as mixed design and is solved by using the mixed ANOVA. Between-groups design with one and two factors shall be discussed in this chapter, whereas repeated measures design shall be explained in detail in Chapter 6. The mixed design is outside the purview of this book. For mixed design, readers are advised to refer to the book titled *Repeated Measures Design for Empirical Researchers* by Verma (2015).

5.2   ONE-WAY ANALYSIS OF VARIANCE

Three group means can be compared by using three t-tests. At the same time using multiple t-tests inflates Type I error rate as well. Thus, if a hypothesis is to be tested at the significance level 0.05, the actual error would be much higher than this; and therefore, the conclusion drawn in this manner may not be reliable. To overcome this problem, some correction is required to be made in the p value associated with t-test. But this problem can be better managed by using the analysis of variance (ANOVA) technique discussed in this chapter.

   The terms involved in ANOVA shall be discussed in reference with the following hypothetical experiment. Consider a study in which the effect of three different treatments (low, medium, and high intensity of circuit training program) on muscular strength is to be compared. The treatments have been randomly allocated to the subjects in such a manner that each treatment is received by an equal number of subjects. Table 5.1 shows the data obtained in this study.

TABLE 5.1   Data on Muscular Strength in Three Different Treatment Groups

Low (X1)	Medium (X2)	High (X3)
60	80	65
65	75	70
60	70	65
70	75	70
65	80	75
45	70	55

One-way ANOVA model shall be constructed to understand the concept involved in hypothesis testing in the analysis.

5.2.1   One-Way ANOVA Model

In this experiment, muscular strength and circuit training are the dependent and the independent variables, respectively. A model as given below may be developed to explain total variability in the dependent variable

$$TSS = SSB + SSE$$

where TSS is the total variability among scores, SSB is the variability between groups, and SSE is the variability within groups.

In ANOVA, we try to compare between-group variability with that of within-group variability. This comparison is done by using F-statistic. Significant value of F indicates that group means are heterogeneous. In other words, it may be inferred that the means of the three groups are not same. Significance of F-statistic can be tested by using p value. F-statistic will be significant at 5% level if its associated p value is less than 0.05, and nonsignificant otherwise.

If F value is significant, the next question comes as to which group mean is the largest. Thus, in ANOVA we test the null hypothesis

$$H_0 : \mu_{Low} = \mu_{Medium} = \mu_{High}$$

against the alternative hypothesis that at least one group mean differs.

5.2.2   Post Hoc Test

Post hoc test is used for testing the significance of mean difference between groups. It is used when the null hypothesis of equality of means is rejected. There are many post hoc tests available to compare the group means such as least significance difference (LSD), Scheffe, Tukey, Bonferroni, Sidak, Duncan, etc. Tukey and Sidak are the most widely used tests by the researchers. Readers are advised to read the details of other post hoc tests from any other standard text on statistics.

In all the post hoc tests, a critical difference is computed at a particular level of significance. If the difference of any pair of means is greater than critical difference, group means differ significantly, otherwise not.

The SPSS output provides p value (significant value) for each pair of means to test the significance of difference between them. If p value for any pair of means is less than 0.05, it indicates significant difference at 5% level, otherwise not.

5.2.3 Application of One-Way ANOVA

One-way ANOVA is used when more than two group means are compared. Such situations are very frequent in research where a researcher may like to compare the effect of more than two treatments. For instance, one may like to compare the reaction time of basketballers, boxers, and sprinters, or one may wish to compare the effects of breaststroke, butterfly stroke, and free stroke in swimming learning.

One-way ANOVA should be used in comparing the effectiveness of treatments when treatments are randomly allocated to the subjects. However, if the effectiveness of treatments is to be compared in intact groups without treatments being randomly allocated to the subjects, the analysis of covariance should be used. Consider an experiment where it is desired to compare the effect of different types of warm-up exercises on 400-meter performance. The three exercises namely warm-up with hot pack, cold pack, and mud pack may be taken as treatments in three intact groups of athletes. In this situation, one may take the difference of post- and preperformance of 400-meter in each of the three treatment groups and then apply one-way ANOVA on these differences of three sets of data. In this way, the results obtained in comparing the effectiveness of three treatments will not be reliable because of the fact that all the three groups might not be homogenous initially. Further, homogeneity of the three treatment groups cannot be ensured as there might be other covariates affecting the performance. In such situation where comparative effectiveness is to be seen, the analysis of covariance (ANCOVA) is a better design instead of ANOVA. The ANCOVA has been discussed in Chapter 7.

5.3 ONE-WAY ANOVA WITH SPSS (EQUAL SAMPLE SIZE)

Example 5.1

The data on anxiety obtained on athletes in individual, dual, and team sports and is shown in Table 5.2. Apply one-way ANOVA to find in which sport anxiety is higher. Discuss the findings at 5% level.

Solution: The hypothesis that needs to be tested here is

$$H_0 : \mu_{\text{Ind\_Sp}} = \mu_{\text{Dual\_Sp}} = \mu_{\text{Team\_Sp}}$$

against the alternative hypothesis that at least one group mean differs.

The SPSS output provides F value along with its significance value (p value). The F-statistic would be significant at 5% level if the p value associated with it is less than 0.05. If F is significant, a post hoc test is used to compare the paired means. SPSS provides facility to choose any post hoc test for analysis.

TABLE 5.2   Data on Anxiety

S.N.	Individual Sport	Dual Sport	Team Sport
1	22	25	20
2	21	20	19
3	21	19	22
4	23	20	19
5	22	16	21
6	23	18	19
7	21	21	22
8	24	16	19
9	22	17	20
10	19	19	24
11	21	22	21
12	24	20	24
13	22	19	19
14	23	22	22
15	20	22	20
16	22	19	19
17	21	20	21
18	21	20	21
19	26	21	22
20	24	19	20

In this example, Tukey test shall be used as a post hoc test for comparing the group means. The SPSS output provides the significance value for each pair of group means difference. Thus, by looking at the results of post hoc test, one can determine as to which group mean is higher. The procedure has been discussed while interpreting the output.

5.3.1   Computation in One-Way ANOVA (Equal Sample Size)

5.3.1.1 Preparation of Data File   Before starting the SPSS commands, data file needs to be prepared by selecting the 'Type in data' option for defining variables as discussed in Chapter 1.

5.3.1.2 Defining Variables   There are two variables in this example—namely, anxiety and sport that need to be defined along with their properties. *Anxiety* is a scale variable whereas *Sport* is a nominal variable. The procedure of defining variables and their characteristics in SPSS is as follows:

1. Click on **Variable View** to define variables and their properties.
2. Write short name of the variables as *Anxiety* and *Sport* under the column heading "Name."
3. Under the column heading "Label," full name of the variables may be defined as *Athlete's Anxiety* and *Type of Sport*.

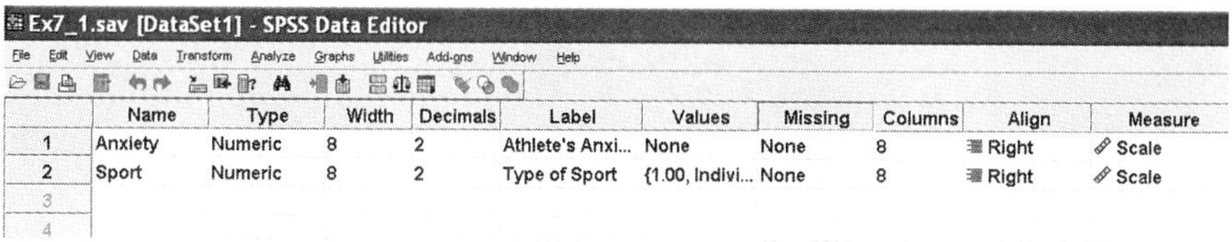

	Name	Type	Width	Decimals	Label	Values	Missing	Columns	Align	Measure
1	Anxiety	Numeric	8	2	Athlete's Anxi...	None	None	8	≡ Right	⟋ Scale
2	Sport	Numeric	8	2	Type of Sport	{1.00, Indivi...	None	8	≡ Right	⟋ Scale
3										
4										

FIGURE 5.1   Defining variables along with their characteristics.

4. Under the column heading "Measure," select the option 'Scale' for the variable *Anxiety* and 'Nominal' for the *Sport*.

5. For the variable *Sport*, double click the cell under the column "Values," and add the following values to different labels:

Value	Label
1	Individual sport
2	Dual sport
3	Team sport

6. Use default entries in rest of the columns.

After defining variables in the **Variable View**, the screen shall look like as shown in Figure 5.1.

Note: More than one dependent variable can be defined in the **Variable View** for doing ANOVA.

5.3.1.3   Entering Data   Once variables are defined in the **Variable View**, click on **Data View** on the left corner in the bottom of the screen shown in Figure 5.1 to open the format for entering data column-wise. After entering the data, the screen will look like as shown in Figure 5.2. Since the data is large, only a portion of the data is shown in Figure 5.2. Save the data file in the desired location before further processing.

5.3.1.4   SPSS Commands   After entering all the data in the **Data View**, do the following steps:

1. *Initiating SPSS commands:* In the **Data View**, click the following commands in sequence:

Analyze → Compare Means → One-Way ANOVA

The screen shall look like as shown in Figure 5.3.

2. *Selecting variables:* After clicking "One-Way ANOVA" option, you will be taken to the next screen for selecting variables. Select the variables *Anxiety* and *Sport* from the left panel, and bring them into the "Dependent list" section and

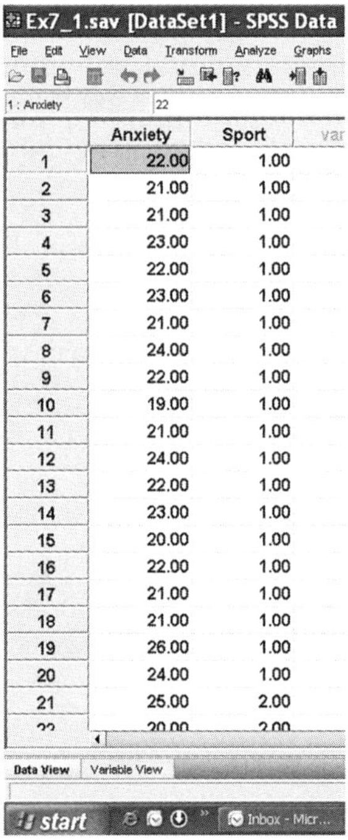

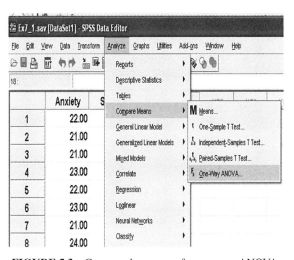

FIGURE 5.2   Data file of anxiety for one-way ANOVA.

FIGURE 5.3   Command sequence for one-way ANOVA.

"Factor" section in the right panel, respectively. The screen will look like as shown in Figure 5.4.

3. *Selecting options for computation:* After selecting variables, option needs to be defined for generating the output in one-way ANOVA. Do the following:

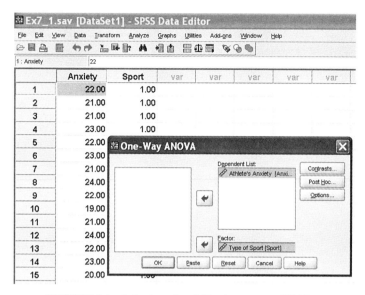

FIGURE 5.4   Selection of variables in one-way ANOVA.

(a) Click **Post Hoc** in the screen shown in Figure 5.4. The screen will look like as shown in Figure 5.5.

(b) Check 'Tukey' option. You may choose any other post hoc test if you so desire.

(c) Write 'Significance level' as 0.05 or 0.01, as the case may be

(d) Click on **Continue**. This will take you back on screen in Figure 5.4.

(e) Click on **Options** and then check 'Descriptive' option as shown in Figure 5.6. Click on **Continue** and then on **OK** for generating the outputs.

4. *Getting the output:* The results of the analysis are generated in the output window. These outputs can be selected by using the right click of mouse and may be copied into the word file. Here the following outputs shall be selected:

(a) Descriptive statistics

(b) ANOVA table

(c) Post Hoc comparison table

5.3.1.5   SPSS Output   In this example, all the outputs so generated by the SPSS will look like as shown in Tables 5.3, 5.4, and 5.5.

5.3.2   Interpretation of Findings

Table 5.3 gives different descriptive statistics that may be used by the readers for their reference and review work. The means of different groups and the results of Table 5.5 have been used to prepare the graphics shown in Table 5.6, which shall be discussed later.

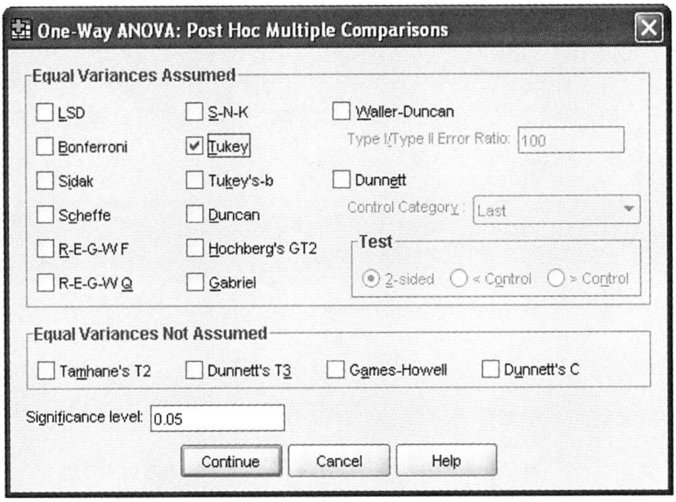

FIGURE 5.5   Selecting option for post hoc test and significance level.

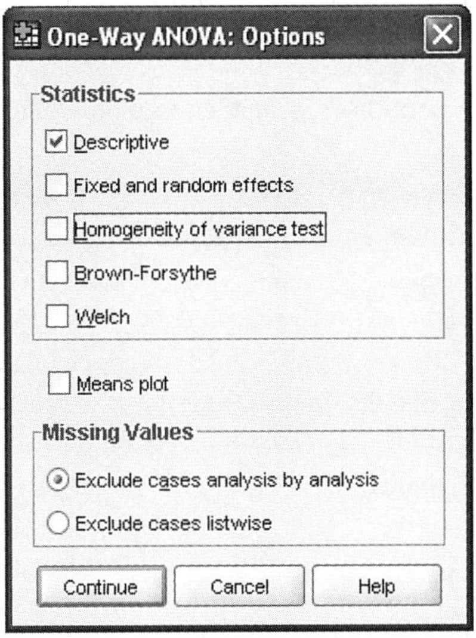

FIGURE 5.6   Option for computing descriptive statistics.

The F value in Table 5.4 is significant as its p value (=0.001) is less than 0.05. Thus, the null hypothesis of no difference among means of the three groups may be rejected at 5% level.

Since F value is significant, post hoc test needs to be applied for comparing means of groups. The SPSS output shown in Table 5.5 provides such

TABLE 5.3   Descriptive Statistics for the Data on Anxiety in Different Sport Group

	N	Mean	SD	SE	95% Confidence Interval for Mean		Min.	Max.
					Lower Bound	Upper Bound		
Individual sport	20	22.10	1.62	0.36	21.34	22.86	19.00	26.00
Dual sport	20	19.75	2.15	0.48	18.74	20.76	16.00	25.00
Team sport	20	20.70	1.59	0.36	19.95	21.45	19.00	24.00
Total	60	20.85	2.02	0.26	20.33	21.37	16.00	26.00

TABLE 5.4   ANOVA Table for the Data on Anxiety

	Sum of Squares	df	Mean Square	F	Sig. (p Value)
Between groups	55.90	2	27.950	8.577	0.001
Within groups	185.75	57	3.259		
Total	241.65	59			

TABLE 5.5   Post Hoc Comparison of Means Using Tukey HSD Test

(I) Type of Sport	(J) Type of Sport	Mean Diff. (I−J)	SE	Sig. (p Value)
Individual sport	Dual sport	2.35*	0.57086	0.000
	Team sport	1.40*	0.57086	0.045
Dual sport	Individual sport	−2.35*	0.57086	0.000
	Team sport	−0.95	0.57086	0.228
Team sport	Individual sport	−1.40*	0.57086	0.045
	Dual sport	0.95	0.57086	0.228

Note: The values of lower bound and upper bound have been omitted from the original output.
*The mean difference is significant at the 0.05 level.

TABLE 5.6   Means of the Groups with Graphics

Individual Sport	Team Sport	Dual Sport
22.10	20.70	19.75

└────────────┘ Represents no significant difference between the means.

comparison. It can be seen that the difference between individual sport and dual sport is significant as the p value for this mean difference is 0.00, which is less than 0.05.

Similarly, the mean difference between individual sport and team sport is also significant as the p value for this difference is 0.045, which is also less than 0.05.

However, there is no difference between the means of the dual sport and team sport. From Table 5.6, it may be seen that the mean anxiety of the individual sport group is significantly higher in comparison to that of the team sport and dual sport groups.

5.4   ONE-WAY ANOVA WITH SPSS (UNEQUAL SAMPLE SIZE)

Example 5.2

The self-concept of different positional players of soccer, that is, defenders, midfielders, and attackers was obtained in a study, which is shown in Table 5.7. Apply one-way ANOVA to find as to which category of players have the highest self-concept.

Solution: Procedure for one-way ANOVA with equal and unequal sample sizes in SPSS is almost same. In case of unequal sample size, one should be careful in feeding the data. The procedure is discussed later. We shall briefly explain the procedure in this case as it is exactly similar to what we have discussed in Example 5.1. Readers are advised to refer to the procedure discussed earlier in case of doubt for solving the ANOVA for unequal sample size.

TABLE 5.7   **Data on Self-Concept**

S.N.	Defenders	Midfielders	Attackers
1	146	210	182
2	139	195	159
3	158	188	169
4	176	198	155
5	185	186	110
6	72	183	150
7	175	178	167
8	162	191	158
9	185	188	149
10	178	185	175
11	165	178	153
12	164	165	159
13	149	164	191
14	154	185	190
15	170	154	167
16	154	170	152
17	166	182	
18	185	182	
19	178		
20	165		

In this example, the null hypothesis that needs to be tested is

$$H_0 : \mu_{\text{Def}} = \mu_{\text{Mid}} = \mu_{\text{Att}}$$

against the alternative hypothesis that at least one group mean differs.

If the null hypothesis is rejected, post hoc test shall be used for comparing group means. Since the sample sizes are different, the Scheffe test shall be used for the post hoc analysis.

5.4.1   Computation in One-Way ANOVA (Unequal Sample Size)

5.4.1.1   Preparation of Data File   Start SPSS and select the 'Type in data' option for defining variables.

5.4.1.2   Defining Variables   There are two variables in this example—namely, *Self-concept* and *Position* that need to be defined along with their properties. *Self-concept* is a 'scale' variable whereas *Position* is a 'nominal' variable. The procedure of defining variables and their characteristics is as follows:

1. Use default entries in rest of the columns.
2. Click on **Variable View** to define variables and their properties.
3. Write short name of the variables as *Self_Concept* and *Position* under the column heading "Name."
4. Under the column heading "Label," full name of the two aforementioned variables may be defined as *Player's self-concept* and *Player's position*.
5. Under the column heading "Measure," select 'Scale' option for the *Self_Concept* and 'Nominal' for the *Position*.
6. For the variable *Position*, double click the cell under the column "Values" and add the following values to different labels:

Value	Label
1	Defenders
2	Midfielders
3	Attackers

7. Instead of 1, 2, and 3, some other numbers may also be chosen to define values for the labels.

5.4.1.3   Entering Data   After defining variables in the **Variable View**, enter the data column-wise in **Data View**. The data feeding format has been shown in Table 5.8.

5.4.1.4 SPSS Commands   After entering all the data in **Data View**, save the data
file in the desired location before further processing. Do the following steps:

1. *Initiating SPSS commands:* In **Data View**, click the following commands in
   sequence:

TABLE 5.8   Format of Data Feeding in Data View

	S.N.	Self-Concept	Position
Defenders $n_1 = 20$	1	146	1
	2	142	1
	3	158	1
	4	176	1
	5	185	1
	6	172	1
	7	175	1
	8	162	1
	9	185	1
	10	178	1
	11	165	1
	12	164	1
	13	149	1
	14	154	1
	15	170	1
	16	154	1
	17	166	1
	18	185	1
	19	178	1
	20	165	1
Midfielders $n_2 = 18$	21	210	2
	22	195	2
	23	188	2
	24	198	2
	25	186	2
	26	183	2
	27	178	2
	28	191	2
	29	188	2
	30	185	2
	31	178	2
	32	165	2
	33	164	2
	34	185	2
	35	154	2
	36	170	2
	37	182	2
	38	182	2

TABLE 5.8 (continued)

	S.N.	Self-Concept	Position
Attackers $n_3 = 16$	39	182	3
	40	159	3
	41	169	3
	42	155	3
	43	110	3
	44	150	3
	45	167	3
	46	158	3
	47	149	3
	48	175	3
	49	153	3
	50	159	3
	51	191	3
	52	190	3
	53	167	3
	54	152	3

Analyze → Compare Means → One-Way ANOVA

2. *Selecting Variables:* After clicking "One-Way ANOVA" option, you will be taken to the next screen for selecting variables. Select variables *Self_Concept* and *Position* from the left panel, and bring them into the "Dependent list" and "Factor" sections in the right panel, respectively. The screen shall look like as shown in Figure 5.7.

3. *Selecting options for computation:* After selecting the variables, option needs to be defined for generating the outputs. Do the following:

   (a) Click on **Post Hoc** in the screen shown in Figure 5.7.

   (b) Check 'Scheffe' option. This test is selected because the sample sizes are unequal. However, you can choose any other test if you so desire.

   (c) Write 'Significance level' as 0.05 or 0.01, as the case may be.

   (d) Click on **Continue.**

   (e) Click on **Options** and then check 'Descriptive' option in statistics section.

   (f) Click on **Continue** and **OK** options for results.

4. *Getting the Output:* The outputs selected from the SPSS window are as follows:

   (a) Descriptive statistics

   (b) ANOVA table

   (c) Post Hoc comparison table

5.4.1.5 SPSS Output The outputs generated in this example are shown in Tables 5.9, 5.10, and 5.11.

5.4.2   Interpretation of Findings

Table 5.9 shows the values of means, SD, SE, and other statistics, which may be of use to the readers. The graphic Table 5.12 has been prepared with the contents of Tables 5.9 and 5.11, which shall be discussed later.

The F value in Table 5.10 is significant as its p value is 0.000, which is less than 0.05. Thus, the null hypothesis of no difference among the means of the three groups, that is, defenders, midfielders, and attackers may be rejected at 5% level.

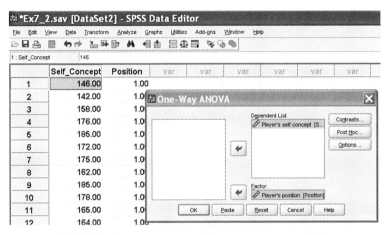

FIGURE 5.7   Selection of variables in one-way ANOVA.

TABLE 5.9   Descriptive Statistics for the Data on Self-Concept of Different Positional Players of Soccer

	N	Mean	SD	SE	95% Confidence Interval for Mean		Min.	Max.
					Lower Bound	Upper Bound		
Defenders	20	166.5	13.06	2.92	160.34	172.56	142.00	185.00
Midfielders	18	182.3	13.21	3.11	175.76	188.90	154.00	210.00
Attackers	16	161.6	19.27	4.82	151.36	171.89	110.00	191.00
Total	54	170.3	17.31	2.36	165.59	175.04	110.00	210.00

TABLE 5.10   ANOVA Table for the Data on Self-Concept

	Sum of Squares	df	Mean Square	F	Sig.
Between groups	4106.95	2	2053.47	8.89	0.000
Within groups	11778.70	51	230.96		
Total	15885.65	53			

TABLE 5.11   Post Hoc Comparison of Means Using Scheffe Test

(I) Position of the Soccer Player	(J) Position of the Soccer Player	Mean Diff. (I−J)	SE	Sig. (p Value)
Defenders	Midfielders	−15.883*	4.937	0.009
	Attackers	4.825	5.097	0.641
Midfielders	Defenders	15.883*	4.937	0.009
	Attackers	20.708*	5.222	0.001
Attackers	Defenders	−4.825	5.097	0.641
	Midfielders	−20.708*	5.222	0.001

Note: The values of lower bound and upper bound have been omitted from the original output.
*The mean difference is significant at the 0.05 level.

TABLE 5.12   Means of the Groups with Graphics

Midfielders	Defenders	Attackers
182.3	166.5	161.6

Represents no significant difference between the means at 0.05 level of significance.

Since the F value is significant, post hoc comparisons need to be done. The SPSS output shown in Table 5.11 provides such comparisons. It can be seen that the difference between self-concept of the defenders and that of the midfielders is significant as the p value for this mean difference is 0.009, which is less than 0.05. Similarly, the mean difference between the self concept of midfielders and that of attackers is also significant as the p value for this difference is 0.001, which is also less than 0.05. However, there is no difference between defenders and attackers in their self-concept because the p value is 0.641.

The results thus obtained can be visualized graphically as shown in Table 5.12. One can see that the self-concept of the midfielders is the best in comparison to that of attackers and defenders.

5.5   TWO-WAY ANALYSIS OF VARIANCE

In one-way ANOVA, we have seen that the dependent variable is affected by the change in the different levels of an independent factor. Consider an example of one-way ANOVA discussed earlier in this chapter where anxiety was influenced by different types of sport, that is, individual, dual, and group. In that study, effect of only factor (*Sport*) on anxiety was investigated. Thus, in one-way ANOVA, the effect of only one factor is studied. On the other hand, in two-way ANOVA effect of two factors on dependent variable is investigated simultaneously. For instance, in studying the effect of different training intensities and weather conditions on muscular strength, the two factors that need to be investigated are training and weather. In this situation, one may conduct few simple experiments by using one-way ANOVA to investigate the following issues:

- Whether the impact of different training intensities on muscular strength is same in each weather condition
- Whether the impact of different weather conditions on muscular strength is same in each training intensity

Thus, if the impact of three training intensities and three weather conditions on muscular strength is to be studied, one has to organize six one-way ANOVA experiments. But, the impact of interaction, that is, joint effect of training and weather cannot be determined in such analysis.

To overcome this problem and to utilize the experimental resources more economically, a two-way ANOVA experiment can be planned in this situation. In two-way ANOVA, there are two independent variables or factors (in this case training and weather) that affect the dependent variable (muscular strength). Further, it may be interesting to know as to which combination of treatment (training × weather) is the most effective proposition to enhance the muscular strength.

A two-way ANOVA can be considered as an extension of one-way ANOVA. In such analysis, the effect of two independent factors on a dependent variable is studied; hence it is named as two-way ANOVA. Application of two-way ANOVA requires certain assumptions to be made about the data.

5.5.1   Assumptions in Two-Way Analysis of Variance

The following assumptions are made while using two-way ANOVA in analyzing the data:

- The population from which the samples have been drawn is normally distributed.
- The samples are independent.
- The population variances are equal.

5.5.2   Hypotheses in Two-Way ANOVA

In two-way ANOVA, the following three null hypotheses are tested:

- The population means of all the levels of the first factor are equal. This is like the one-way ANOVA for the row factor.
- The population means of all the levels of the second factor are equal. This is like the one-way ANOVA for the column factor.
- There is no interaction between the two factors. This is similar to performing a test for independence with contingency table.

5.5.3 Factors

In two-way ANOVA, each of the two independent variables is usually known as factors. The effects of these two factors on the dependent variable are studied. Each of the two factors may have two or more levels, and the degree of freedom for each factor is 1 less than the number of levels.

5.5.4 Treatment Groups

The number of treatment groups in the experiment is equal to the number of combinations of the levels of the two factors. For example, if the first factor has two levels and the second has three, then there will be $2 \times 3 = 6$ different treatment groups.

In the example discussed earlier, let's assume that there are three different intensities of exercise and three different weather conditions. To see the impact of these two factors on muscular strength, there will be nine different treatment groups. Thus, nine samples having the same size need to be identified so that these different combinations of treatments can be administered on them.

5.5.5 Main Effect

The main effect is the effect of one independent variable on the dependent variable at a time. The interaction is ignored for this part. Just the rows or just the columns are used, not mixed. This is the part that is similar to one-way ANOVA. Each of the variances calculated to analyze the main effects (rows and columns) is like between variances.

5.5.6 Interaction Effect

The joint effect of two factors on the dependent variable is known as interaction effect. It can also be defined as the effect that one factor has on the other. The degrees of freedom for the interaction are the product of degrees of freedom of both the factors.

5.5.7 Within-Groups Variation

The within-groups variation is the sum of squares within each treatment group. The total number of treatment groups is the product of the number of levels for each factor. The within variance is equal to within variation divided by its degrees of freedom. The within group is also denoted as an error.

5.5.8 F-Statistic

F-statistic is computed for each source of variation to test its significance. F-value is obtained by dividing the mean sum of squares of main or interaction effect by the mean sum of squares of the error effect. The numerator degrees of freedom comes from each effect, and the denominator degrees of freedom is of the within effect in each case.

5.5.9 Two-Way ANOVA Table

Let us assume that the main effect A has "r" levels and the main effect B has "c" levels, whereas n is the sample size in each treatment group. Thus, the total sample size in the experiment becomes $N = n \times r \times c$. The degrees of freedom for each main effect are 1 less than its level. Similarly, total degrees of freedom are also one less than the total sample size.

Source	SS	df	MSS	F
Main effect A (row)	SSR	$r-1$	$S_R^2 = SSR/(r-1)$	$\text{F for row} = \dfrac{S_R^2}{S_E^2}$
Main effect B (column)	SSC	$c-1$	$S_C^2 = SSC/(c-1)$	$\text{F for column} = \dfrac{S_C^2}{S_E^2}$
Interaction effect	SSI	$(r-1)(c-1)$	$S_I^2 = SSI/(r-1)(c-1)$	$\text{F for interaction} = \dfrac{S_I^2}{S_E^2}$
Within effect	SSE	$N-rc$	$S_E^2 = SSE/(N-rc)$	
Total	TSS	$N-1$		

5.5.10 Interpretation

The SPSS output provides the significance value (p value) for each of the F-statistic computed in two-way ANOVA table. If the p value is less than 0.05, F is significant. Post hoc test for comparing means is applied to those factors and interaction whose F values are significant.

5.5.11 Application of Two-Way Analysis of Variance

Besides investigating main effects, two-way ANOVA facilitates the investigation of interaction effect between the two factors on dependent variable. The following example shall provide an insight to the researchers for appreciating the use of this analysis.

Consider an example where the effect of three circuit training programs needs to be compared under two different intensities of the weight training for investigating the improvement in 100-meter sprinting performance.

		Wt. Training (B)	
		Low (b_1)	Medium (b_2)
Circuit training (A)	I (a_1)	$n = 10$	$n = 10$
	II (a_2)	$n = 10$	$n = 10$
	III (a_3)	$n = 10$	$n = 10$

This is an example of a 3×2 factorial experiment with six treatment groups (or cells) each having 10 subjects. In this example, 100-meter sprinting performance is the dependent variable. If 60 college students are randomly selected in the study, then six treatments shall be randomly allocated to these subjects in such a manner that each subject gets one and only one treatment. Thus, each treatment group will have 10 subjects. These six treatment combinations can be represented by a_1b_1, a_1b_2, a_2b_1, a_2b_2, a_3b_1, and a_3b_2.

The purpose of this experiment is to find the best combination of treatment suitable for enhancing the performance in 100-meter event.

Now let's discuss the type of information this analysis can yield. The following three types of information may be achieved here:

1. *Factor A effect*: addresses whether circuit training affects 100-meter performance.
2. *Factor B effect*: addresses whether weight training affects 100-meter performance.
3. *Interaction effect $(A \times B)$*: addresses whether the effects of circuit training depend on the intensities of weight training in improving 100-meter performance of an athlete.

Thus, the following three hypotheses may be tested in this analysis:

1.
$$H_0 : \mu_{I\_CT} = \mu_{II\_CT} = \mu_{III\_CT}$$

All the three circuit training programs are equally effective in improving 100-meter performance (both the intensities of weight training program combined).

2.
$$H_0 : \mu_{LowWT} = \mu_{MediumWT}$$

Both intensities of the weight training programs are equally effective (all circuit training programs combined).

3. H_0: No interaction between weight training and circuit training.

Effect of circuit training program on 100-meter performance is independent to the weight training program.

Thus, in a two-way factorial experiment we investigate two main effects and also the interaction effect between the factors. If interaction effect is significant, then simple effects are investigated.

5.6 TWO-WAY ANOVA USING SPSS

Example 5.3

Fifteen wrestlers and fifteen Gymnasts were randomly chosen for the study. In each category, the subjects were divided into three equal groups. Three different types of diets were randomly administered to these three groups of subjects for 4 weeks. After four weeks of treatment, these subjects were given a fitness test, high score representing better performance. Test scores so recorded is shown in Table 5.13. Let us see how to apply two-way ANOVA and interpret the findings:

Solution: Here two main factors, namely, *Sport* (factor A) and *Diet* (factor B) as well as *Interaction* between *Sport* and *Diet* (A × B) need to be studied. Thus, the following three hypotheses shall be tested:

1. $$H_0 : \mu_{\text{Wrestlers}} = \mu_{\text{Gymnasts}}$$

   [Fitness levels of the wrestlers and gymnasts are same (all diet groups combined)].

2. $$H_0 : \mu_{\text{High\_Diet}} = \mu_{\text{Medium\_Diet}} = \mu_{\text{Low\_Diet}}$$

   [Fitness levels of all the three diet groups are same (both sport groups combined)].

3. H_0: No interaction exists between *Sport* and *Diet*.

The SPSS output for two-way ANOVA provides F value for *Sport* (Factor A), *Diet* (Factor B), and *Interaction* (*Sport* × *Diet*) along with their significance values (p values). In case F is significant for any factor or interaction, then a post hoc test shall be conducted to compare the paired means. SPSS provides option for many post hoc tests for testing the significance of mean difference.

In this example, Tukey test shall be used as a post hoc test for comparing group means. The SPSS output provides significance value for the difference of each pair of group means.

TABLE 5.13   Adolescents' Data on Fitness Test

	Group	Diet		
		High Protein	Medium Protein	Low Protein
Sport	Wrestlers	10	8	5
		7	6	4
		9	8	7
		6	5	4
		8	6	5
	Gymnasts	4	5	3
		4	4	3
		5	6	4
		2	7	2
		2	4	1

5.6.1 Computation in Two-Way ANOVA

5.6.1.1 Preparation of Data File

After preparing the data file, SPSS commands can be used for two-way ANOVA. After starting SPSS package as discussed in Chapter 1, select the 'Type in data' option. The sequence of commands to start SPSS is as follows:

Start → All Programs → SPSS Inc → SPSS 20.0 → Type in Data

Now you are ready for defining variables row-wise.

5.6.1.2 Defining Variables

There are three variables in this example, namely, *Fitness Score*, *Sport*, and *Diet* that need to be defined along with their properties. *Fitness Score* is a scale variable, whereas *Sport* and *Diet* are nominal variables. The procedure for defining variables and their characteristics in SPSS is as follows:

1. Click on **Variable View** to define variables and their properties.
2. Write short name of the variables as *Fitness_score, Sport*, and *Diet* under the column heading "Name."
3. Under the column heading "Label," full name of these variables may be defined as *Fitness test score, Sport of the subject*, and *Diet* type. Alternate names may also be chosen for describing the variables.
4. Under the column heading "Measure," select 'Scale' option for the variable *Fitness_score* and 'Nominal' for *Sport* and *Diet* variables.
5. For *Sport*, double click the cell under the column 'Values' and add following values to different labels:

Value	Label
1	Wrestler
2	Gymnast

6. Similarly for *Diet*, add the following values to different labels.

Value	Label
3	High-protein diet
4	Medium-protein diet
5	Low-protein diet

7. Use default entries in rest of the columns.

After defining variables in the **Variable View**, the screen shall look like as shown in Figure 5.8.

5.6.1.3 Entering Data

Once variables are defined in the **Variable View**, click on **Data View** on the left corner in the bottom of the screen shown in Figure 5.8 to open the format for entering data column-wise.

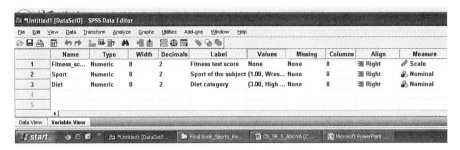

FIGURE 5.8   Defining variables along with their characteristics.

One should note the procedure of data feeding carefully in this example. First 15 fitness scores of wrestlers of Table 5.8 are entered in the column of *Fitness_score* after which 15 fitness scores of the gymnasts are entered in the same column. Under the column *Sport*, first 15 scores are entered as 1 (denotes wrestler) and next 15 scores are entered as 2 (denotes gymnast). Under the column *Diet*, first five scores are entered as 3 (denotes high protein), next five scores as 4 (denotes medium protein), and subsequent five scores as 5 (denotes low protein). These 15 data belong to wrestler's group. Similarly, next 15 scores of diet can be just the repetition of the wrestler's group data.

After entering the data, the screen will look like as shown in Figure 5.9. Save the data file in the desired location before further processing.

5.6.1.4   SPSS Commands   After entering all the data in the **Data View**, the following steps must be followed:

1. *Initiating SPSS commands:* In the **Data View**, click the following commands in sequence

   Analyze → General Linear Model → Univariate

   The screen shall look like as shown in Figure 5.10.

2. *Selecting variables for two-way ANOVA:* After clicking the "Univariate" option, you will be taken to the next screen for selecting variables. Select the variable *Fitness test score* from left panel, and bring it to the "Dependent variable" section in the right panel. Similarly, select the *Sport* and *Diet* variables from the left panel and bring them into the "Fixed Factor(s)" section in the right panel. The screen will look like as shown in Figure 5.11.

3. *Selecting option for computation:* After selecting variables, various options need to be defined for generating the outputs. Do the following:

   (a) Click on **Post Hoc** in the screen shown in Figure 5.11.

   (b) Select the factors *Sport* and *Diet* from the left panel, and bring them into the "Post Hoc Tests for" panel in the right side by using the arrow key.

   (c) Check 'Tukey' option. The screen will look like as shown in Figure 5.12.

   (d) Click on **Continue**, this will again take you back to the screen shown in Figure 5.11.

   (e) Now click on **Options** command and then check 'Descriptive Statistics,' 'Estimates of effect size,' and 'Homogeneity test' options.

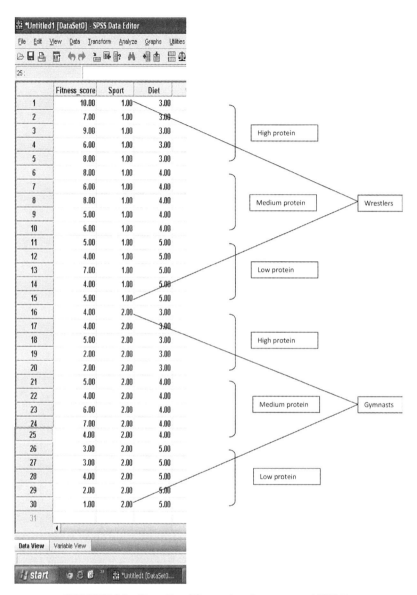

FIGURE 5.9   Data file of fitness data for two-way ANOVA.

(f) Select variables *Sport, Diet,* and *Sport * Diet* from the left panel, and bring them into the "Display Means for" section in the right panel.

(g) Check 'Compare main effects' option.

(h) Ensure that the value of significance level is 0.05 in the box. The screen for these options shall look like as shown in Figure 5.13.

(i) Click on **Continue** to go back to the main screen shown in Figure 5.11.

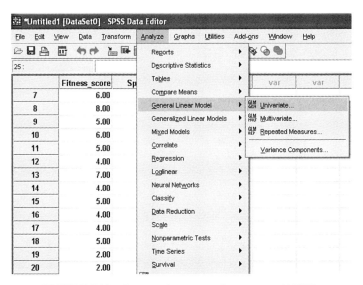

FIGURE 5.10   Command sequence for two-way ANOVA.

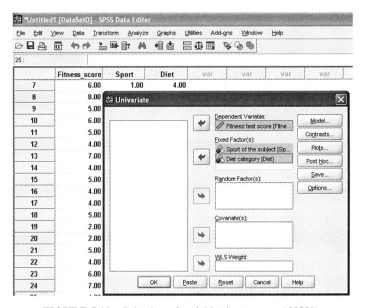

FIGURE 5.11   Selection of variables in two-way ANOVA.

4. *Selecting option for means plot:* After selecting variables, option needs to be defined for generating means plots. Click on **Plots** command to get the screen as shown in Figure 5.14. Do the following:

   (a) Select *Sport* variable from the "Factors" section and bring it to the "Horizontal Axis" area for generating means plot of the main effect *Sport*. This plot is used to compare the means of sport groups. Click on **Add.**

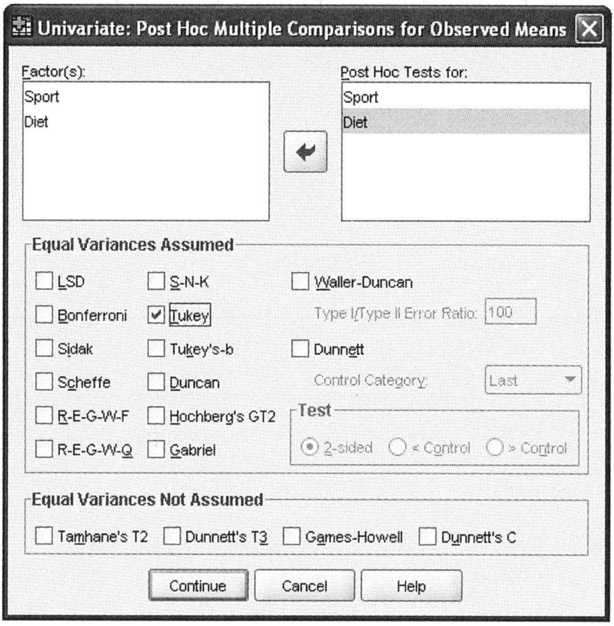

FIGURE 5.12 Options for post hoc test results.

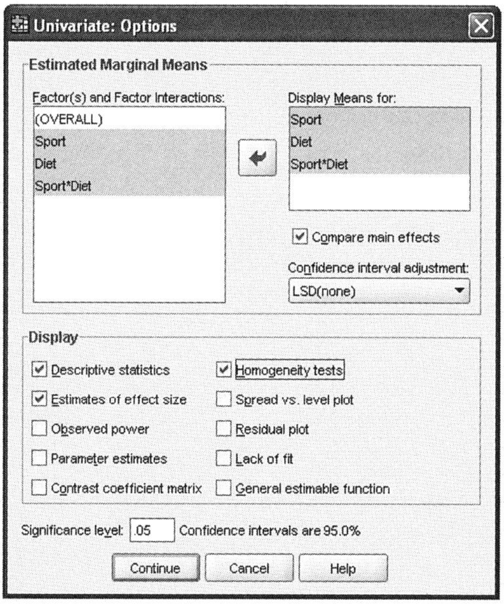

FIGURE 5.13 Options for various outputs in two-way ANOVA.

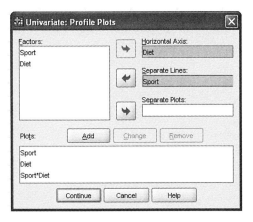

FIGURE 5.14   Options for generating means plot.

(b) Select *Diet* variable from the "Factors" section and bring it into the "Horizontal Axis" area for generating means plot of the main effect *Diet*. This plot is used to compare the main effect of *Diet* factor on fitness. Click on **Add**.

(c) For generating the mean plots of interaction, bring the *Sport* and *Diet* variables from the "Factors" section to the "Horizontal Axis" and "Separate Lines" areas, respectively. This plot is helpful in comparing simple effect of sport in each level of the diet. Click on **Add** to get the means plot in the output.

(d) Similarly for comparing the simple effect of diet in each level of the sport enter *Diet* and *Sport* variables from the "Factors" section to the "Horizontal Axis" and "Separate Lines" areas, respectively. Click on **Add.**

(e) Click on **Continue** and then on **OK** for generating outputs.

5.6.2   Interpretation of Findings

The following outputs have been selected in this analysis from the output windows for discussion:

1. Descriptive statistics
2. Two-way ANOVA table
3. Pair-wise comparisons of sport groups (all diet groups combined)
4. Pair-wise comparisons of different diet groups (both sport groups combined)
5. Means plots for interaction analysis

Table 5.14 shows the descriptive statistics. These values are used to generate means plot for understanding the simple effect of each factor.

TABLE 5.14 Descriptive Statistics

	Dependent Variable: Fitness Score			
Sport of the Subjects	Diet Category	Mean	SD	N
Wrestlers	High diet	8.0000	1.58114	5
	Medium diet	6.6000	1.34164	5
	Low diet	5.0000	1.22474	5
	Total	6.5333	1.80739	15
Gymnasts	High diet	3.4000	1.34164	5
	Medium diet	5.2000	1.30384	5
	Low diet	2.6000	1.14018	5
	Total	3.7333	1.62422	15
Total	High diet	5.7000	2.79086	10
	Medium diet	5.9000	1.44914	10
	Low diet	3.8000	1.68655	10
	Total	5.1333	2.20866	30

TABLE 5.15 Levene's Test of Equality of Error Variances[a]

Dependent Variable: Fitness Test Data			
F	df1	df2	Sig.
0.284	5	24	0.917

Tests the null hypothesis that the error variance of the dependent variable is equal across groups.

[a] Design: *Intercept + Sport + Diet + Sport * Diet*.

In two-way ANOVA, one of the main assumptions is that the variance of the dependent scores across entire cell should be same. This can be tested by the Levene's test shown in Table 5.15. This table reveals that the F value is not significant; hence the variability across all the cells is same. Thus, this assumption is satisfied.

5.6.2.1 Testing Main Effects The output of Table 5.16 may be truncated and shown in more readable format in Table 5.17. This table shows that the F values for *Sport*, *Diet*, and *Interaction* are all significant because their associated values of p are less than 0.05. Since interaction is significant, analyzing main effects of *Sport* and *Diet* becomes meaningless. However, just to show the procedure, we shall discuss testing significance of main effects as well.

5.6.2.1.1 Main Effect of Sport Since F for sport is significant, pair-wise comparison shall be done by using the contents in Table 5.18. By using the information given in Tables 5.14 and 5.18, the means plot as shown in Figure 5.15 can be obtained. In fact, this plot is generated in the SPSS output. It can be seen

TABLE 5.16   Two-Way ANOVA Table Generated by the SPSS

	Dependent Variable: Fitness Score				
Source	Type III Sum of Squares	df	Mean Square	F	Sig.
Corrected model	99.067[a]	5	19.813	11.215	0.000
Intercept	790.533	1	790.533	47.472	0.000
Sport	58.800	1	58.800	33.283	0.000
Diet	26.867	2	13.433	7.604	0.003
Sport*Diet	13.400	2	6.700	3.792	0.037
Error	42.400	24	1.767		
Total	932.000	30			
Corrected total	141.467	29			

[a] $R^2 = 0.700$ (adjusted $R^2 = 0.638$).

TABLE 5.17   Two-Way ANOVA Table for the Data on Fitness Score

Source of Variation	Sum of Squares (SS)	df	Mean Sum of Squares (MSS)	F	p Value (Sig.)
Sport	58.80	1	58.80	33.28	0.000
Diet	26.87	2	13.43	7.60	0.003
Interaction (Sport*Diet)	13.40	2	6.70	3.79	0.037
Error	42.40	24	1.77		
Corrected total	141.47	29			

TABLE 5.18   Pairwise Comparison of Sport Groups

	Dependent Variable: Fitness Test Data					
					95% Confidence Interval for Difference[a]	
(I) Sport of the Subjects	(J) Sport of the Subjects	Mean Diff. (I−J)	SE	Sig.[a]	Lower Bound	Upper Bound
Wrestlers	Gymnasts	2.800*	0.485	0.000	1.798	3.802
Gymnasts	Wrestlers	−2.800*	0.485	0.000	−3.802	−1.798

Based on estimated marginal means.
[a] Adjustment for multiple comparisons: Least Significant Difference (equivalent to no adjustments).
*The mean difference is significant at the 0.05 level.

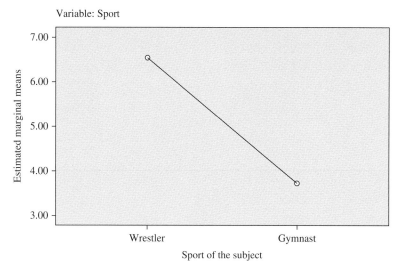

FIGURE 5.15   Marginal means plot of *Sport*.

TABLE 5.19   Pairwise Comparison of Different Diet Groups

Dependent Variable: Fitness Test Score

(I) Diet Group	(J) Diet Group	Mean Diff. (I−J)	SE	Sig.[a]	95% Confidence Interval for Difference[a] Lower Bound	Upper Bound
High protein	Medium protein	−0.200	0.594	0.982	−1.725	1.325
	Low protein	1.900*	0.594	0.012	0.375	3.425
Medium protein	High protein	0.200	0.594	0.982	−1.325	1.725
	Low protein	2.100*	0.594	0.005	0.575	3.625
Low protein	High protein	−1.900*	0.594	0.012	−3.425	−0.375
	Medium protein	−2.100*	0.594	0.005	−3.625	−0.575

Based on estimated marginal means.

[a] Adjustment for multiple comparisons: Least Significant Difference (equivalent to no adjustments).

*The mean difference is significant at 0.05 level.

from this figure that the average fitness score of wrestlers is significantly higher than that of gymnasts irrespective of the diet types.

5.6.2.1.2   Main Effect of Diet   It can be seen from Table 5.17 that the effect of *Diet* on fitness is significant; hence pair-wise comparison shall be done by using the contents of Table 5.19. By using the information given in Tables 5.14 and 5.19, the means plot as shown in Figure 5.16 can be obtained. This plot is generated in the SPSS output. This figure shows that the diet with high protein is more effective and

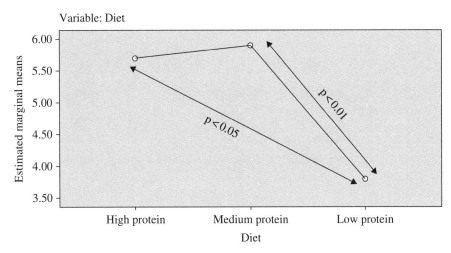

FIGURE 5.16   Marginal means plot of *Diet*.

that with low protein is least effective for fitness irrespective of the sports. However, diet with high and medium protein is equally effective.

5.6.2.2 Interaction Analysis   Since interaction effect between sport and diet is significant in Table 5.17, it would be interesting to investigate the simple effect. In fact, the main purpose of factorial experiment using two-way ANOVA is to test whether the interaction effect is significant or not. Results of the simple effect are not obtained in the SPSS outputs; hence, some extra work is required to get the outputs for simple effects of sport and diet. The detailed procedure is shown in the following sections:

5.6.2.2.1   Simple Effect of Diet   To find the simple effect of *Diet*, all three diet groups need to be compared in each sport category separately. To do so, two separate one-way ANOVA need to be applied. This can be done by splitting the data file (developed in this example as shown in Figure 5.9) into SPSS by using the following sequence of commands:

Data → Split File

The screen shall look like as shown in Figure 5.17. Choose the radio button 'Organize output by groups' and bring the variable *Sport* from left panel into the area marked with "Grouped based on" in the right panel. Ensure that the radio button 'Sort the file by grouping variables' is selected. This option is in fact selected by default. Click on **OK** to get the data file split as per the *Sport* category. The SPSS will show the following message in the output dialog box:

SORT CASES BY *Sport*.
SPLIT FILE SEPARATE BY *Sport*.

Go back to the data file and click on the following commands in sequence for one-way ANOVA:

Analyze → Compare Means → One-Way ANOVA

After clicking on "**One-Way ANOVA**" option, you will be directed to the next screen for selecting variables as shown in Figure 5.18. Select the *Fitness_score* and *Diet* from left panel, and bring them to the "Dependent list" and "Factor" sections in the right panel, respectively. This will provide the outputs for investigating the simple effect of *Diet* in each *Sport* category.

After selecting variables, option needs to be defined for generating the output in one-way ANOVA. Click on **Post Hoc** command and check the option 'Tukey.' The screen will look like as shown in Figure 5.19. Click on **Continue** to go back to the screen as shown in Figure 5.18.

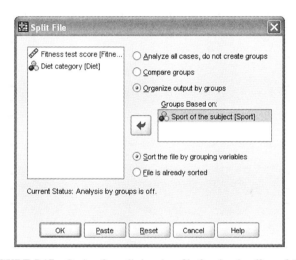

FIGURE 5.17   Option for splitting data file for simple effect of *Diet*.

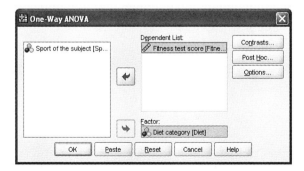

FIGURE 5.18   Selection of variables for generating simple effect of *Diet*.

Click on **Options** command in the screen shown in Figure 5.18 and then check 'Descriptive' option (Fig. 5.20). Click on **Continue** and **OK** commands for generating outputs as shown in Tables 5.20 and 5.21. The SPSS outputs for sports group have been shown in these tables.

Table 5.20 shows that the F values for *Diet* in wrestling (p = 0.017) and in gymnastics (p = 0.05) are significant as their associated p values are less than 0.025 (value of

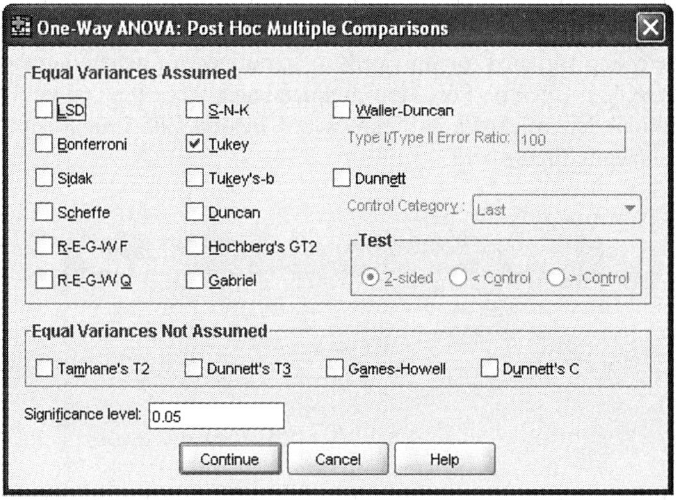

FIGURE 5.19   Options for post hoc test and significance level.

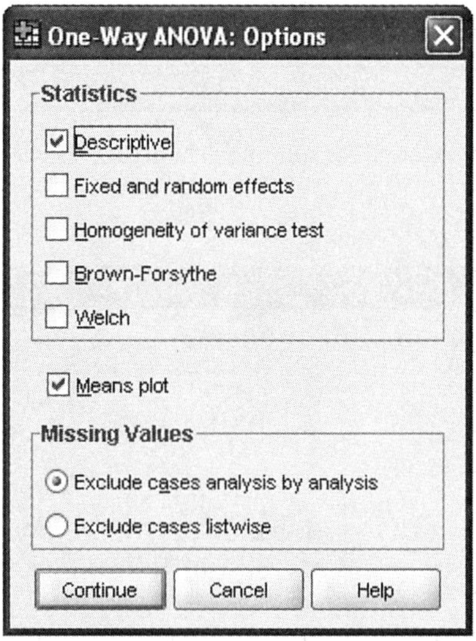

FIGURE 5.20   Options for descriptive statistics.

TABLE 5.20   F-Table for Testing the Effect of Diet in Each Sport Category

		Measure: Fitness Test Data				
Sport		Sum of Squares	df	Mean Square	F	Sig. (p Value)
Wrestling	Between groups	22.533	2	11.267	5.828	0.017
	Within groups	23.200	12	1.933		
	Total	45.733	14			
Gymnastics	Between groups	17.733	2	8.867	5.542	0.020
	Within groups	19.200	12	1.600		
	Total	36.933	14			

α, 0.05 has been divided by 2 as two ANOVA's have been computed). Thus, the null hypothesis of no difference in mean fitness scores among the three diet groups is rejected in each sport category. Since the effect of *Diet* is significant in each sport category, it is important to do the pair-wise comparison of means among three levels of diet in each sport category.

5.6.2.2.1.1   PAIR-WISE COMPARISON OF MEANS IN EACH SPORT CATEGORY   Pair-wise comparison of means among three levels of diet in each sport category has been shown in Table 5.21. The following conclusions can be drawn:

In wrestling category, there is a significant difference ($p<0.025$) between high- and low-protein diet groups.

In gymnastics category, there is a significant difference between medium- and low-protein diet groups. ($p<0.025$).

In order to know in which diet group average fitness score is more a means plot has been shown in Figure 5.13. This has been obtained in the main output of the SPSS during the analysis of the main effects.

5.6.2.2.1.2   MEANS PLOT (*SPORT × DIET*)   The contents of Tables 5.14 and 5.21 can be used to show the means plots of different diet groups in each *Sport* category as shown in Figure 5.21. This means plot provides a clear picture about the analysis. It shows that the fitness improves if the high protein diet is taken instead of low protein diet among the wrestlers.

In gymnastics, medium intake of protein diet improves fitness significantly in comparison to low-protein diet.

5.6.2.2.2   Simple Effect of Sport   To investigate the simple effect of *Sport*, scores of both the sports groups need to be compared in each diet category separately. Since sport has two groups, it can easily be known as to which sport group's fitness is better in each diet category. However, we shall discuss the procedure so that the readers can use if there are more than two categories of this factor (*Sport*). Thus, to investigate the simple effect of sport, two separate one-way ANOVA need to be applied. This can be done by splitting the data file (developed in this example as shown in Fig. 5.9) in SPSS by using the following sequence of commands:

TABLE 5.21 Pairwise Comparison of Means in Sport Category

| | | | Fitness Test Data | | | | |
| | | | Tukey HSD | | | 95% Confidence Interval | |
Dependent Variable	(I) Diet Category	(J) Diet Category	Mean Diff. (I–J)	SE	Sig.	Lower Bound	Upper Bound
Wrestling	H_prot	M_prot	1.40000	0.87939	0.286	−0.9461	3.7461
		L_prot	3.00000*	0.87939	**0.013**	0.6539	5.3461
	M_prot	H_prot	−1.40000	0.87939	0.286	−3.7461	0.9461
		L_prot	1.60000	0.87939	0.205	−0.7461	3.9461
	L_prot	H_prot	−3.00000*	0.87939	**0.013**	−5.3461	−0.6539
		M_prot	−1.60000	0.87939	0.205	−3.9461	0.7461
Gymnastics	H_prot	M_prot	−1.80000	0.80000	0.103	−3.9343	0.3343
		L_prot	0.80000	0.80000	0.591	−1.3343	2.9343
	M_prot	H_prot	1.80000	0.80000	0.103	−0.3343	3.9343
		L_prot	2.60000*	0.80000	**0.018**	0.4657	4.7343
	L_prot	H_prot	−0.80000	0.80000	0.591	−2.9343	1.3343
		M_prot	−2.60000*	0.80000	**0.018**	−4.7343	−0.4657

*The mean difference is significant at the 0.05 level.

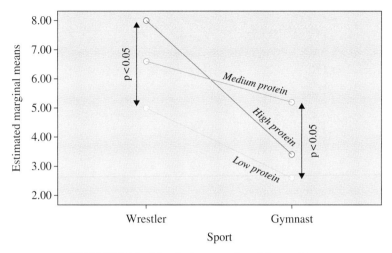

FIGURE 5.21   Marginal means plot of *Sport × Diet*.

Data → Split File

The screen shall look like as shown in Figure 5.22. Choose the radio button 'Organize output by groups' and bring the variable *Diet* this time from left panel into the area marked with "Grouped based on" in the right panel. Ensure that the radio button 'Sort the file by grouping variables' is selected. This option is in fact selected by default. Click on **OK** to get the data file split as per the sport category. The SPSS will show the following message in the output dialog box:

SORT CASES BY *Diet*.
SPLIT FILE SEPARATE BY *Diet*.

Go back to the data file and use the commands for one-way ANOVA as we did earlier. After clicking on "One-Way ANOVA" option, you will be directed to the next screen for selecting variables as shown in Figure 5.23. Now select *Fitness test score* and *Sports* variables from left panel and bring them to the "Dependent list" and "Factor" sections, respectively, in the right panel. This will provide the outputs for investigating the simple effect of sport in each diet category.

After selecting variables and choosing 'Tukey' option for the post hoc test, the outputs have been generated. The SPSS outputs of all the three diet groups have been combined in Table 5.22.

Since F value for high-protein and low-protein groups are significant ($p < 0.017$), mean fitness scores of the two sports shall be compared only in these two groups. This can be done by using the means plot. Here significance of F has been tested at 0.017 (=0.05/3) because three one-way ANOVA have been computed on the same data.

5.6.2.2.2.1   MEANS PLOT (*DIET × SPORT*)   The means plot Diet × Sport is generated in the main analysis by the SPSS. This plot is shown in Figure 5.24. It indicates that

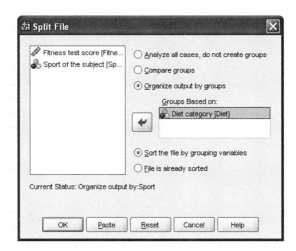

FIGURE 5.22   Option for splitting data file for simple effect of *Sport*.

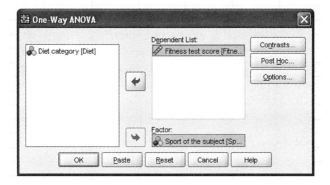

FIGURE 5.23   Selection of variables for simple effect of *Sport*.

TABLE 5.22   F-Table for Testing the Effect of Sport in Each Diet Category

Diet		Sum of Squares	df	Mean Square	F	Sig. (p Value)
			Measure: Fitness Test Data			
High protein	Between groups	52.900	1	52.900	24.605	0.001
	Within groups	17.200	8	2.150		
	Total	70.100	9			
Medium protein	Between groups	4.900	1	4.900	2.800	0.133
	Within groups	14.000	8	1.750		
	Total	18.900	9			
Low protein	Between groups	14.400	1	14.400	10.286	0.012
	Within groups	11.200	8	1.400		
	Total	25.600	9			

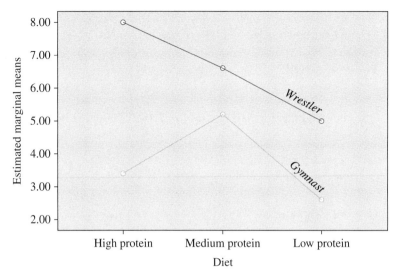

FIGURE 5.24 Marginal means plot of *Diet* × *Sport*.

fitness for the wrestler is significantly higher than that of gymnasts in the high-protein diet category. This trend is also followed in low-protein diet category as well.

5.7   SUMMARY OF THE SPSS COMMANDS

5.7.1   One-Way ANOVA

1. Start SPSS by using the following commands:

    Start → All Programs → SPSS Inc → SPSS 22.0

2. Click on **Variable View** and define *Anxiety* and *Sport* as a scale and nominal variables, respectively.
3. Under the column heading "Values," define '1' for Individual Sport, '2' for Dual Sport, and '3' for Team Sport.
4. Once variables are defined, type the data for these variables by clicking on **Data View** button.
5. In **Data View**, for the computation involved in one-way ANOVA, the following commands must be followed in sequence:

    Analyze → Compare Means → One-Way ANOVA

6. Select variables *Anxiety* and *Sport* from left panel and bring them into "Dependent list" section and "Factor" section in the right panel, respectively.
7. Click on **Post Hoc** command and select 'LSD' option and write the value of 'Significance level' as 0.05. Click on **Continue**.

8. Click on **Options** command and then check 'Descriptive.' option.

9. Click on **Continue** and then on **OK** to generate outputs.

5.7.2   Two-Way ANOVA

1. Start SPSS by using the following commands in sequence:

   Start → All Programs → SPSS Inc → SPSS 22.0 → Type in Data

2. Click on **Variable View** and define *Fitness_Score* as a scale variable and *Sport* and *Diet* as nominal variables.

3. Once variables are defined, type the data for these variables by clicking on **Data View.**

4. In the **Data View**, use the following commands in sequence:

   Analyze → General Linear Model → Univariate

5. Select *Fitness_Scores* variable from the left panel and bring it to the "dependent variable" section in the right panel. Similarly, select the variables *Sport* and *Diet* from left panel and bring them to the "Fixed Factor(s)" section in the right panel.

6. Click on **Post Hoc** command and select the factors *Sport* and *Diet* from the left panel and bring them to the "Post Hoc test" panel on the right side. Check the option 'Tukey' and then click on **Continue**.

7. Click on **Options** command. Select *Sport, Diet*, and *Sport*Diet* variables from left panel and bring them into the right panel. Select 'Compare main effects' and 'Descriptive statistics' options and ensure that the value of significance is 0.05. Click on **Continue**.

8. Select option for means plots for main and simple effects.

9. Click on **OK** for output.

10. For simple effect, split the data file by using the following commands in sequence:

    Data → Split File

11. Apply one-way ANOVA for generating outputs for the simple effect of diet and sport

5.8   EXERCISE

5.8.1   Short Answer Questions

Note: Write answer to each of the following questions in not more than 200 words.

Q.1   In an experiment, it is desired to compare the reaction time of basketballers, gymnasts, and volleyballers. Write the null hypothesis as well as all possible types of alternative hypotheses.

Q.2   Explain a situation where one-way ANOVA can be applied. Which variances are compared in one-way ANOVA?

Q.3   ANOVA is used for comparing means of different groups but it uses F-test that is a test of significance for comparing variances of two groups. Discuss this anomaly.

Q.4   What do you mean by the post hoc test? Explain its procedure.

Q.5   What is p value? In what context is it used?

Q.6   What do you mean by interaction? Explain it by describing an experimental situation.

Q.7   Justify the name "two-way ANOVA." Discuss the advantages of two-way ANOVA over one-way ANOVA.

Q.8   In an experiment, the effects of three circuit training programs were compared under three weather conditions. Thus, nine treatment groups were studied with five samples in each. With the help of the given results like SS (Training) = 234, SS (Weather) = 145, SS (Interaction) = 101, and TSS = 705, complete two-way ANOVA table.

Q.9   While using two-way ANOVA, what assumptions need to be made about the data?

Q.10 Describe an experimental situation where two-way ANOVA can be used. Discuss different types of hypotheses that you would like to test.

Q.11 What do you mean by 'Factors' in two-way ANOVA? Explain the same by means of examples.

Q.12 What is main effect? How is it different from interaction effect?

5.8.2   Multiple Choice Questions

Note: Questions 1–10 have four alternative answers for each question. Tick mark the one that you consider the closest to the correct answer.

1   Choose the correct statement.
    (a) Total sum of square is additive in nature.
    (b) Total mean sum of square is additive in nature.
    (c) Total sum of square is nonadditive.
    (d) Total mean sum of square is equivalent to the total sum of square.

2   In ANOVA experiment if the variability due to chance decreases the F value will
    (a) remains same.
    (b) decreases.
    (c) increases.
    (d) can't say with this information.

3 Choose the correct statement
   (a) If F-statistic is significant at 0.05 level, it will also be significant at 0.01 level.
   (b) If F-statistic is significant at 0.01 level, it may not be significant at 0.05 level.
   (c) If F-statistic is significant at 0.01 level, it will necessarily be significant at 0.05 level.
   (d) If F-statistic is not significant at 0.01 level, it will not be significant at 0.05 level.

4 Choose the correct statement.
   (a) If p value is 0.02, F-statistic shall be significant at 5% level.
   (b) If p value is 0.02, F-statistic shall not be significant at 5% level.
   (c) If p value is 0.02, F-statistic shall be significant at 1% level.
   (d) None of the above is correct.

5 In comparing the IQ among three classes using one-way ANOVA in SPSS, choose the correct statement about the variable types.
   (a) IQ is a 'nominal' variable and Class is a 'scale' variable.
   (b) Both IQ and Class are the scale variables.
   (c) IQ is a 'scale' variable and Class is a 'nominal' variable.
   (d) Both IQ and Class are 'nominal' variables.

6 If coordinative ability is to be compared among three sport groups, then choose the valid variable names in SPSS.
   (a) Coord_Abil and Sport
   (b) Coord-Abil and Sport
   (c) Coord-Abil and Group_Sport
   (d) Coord_Abil and Group-Sport

7 If three groups of students are compared on their physical fitness index and in each group there are 12 subjects, what would be the degrees of freedom for the within group in one-way ANOVA?
   (a) 30
   (b) 31
   (c) 32
   (d) 33

8 Choose the correct model in one-way ANOVA.
   (a) $TSS = (SS)_b + (SS)_w$
   (b) $TSS = (SS)_b - (SS)_w$
   (c) $TSS = (SS)_b \times (SS)_w$
   (d) $TSS = (SS)_b / (SS)_w$

9 In one-way, four groups were compared for their memory retention power. These four groups had 8, 12, 10, and 11 subjects, respectively. What shall be the degree of freedom of between groups?
   (a) 41
   (b) 37
   (c) 3
   (d) 40

10 If anxiety has to be compared in three different sport groups using one-way ANOVA, then *Anxiety* and *Sport* variables need to be selected in SPSS. Choose the correct selection strategy.
(a) *Anxiety* in "Factor" section and *Sport* in "Dependent list" section.
(b) *Anxiety* in "Dependent list" section and *Sport* in "Factor" section.
(c) Both *Anxiety* and *Sport* in "Dependent list" section.
(d) Both *Anxiety* and *Sport* in "Factor" section.

11 In applying two-way ANOVA in an experiment, *r* levels of factor *A* and *c* levels of factor *B* are studied. What will be the degrees of freedom for interaction?
(a) rc
(b) $r+c$
(c) $rc-1$
(d) $(r-1)(c-1)$

12 In an experiment, "*r*" levels of factor *A* are compared in "*c*" levels of factor *B*. There are *N* scores in this experiment. What will be the degree of freedom for within group?
(a) $N-rc$
(b) $N+rc$
(c) $N-rc+1$
(d) $Nrc-1$

13 While using two-way ANOVA, certain assumptions are taken. Choose the correct assumption.
(a) The population variances must be different.
(b) The sample must be dependent.
(c) The populations from which the samples were drawn must have binomial distribution.
(d) The sample size in all the groups must be same.

14 Consider an experiment in which the hemoglobin (Hb) contents of different sportsmen are to be compared under three different exercise programs. Choose the correct statement in defining three variables *Sport*, *Exercise*, and *Hb* in SPSS.
(a) *Sport* and *Hb* are Scale variables and *Exercise* is the Nominal variable.
(b) *Sport* and *Exercise* are Nominal variables and *Hb* is the Scale variable.
(c) *Sport* and *Exercise* are Scale variables and *Hb* is the Nominal variable.
(d) *Exercise* and *Hb* are Scale variables and *Sport* is the Nominal variable.

15 Command sequence in SPSS for starting two-way ANOVA is
(a) Analyze → General Linear Model → Univariate
(b) Analyze → General Linear Model → Multivariate
(c) Analyze → General Linear Model → Repeated Measures
(d) Analyze → Univariate → General Linear Model

16   In two-way ANOVA, Fixed Factors refer to
     (a) Dependent variables
     (b) Independent variables
     (c) Both dependent and independent variables
     (d) None of the above

17   If there are N scores in a two-way ANOVA experiment, the total degree of free-dom would be
     (a) $N + 1$
     (b) $N - 1$
     (c) N
     (d) $N - 2$

18   If three levels of factor A are compared among the four levels of factor B, how many treatment groups will have to be created?
     (a) 7
     (b) 1
     (c) 12
     (d) 11

5.8.3   Assignment

1. A study was conducted on cricketers to compare the shoulder flexibility of bowlers, batsmen, and all-rounders. The data so obtained is shown in Table 5.23. Apply one-way ANOVA and discuss your findings at 5% level.

2. A study was conducted on the lifestyle of young, middle-aged, and old-aged executives of production and marketing division of an industry. A lifestyle inventory was administered on each individual who participated in the study. A high score on the test indicates a better lifestyle. Test scores are shown. Analyze the data given in Table 5.24 by using two-way ANOVA and discuss your findings at 5% level.

TABLE 5.23   Data on Shoulder Flexibility in Inches

Batsman	Bowlers	All-Rounder
10	18	12
14	17	15
11	15	11
15	16	13
13	16	12
13.5	18	17
10.5	17	13
9.5	17	13
9.6	13	14
15.3	17	14

TABLE 5.24 Data on Lifestyle Evaluation

Group	Young Executives	Middle-Aged Executives	Old-Aged Executives
Production	3	7	11
	2	4	7
	2	7	9
	4	6	8
	2	6	10
Marketing	8	8	11
	4	10	9
	3	7	11
	5	7	12
	5	8	12

5.9 CASE STUDY ON ONE-WAY ANOVA DESIGN

Objective

While developing weight training schedule, a coach wanted to know whether back strength differs among the athletes playing soccer, wrestling, and hockey. He organized an experiment in which 10 soccer players, 14 wrestlers, and 12 hockey players were selected. Back strength for these subjects was tested by using the leg dynamometer. The data so obtained is shown in Table 5.25.

Research Questions

The following research questions were investigated:

1. Whether back strength has anything to do with the type of sports one play.
2. Whether back strength of any one sport is significantly different than others

Data Format

The format used for preparing data file in SPSS is shown in Table 5.26.

Analyzing Data

To investigate the research issues, one-way ANOVA was applied for testing the null hypothesis that the mean difference among the three sports group is same against the alternative hypothesis that at least one group mean differs. The F value in the ANOVA table was found to be significant; hence, a post hoc analysis was carried out by using the Tukey HSD test. The one-way ANOVA was applied in SPSS by using the following commands in sequence: **Analyze, Compare Means**, and **One-Way ANOVA**.

TABLE 5.25   Data on Back Strength in kg

Soccer	Wrestling	Hockey
68	122	78
88	88	82
100	94	96
116	100	110
72	110	120
66	120	88
88	88	92
78	82	98
90	104	88
92	110	110
	98	88
	105	86
	102	
	95	

The output was obtained by placing the dependent variable and group variable in the appropriate locations in the dialog box, checking 'Tukey' as a post hoc test and 'Means Plot' options. The results so obtained are shown in Table 5.27.

Interpreting Findings

Table 5.27 shows that the F value is significant at 0.05 significance level; hence the null hypothesis is rejected. Since null hypothesis was rejected, a Tukey post hoc test was applied whose results are shown in Table 5.28. It can be seen from this table that the mean difference between soccer and wrestling groups is significant ($p = 0.020$), whereas all other mean differences are nonsignificant.

Means Plot

Figure 5.25 indicates the means plot. On the basis of the sampled data, means plot shows that the mean back strength of soccer and wrestling groups differs significantly. Further, there is no difference between soccer and hockey groups and that of wrestling and hockey groups.

Reporting

- Since F (=4.049) is significant ($p = 0.027$), the null hypothesis that the mean back strength is same among all the three groups is rejected. Thus, on the basis of the sampled data, it can be concluded that the back strength is related with the type of sports one play.
- Tukey post hoc test indicates that there is a significant difference between soccer and wrestling groups in relation to back strength.
- The means plot indicates that the back strength of the wrestling group is significantly higher than that of the soccer group.

TABLE 5.26 Data Format used in SPSS for Back Strength (in kg)

Back Strength	Sports Group
68	1
88	1
100	1
116	1
72	1
66	1
88	1
78	1
90	1
92	1
122	2
88	2
94	2
100	2
110	2
120	2
88	2
82	2
104	2
110	2
98	2
105	2
102	2
95	2
78	3
82	3
96	3
110	3
120	3
88	3
92	3
98	3
88	3
110	3
88	3
86	3

Group code: 1, soccer; 2, wrestling; 3, hockey.

TABLE 5.27 ANOVA

	Back Strength				
	Sum of Squares	df	Mean Square	F	Sig.
Between groups	1399.098	2	699.549	4.049	0.027
Within groups	5701.124	33	172.761		
Total	7100.222	35			

TABLE 5.28 Multiple Comparisons

| | | Back Strength | | | 95% Confidence Interval | |
| | | Tukey HSD | | | | |
(I) Sports Group	(J) Sports Group	Mean Diff. (I−J)	SE	Sig.	Lower Bound	Upper Bound
Soccer	Wrestling	−15.48571*	5.44208	**0.020**	−28.8395	−2.1320
	Hockey	−8.86667	5.62787	0.270	−22.6763	4.9430
Wrestling	Soccer	15.48571*	5.44208	0.020	2.1320	28.8395
	Hockey	6.61905	5.17077	0.416	−6.0690	19.3071
Hockey	Soccer	8.86667	5.62787	0.270	−4.9430	22.6763
	Wrestling	−6.61905	5.17077	0.416	−19.3071	6.0690

*The mean difference is significant at the 0.05 level.

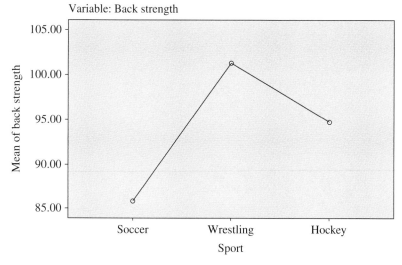

FIGURE 5.25 Means plots.

5.10   CASE STUDY ON TWO-WAY ANOVA

Objective

An exercise scientist wanted to evaluate the effect of gender (male and female) and music (jazz, classical, and opera) on mood of the subjects during treadmill exercise. He conducted a 2×3 factorial study in which 15 male and 15 female participated. Male and female were randomly divided into three groups. These groups were randomly assigned the music treatment in the background while doing the exercise for 30 min on treadmill with a particular load. After the workout, their mood score was recorded by means of a questionnaire. The data so obtained are shown in Table 5.29.

Research Questions

The following research questions were investigated:

1. Whether gender affects the mood during exercise irrespective of the background music
2. Whether music affects the mood during exercise irrespective of the gender
3. Whether interaction between gender and mood exists

Data Format

The format used for preparing data file in SPSS is shown in Table 5.30.

TABLE 5.29   Data on Mood After the Treadmill Exercise in Each Treatment Group

Group	Jazz	Classical	Opera
Female	20	8	27
	24	10	26
	21	11	31
	16	6	24
	21	9	26
Male	23	15	15
	20	18	19
	26	12	20
	19	10	12
	20	13	18

Analyzing Data

For investigating all the three research questions, a two-way ANOVA was carried out by using SPSS. The F for *Gender*, *Music*, and *Interaction* was tested for their significance. Post hoc test was applied if F was significant for the component. The two-way ANOVA was applied in SPSS by using the following commands in sequence: **Analyze, General Linear Model**, and **Univariate**. *Mood* variable was placed in the dependent variable section, whereas gender and music were inserted in the fixed factor. Appropriate options were defined for generating the means plot. Tukey was selected as a post hoc test and by checking 'Descriptive statistics' and 'Homogeneity test' various outputs were generated, which are shown in Tables 5.30, 5.31, 5.32, 5.33, and 5.34.

Testing Assumption

One of the main assumptions in two-way ANOVA is that the variance of the dependent scores across the entire cell should be same. To test this hypothesis, SPSS provides Levene's test in its output, which is shown in Table 5.31. This table shows that the F value is not significant. Therefore, the variability across all the cells is same; hence this assumption is satisfied.

Testing Significance of Different Effects

Table 5.32 shows that the F values for *Music* (p = 0.000) and *Interaction* (p = 0.000) are significant; hence post hoc analysis was done for getting the correct picture. Since interaction effect was significant, no post hoc analysis was done for the main effect, music. The whole concentration was on investigating the interaction effect. Since interaction effect was significant, simple effects of *Gender* and *Music* were investigated.

TABLE 5.30   Data Format used in SPSS for Back Strength (in kg)

Gender	Music	Mood_Score
1	1	20
1	1	24
1	1	21
1	1	16
1	1	21
1	2	8
1	2	10
1	2	11
1	2	6
1	2	9
1	3	27
1	3	26
1	3	31
1	3	24
1	3	26
2	1	23
2	1	20
2	1	26
2	1	19
2	1	20
2	2	15
2	2	18
2	2	12
2	2	10
2	2	13
2	3	15
2	3	19
2	3	20
2	3	12
2	3	18

Gender code: 1, male; 2, female.
Music code: 1, jazz; 2, classical; 3, opera.

TABLE 5.31   Levene's Test of Equality of Error Variances[a]

Dependent Variable: Mood_Score			
F	df1	df2	Sig.
0.421	5	24	0.829

Tests the null hypothesis that the error variance of the dependent variable is equal across groups.

[a] Design: *Intercept + Gender + Music + Gender * Music*.

TABLE 5.32   Tests of Between-Subjects Effects

Source	Type III Sum of Squares	df	Mean Square	F	Sig.
Dependent Variable: Mood_Score					
Corrected model	1008.000[a]	5	201.600	25.736	0.000
Intercept	9720.000	1	9720.000	1.241E3	0.000
Gender	13.333	1	13.333	1.702	0.204
Music	696.800	2	348.400	44.477	**0.000**
Gender*Music	297.867	2	148.933	19.013	**0.000**
Error	188.000	24	7.833		
Total	10916.000	30			
Corrected total	1196.000	29			

[a] $R^2 = 0.843$ (adjusted $R^2 = 0.810$).

TABLE 5.33   Descriptive Statistics

Gender	Music	Mean	SD	N
Dependent Variable: Mood_Score				
Male	Jazz	20.4000	2.88097	5
	Classical	8.8000	1.92354	5
	Opera	26.8000	2.58844	5
	Total	18.6667	8.05044	15
Female	Jazz	21.6000	2.88097	5
	Classical	13.6000	3.04959	5
	Opera	16.8000	3.27109	5
	Total	17.3333	4.43471	15
Total	Jazz	21.0000	2.78887	10
	Classical	11.2000	3.48967	10
	Opera	21.8000	5.95912	10
	Total	18.0000	6.42195	30

TABLE 5.34   Mean Mood Scores for Different Music Groups in Each Gender Group

Gender Group				CD at 5% level
Male	26.8 (Opera)	20.4 (Jazz)	8.8 (Classical)	3.65
Female	21.6 (Jazz)	16.8 (Opera)	13.6 (Classical)	3.65

" |_____| " Denotes no difference between the means at 0.05 level of significance.

Interaction Analysis

Table 5.33 shows the mean of each cell. To compare these cell means among male and female and among different music groups, a critical difference was computed as follows:

$$\text{CD for Interaction} = t_{0.05}(24)\sqrt{\frac{2(\text{MSS})_E}{n}}$$

$$= 2.06\sqrt{\frac{2 \times 7.833}{5}} = 3.65$$

If the difference between two cells' mean is higher than 3.65, significant difference exists, otherwise not.

Simple Effect of Music

Simple effect of the music can be investigated by using the contents of Table 5.34. This table has been obtained by using the critical difference and the mean values of different cell. By looking to Table 5.34, it can be inferred that among male, opera music enhances the mood significantly during exercise; whereas in female, section jazz music is more effective.

Simple Effect of *Gender*

Looking to the results of Table 5.35, it can be inferred that with the classical music in the background female subject's mood was significantly better in comparison to male; whereas in opera music, male's mood was found to be significantly better in comparison to that of female.

Reporting

- Since F ratio for the *Music* was significant (p=0.000), it can be inferred that the *Music* has a significant impact on the mood of the subjects while doing the exercise irrespective of the gender.

TABLE 5.35 Mean Mood Scores for Different Gender Groups in Each Music Group

Music Group	Male	Female	CD at 5% level
Jazz	20.4	21.6	3.65
Classical	8.8	13.6	3.65
Opera	26.8	16.8	3.65

"⌐_____⌐ " Denotes no difference between the means at 0.05 level.

- Since F ratio for the interaction was significant ($p = 0.000$), it may thus be concluded that the interaction effect was significant.
- Interaction analysis showed that opera music was more suitable for male and jazz for female in enhancing their mood while exercising.

Further female's mood was elevated while exercising with classical music in the background, whereas male liked the opera music for mood enhancement.

6

REPEATED MEASURES ANOVA

LEARNING OBJECTIVES

After completing this chapter, you should be able to do the following:

- Understand the difference between independent measures ANOVA and repeated measures ANOVA
- Know the assumptions that are required to satisfy in repeated measures ANOVA
- Learn the procedure of solving one-way repeated measures design and mixed design with SPSS.
- Describe the output generated in repeated measures designs

6.1 INTRODUCTION

Experimental studies are conducted to investigate the effect of one or more factors on some variable of interest. These studies are designed in such a manner so as to ensure the validity of findings. In experimental studies, a researcher manipulates an independent variable to see its effect on a dependent variable. It is important that a researcher controls the effect of extraneous factors. Effect of extraneous factors can be controlled be using nonstatistical or statistical methods. The nonstatistical methods include randomization, elimination, and matching. The randomization method ensures normality of data and enhances external and internal validity. It refers to random selection of sample from the population of interest and allocating

Sports Research with Analytical Solution using SPSS®, First Edition. J. P. Verma.
© 2016 John Wiley & Sons, Inc. Published 2016 by John Wiley & Sons, Inc.
Companion website: www.wiley.com/go/Verma/Sportsresearch

treatments randomly to the subjects in the sample. On the other hand, elimination method refers to stabilizing a covariate if it affects an experiment. For instance, if the effect of three different intensities of a circuit training program on muscular strength is to be compared in a sample of subjects consisting both male and female, then the female subjects can be eliminated from the experiment. This is because male and female react differently in the experiment and the effect of gender might be confounded in the result. But in that case, the findings will only be applicable to the male subjects. Another nonstatistical procedure of controlling the effect of extraneous factor is matching. It refers to dividing the subjects in different treatment groups based on some criteria. For instance, in investigating the effect of training intensity on shooting accuracy in basketball, one may think that the performance during experiment depends upon the height of the players and therefore the subjects may be matched on the basis of their height. In such case, subjects' heights can be arranged in ascending order and then first three subjects may be randomly allocated in the three different treatment groups if there are three levels of training. Thereafter, next three subjects may be randomly allocated to the three treatment groups. This process continues till all subjects are allocated to different treatment groups. Validity of findings can be ensured by following any of these three nonstatistical procedures. However, in many situations these methods are not sufficient to control internal validity; hence, some statistical methods are used to enhance the validity of findings. These methods include independent measures design, repeated measures design, and analysis of covariance (ANCOVA) design. In independent measures design, each subject received one and only one treatment, whereas in repeated measures each subject receives all treatments. On the other hand, ANCOVA design is used when randomization of treatments is not possible and the treatments are allocated to the intact group.

The one-way ANOVA and two-way ANOVA methods discussed in Chapter 5 are the independent measures design. This chapter specifically deals with the repeated measures designs. Here we shall discuss the repeated measures design with one-way and two-way classification by using the SPSS software. In repeated measures design, one of the advantages is that variation due to subjects in different treatment groups is eliminated because each subject receives all the treatments. Another advantage of these designs is that less number of subjects are required to perform the experiment.

6.2   ONE-WAY REPEATED MEASURES ANOVA

In one-way repeated measures ANOVA, an experimenter manipulates an independent variable to see the effect on some dependent variable where all the subjects participate in all the treatment conditions. Consider an experiment in which the effect of different intervention on the recovery pattern after the match is investigated among football players. The researcher may identify three different interventions (autogenic relaxation, aqua therapy, and yoga exercises) for a particular duration. In this design, same subjects are tested under each treatment condition to avoid the individual variation.

In repeated measures design, subjects serve their own control. In order do away with the learning or fatigue effect, sufficient time gap is maintained between any two treatments. Sometimes, a researcher may be interested to investigate the impact of training on the performance in different durations. For instance, one might be interested to know the effect of aerobic program on the VO_2 max after two, four, and six weeks, respectively. The purpose of such experiment is to know the pattern of improvement among the subjects over a period of time. Such designs are also treated as repeated measures design. Repeated measures design is also known as within-group design.

6.2.1 Assumptions in One-Way Repeated Measures ANOVA

Using repeated measures design requires certain assumptions to be satisfied. It is essential to test these assumptions before using this design. If assumptions violates, the level of significance inflates in the experiment; hence, the following assumptions should hold in repeated measures designs:

1. The independent variable should be categorical and the dependent variable should be measured on interval or ratio scale.
2. Observations obtained on the dependent variable must be independent from each other.
3. The data on the dependent variable obtained on the subjects in each treatment condition must follow normal distribution.
4. The sphericity should not exist among the data. Sphericity assumption is satisfied if correlations among the repeated measures on the dependent variable are all equal.

6.2.2 Application in Sports Research

There may be numerous situations in which one-way repeated measures ANOVA can be used. This design should be used in a situation where it is difficult to control the variation in the treatment groups due to individual variation. Some of these situations are as follows:

1. A researcher may wish to investigate the effect of different warming-up exercises on 400 meter event. A group of randomly selected athletes may be tested for their performance on 400 meter in each of the three treatment conditions; warm-up exercise with cold pack, hot pack, and mix of both on the abdomen. These within-group data may be compared by using the single-group repeated measures design.
2. An investigator may study the effect of angle of release on shooting performance in basketball. A group of subjects may be tested for their performance on basketball shooting from a specific distance using three different angles: 45°, 50°, and 55°.

3. The effect of conditioning program on fitness index may be studied on the subjects over a period of time. The purpose of such studies is to identify the time period in which significant improvement in the criterion variable occurs and also to know the time period after which the improvement stops increasing. The study may be planned in such a manner that each subject is tested for fitness index at 0 days and after 2, 4, 6, 8, and 10 weeks while undergoing the conditioning program.

4. An exercise scientist may like to investigate the effect of a low intensity exercise intervention on the cardio-respiratory endurance on overweight subjects. A random sample of subjects having weight 200 lb or more may be selected for the study on which the low intensity exercise program may be implemented. The performance of these subjects on cardio-respiratory endurance may be measured at 0 days and after 3, 6, 9, and 12 weeks of exercise intervention to identify the minimum duration for significant improvement. The investigator may further be interested to know the pattern of improvement in cardio-respiratory endurance during different time periods while undergoing the exercise intervention program.

6.2.3 Steps in Solving One-Way Repeated Measures ANOVA

One of the main assumptions in the repeated measures design is sphericity. If the assumption of sphericity is violated, the correction is required to be made in the degrees of freedom attached to the computed values of F. The following steps are used in solving one-way repeated measures ANOVA in SPSS:

1. Check the assumption of normality of the data in all the treatment conditions. (You may refer to the Chapter 2 for the detailed procedure.)
2. Formulate the hypothesis to be tested.
3. Use SPSS to generate the following output:
   (a) Descriptive statistics
   (b) Mauchly's test of sphericity including estimated value of epsilon
   (c) F-table for testing within-subjects effect
   (d) Pair-wise comparisons
   (e) Means plot
4. If Mauchly's test is significant ($p < 0.05$), sphericity assumption is violated and in that case correction in the degrees of freedom for F statistic is applied; whereas if the sphericity is not violated, no correction is applied to the degrees of freedom attached to the F statistic.
5. In case sphericity is violated, look for the value of epsilon (ε). If its value is less than 0.75, apply Greenhouse-Geisser correction. Otherwise, apply Huynh-Feldt correction in the degrees of freedom and then test the significance of F by looking to the p value attached to it.

6. If F ratio is significant, do the pair-wise comparisons among group means by applying the Bonferroni correction.

7. Report the findings.

6.3 ONE-WAY REPEATED MEASURES ANOVA USING SPSS

Example 6.1

An exercise scientist used a cardio intervention program on 10 randomly selected sedentary male subjects, aged 41–50 years, to see its impact on VO_2 max for assessing the cardio-respiratory efficiency. Repeated measures of VO_2 max were obtained on each subject at zero, two, four, and six weeks which is shown in Table 6.1. Apply repeated measures ANOVA to report its findings at the significance level 0.05.

Solution: Here it is required to test whether VO_2 max of the subjects differs in all the four time periods of testing during cardio-intervention program. To test this research hypothesis, the following null hypothesis shall be tested against alternative hypothesis that at least one group mean differs $H_0 : \mu_{Zero\_week} = \mu_{Two\_week} = \mu_{Four\_week} = \mu_{Six\_week}$.

TABLE 6.1 Data on VO_2 max (in ml/kg/min) Obtained on the Subjects at Different Duration During Cardio-Intervention Program

Zero Week	Two Weeks	Four Weeks	Six Weeks
31	36	35	37
31	34	34	35
32	31	37	35
30	32	36	35
34	33	37	37
35	34	36	38
36	31	31	38
36	35	30	40
32	31	35	36
33	32	34	36

6.3.1 Computation in the One-Way Repeated Measures ANOVA

6.3.1.1 Preparation of Data File   To solve repeated measures ANOVA in SPSS, the first step is to prepare a data file. The readers who are using SPSS for the first time are advised to refer to the Chapter 1 for the detailed procedure in preparing data file. The data file will look like as shown in Figure 6.1.

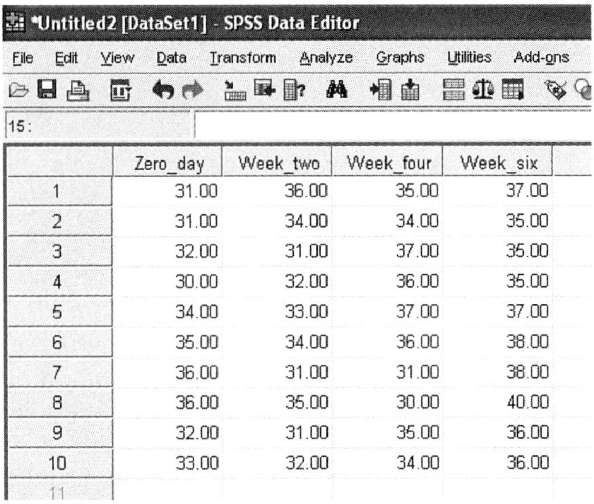

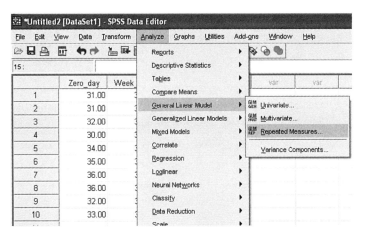

FIGURE 6.1   Data file of VO$_2$ max in one-way repeated measures ANOVA.

FIGURE 6.2   Command sequence in one-way repeated measures ANOVA.

6.3.1.2   SPSS Commands   After preparing the data file, save it in the desired location before further processing. Do the following steps:

1. *Initiating SPSS commands*: While being in the **Data View**, click the following commands in sequence.

    Analyze → General Linear Model → Repeated Measures

    The screen shall look like as shown in Figure 6.2.
2. *Selecting variables for analysis:* After clicking **Repeated Measures** command, the screen shown in Figure 6.3 shall be obtained to define the variables. By default, the "Within-Subject Factor Name" is written as factor 1. Change this by *Time* because this is the independent (within-subjects) variable in this

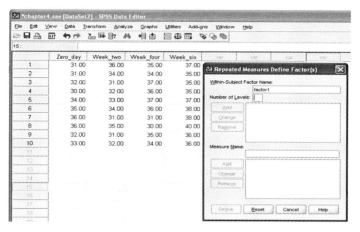

FIGURE 6.3 Screen for defining variables.

example. Write the number of levels as 4 as there are four time periods in which the data has been obtained. Click **Add**. In the "Measure Name" area type 'VO$_2$ max.' Click **Add**. Please note that the name of the independent and dependent variables should start only from alphabet, and no gap should be there in between the two words in defining these names. If name contains two or more words, they must be joined by using the underscore. You should get the two screens as shown in Figures 6.3 and 6.4 before and after clicking **Add**, respectively.

3. *Selecting options for computation:* Clicking **Define** in the screen shown in Figure 6.4 will take you to the screen as shown in Figure 6.5 for selecting the within-subjects variables. Select all four variables from the left panel and bring them to the "Within-Subjects Variables" section of the screen. After selecting the variables, option needs to be defined for generating the output. Do the following:

(a) Click **Plots** command and transfer the variable 'Time' from the "Factor" section into the "Horizontal Axis" area. Click **Add** to get the means plot in the output.

(b) Click **Continue** to get the screen as shown in Figure 6.6 for selecting further options in the design.

(c) Click **Option** and transfer the variable 'Time' from the "Factor(s) and Factor Interactions" section into the "Display Means for" section. Do the following:

(i) Check 'Compare main effects' option.

(ii) Select Bonferroni correction by clicking on the sign ▼ in "Confidence interval adjustment" drop down menu.

(iii) Check 'Descriptive statistics' option for computing mean and standard deviation in each group. Ensure that the level of significance is selected as 0.05. In fact by default it is selected as 0.05. Let all other options remain as it is.

(iv) Click **Continue** and **OK** to get the outputs.

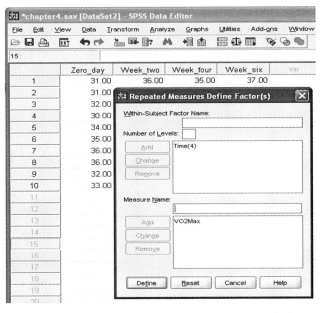

FIGURE 6.4   Screen for adding variables in the analysis.

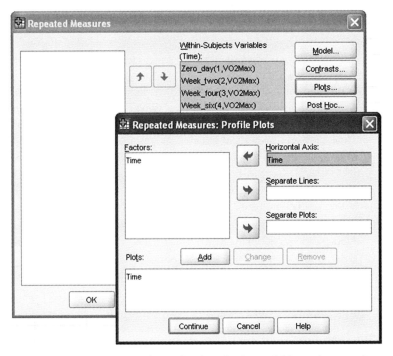

FIGURE 6.5   Screen showing option for selecting variables and means plot.

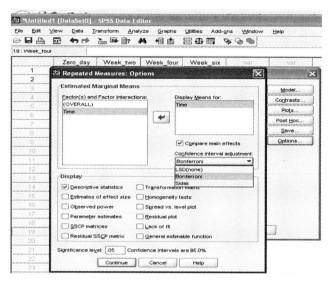

FIGURE 6.6 Option for computing descriptive statistics and pair-wise comparison of means using Bonferroni correction.

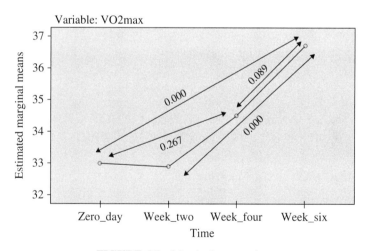

FIGURE 6.7 Marginal means plot.

6.3.1.3 SPSS Output In SPSS, all the outputs are generated in the output panel. Only relevant outputs are selected for the discussion. Right click the mouse over the output which is required to be selected, copy it, and paste it in your word document. The outputs selected in this analysis are shown in Tables 6.3, 6.4, 6.5, 6.6, and 6.7 and in Figure 6.7.

6.3.2 Interpretation of Findings

Before interpreting the outputs of this analysis, let us first investigate the assumptions of this design.

6.3.2.1 Testing Assumptions   Let's see whether all the assumptions required for this repeated measures design hold true.

1. Since the independent variable 'Time' is categorical and the dependent variable 'VO$_2$ max' is measured on ratio scale, the assumption about the data type holds true.
2. Since subject's performance on VO$_2$ max has been independently measured, the data can be considered independent to each other.
3. The assumption about the normality of data is also satisfied as Shapiro–Wilk statistic is not significant for any of the data set in different treatment groups as shown in the Table 6.2. Readers are advised to test this normality assumption by referring to the procedure discussed in Chapter 2.
4. Assumption about the sphericity will be tested using the output generated in the SPSS later in this chapter for further action in case if it is violated.

6.3.2.2 Outputs Selected   Following outputs have been selected from the output window of SPSS for interpretation:

- Descriptive statistics (Table 6.3)
- Mauchly's test of sphericity (Table 6.4)
- F-table for testing within-subjects effects (Table 6.5)
- Pair-wise comparison of means (Table 6.6)
- Marginal means plot (Fig. 6.7)

6.3.2.3 Descriptive Statistics   The first output in Table 6.3 shows descriptive statistics in all the treatment conditions. One can show these results in their project in

TABLE 6.2   Test of Normality

Treatment Groups	Shapiro–Wilk Statistic	df	Sig.
Zero week	0.924	10	0.393
Two weeks	0.905	10	0.246
Four weeks	0.879	10	0.128
Six weeks	0.902	10	0.228

TABLE 6.3   Descriptive Statistics

	Mean	SD	N
Zero week	33.0000	2.16025	10
Two weeks	32.9000	1.79196	10
Four weeks	34.5000	2.36878	10
Six weeks	36.7000	1.63639	10

TABLE 6.4   Mauchly's Test of Sphericity[a]

Measure: VO_2 max

Within-Subjects Effect	Mauchly's W	Approx. Chi-Square	df	Sig.	Epsilon[a]		
					Greenhouse-Geisser	Huynh-Feldt	Lower Bound
Time	0.062	21.441	5	0.001	0.546	0.650	0.333

[a] Design: intercept.
Within-subjects design: time.

TABLE 6.5   F-Table for Testing Significance of Within-Subjects Effects

Measure: VO_2 max

Source		Type III SS	df	Mean Square	F	Sig.	Partial Eta Squared
Time	Sphericity assumed	94.475	3.000	31.492	7.281	0.001	0.447
	Greenhouse-Geisser	94.475	**1.637**	57.725	**7.281**	**0.009**	0.447
	Huynh-Feldt	94.475	1.951	48.423	7.281	0.005	0.447
	Lower bound	94.475	1.000	94.475	7.281	0.024	0.447
Error	Sphericity assumed	116.775	27.000	4.325			
(Time)	Greenhouse-Geisser	116.775	**14.730**	7.928			
	Huynh-Feldt	116.775	17.559	6.650			
	Lower bound	116.775	9.000	12.975			

TABLE 6.6   Pair-Wise Comparison of Marginal Means

Measure: VO_2 max

(I) Time	(J) Time	Mean Difference (I−J)	Std. Error	Sig[a]	95% CI for Difference[a]	
					Lower Bound	Upper Bound
Zero week	Two weeks	0.100	0.875	1.000	−1.879	2.079
	Four weeks	−1.500	1.267	1.000	−4.366	1.366
	Six weeks	−3.700*	0.367	0.000	−4.529	−2.871
Two weeks	Zero week	−0.100	0.875	1.000	−2.079	1.879
	Four weeks	−1.600	1.013	0.893	−3.892	0.692
	Six weeks	−3.800*	0.573	0.001	−5.097	−2.503
Four weeks	Zero week	1.500	1.267	1.000	−1.366	4.366
	Two weeks	1.600	1.013	0.893	−0.692	3.892
	Six weeks	−2.200	1.153	0.532	−4.808	0.408
Six weeks	Zero week	3.700*	0.367	0.000	2.871	4.529
	Two weeks	3.800*	0.573	0.001	2.503	5.097
	Four weeks	2.200	1.153	0.532	−0.408	4.808

Based on estimated marginal means.
[a] Adjustment for multiple comparisons: Bonferroni.
* The mean difference is significant at the 0.05 level.

order to have an idea about the central location and measure of spread in the data of different groups. These values of means may be used to compare the marginal means.

6.3.2.4   Testing Sphericity
Table 6.4 is the output for Mauchly's test of sphericity and shows the estimates of epsilon (ε) required for correcting the degrees of freedom in testing the significance of F value. It may be seen from this table that the Mauchly's test is significant as the significance level for the chi-square statistic is 0.001 which is less than 0.05. Since Mauchly's test is significant, this indicates that the sphericity assumption violates. For sphericity assumption to be satisfied, the Mauchly's test should not be significant. Since sphericity assumption is violated, some correction is required to be made in the degrees of freedom for the treatment and the error components before testing the significance of F.

6.3.2.5   F-Table for Testing Within-Subjects Effects
Two different corrections namely Greenhouse-Geisser and the Huynh-Feldt are usually applied if the sphericity assumption is violated. Since the value of epsilon (ε) estimated by the Greenhouse-Geisser is 0.546 as shown in Table 6.4, which is less than 0.75, the Greenhouse-Geisser estimate shall be used for correcting degrees of freedom. Had the sphericity assumption satisfied, the degrees of freedom for the treatment (Time) and Error would have been as usual 3 and 27 as shown in Table 6.5. Since sphericity assumption has been violated, these degrees of freedom shall not be used to find the p value associated with the F. Instead, the significance of F shall be tested at the degrees of freedom (1.637, 14.730). In SPSS, the significance of F value is tested by means of p value, and therefore you can notice that the p value differs in a situation where Greenhouse-Geisser correction has been made (p=0.009) with that of a situation where sphericity is assumed (p=0.001). In other words the Greenhouse-Geisser correction simply changes the value of p and nothing more.

From Table 6.5, it can be seen that after applying the Greenhouse-Geisser correction, the F value is significant because associated p value of F is 0.009 which is less than 0.05. In fact, the F is significant in all the situations and no difference in findings occurs due to violation of the sphericity assumption.

6.3.2.6   Pair-Wise Comparison of Means
In repeated measures design post hoc test cannot be used because the data in each group is related with each other. Because of this reason, no option for the post hoc is shown in SPSS while solving one-way repeated measures ANOVA. In this design if F is found to be significant the paired t-test is used for pair-wise comparison of group means. Due to multiple comparisons of pair group means, the level of significance inflates and therefore Bonferroni correction is used to compensate for this error.

SPSS uses paired t-test for each comparison of paired group means by using the Bonferroni correction and provides significance value (p) as shown in Table 6.6. The group means will differ if the significance value (p) attached to the mean difference is less than 0.05. It can be seen that the difference between the group means of zero and six weeks and that of between two and six weeks are significant because the p values associated with these mean differences are less than 0.05. However, no

TABLE 6.7 Mean Score of VO_2 max in Different Time Period

Six Weeks	Four Weeks	Zero Week	Two Weeks
36.7	34.5	33.0	32.9

"⌣‾‾‾‾⌣" represents no significant difference between the means at 0.05 level.

difference is found between the group means of zero and two weeks, zero and four weeks, and two and four weeks.

Pair-wise comparison of marginal means can also be shown by the Table 6.7 which can be obtained by using the information listed in Tables 6.3 and 6.6. Arrange marginal means in decreasing order and indicate the nonsignificance difference between the two group means by joining them by line as shown in the table.

6.3.2.7 *Marginal Means Plot*

The marginal means plot of VO_2 max measured in different time periods can be shown graphically as depicted in Figure 6.7. This output is generated by the SPSS. Additional information about the significance level (as shown in Table 6.6) between the two group means may be added in this figure. It may be noticed from the Figure 6.7 that the value of VO_2 max increases in general with the passage of time during cardio-intervention program. However, there was no significant increase in VO_2 max till four weeks of the training because the p value between zero and four weeks is 0.267, but significant increase has been observed in the six weeks because the p value between zero and six weeks is 0.000. Similarly, the mean value between two and six weeks is also significant because the p value for this difference is 0.000. Thus, based on the sampled data, it may be concluded from this figure that the significant increase in the VO_2 max is observed only in six weeks, and therefore the endurance program should be implemented at least for six weeks to get the significant increase in the VO_2 max.

6.3.3 Findings of the Study

In reporting the findings in one-way repeated measures ANOVA, the outputs shown in Tables 6.3, 6.4, 6.5, 6.6, and 6.7 and Figure 6.7 should normally be mentioned. In this illustration the findings have been reported as follows:

Since the Mauchly's test is significant in Table 6.4, sphericity assumption is violated. Since the Greenhouse-Geisser estimate of epsilon (ε) is 0.546 which is less than 0.75, this estimate was used to correct the degrees of freedom. After the correction, the degrees of freedom for finding the significance value of F has become (1.637, 14.730) instead of (3, 27). From Table 6.5, it can be seen that after applying the Greenhouse-Geisser correction the F value is significant (p=0.009).

The results of the pair-wise comparison of means show that the significant increase in the VO_2 max due to cardio-intervention program has significantly increased only after six weeks of intervention. However, no significant difference has been observed in VO_2 max measured at two, and four weeks.

6.3.4   Inference

On the basis of the sampled data, it may be concluded that the cardio-intervention program significantly affects the cardio-respiratory efficiency of the subjects. However, the significant effect has been observed only after six weeks of the intervention program.

6.4   TWO-WAY REPEATED MEASURES ANOVA

In two-way repeated measures ANOVA, effect of two factors on some dependent variable is investigated simultaneously where both factors are within-subjects. Since in within-subjects factor all subjects are tested under all treatment conditions, in two-way repeated measures design all subjects are tested in each level of both the factors. If a two-way repeated measures ANOVA is planned where first factor has two levels and the second has three, then in the experiment all the subjects shall be tested under each of the six treatment conditions. Two-way repeated measures ANOVA is also known as two-factorial ANOVA with repeated measures. Consider an experiment in which a researcher wishes to see the effect of *temperature* (20° and 30°) and *exercise machine* (treadmill, cycle, and stepper) on sweating loss. Here both factors, temperature and exercise machine, are within-subjects having levels 2 and 3, respectively. If temperature levels are denoted by A_1 (20°) and A_2 (30°) and exercise machine levels are denoted by B_1 (treadmill), B_2 (cycle), and B_3 (stepper), then each subject shall be tested in all the six treatment conditions: A_1B_1, A_1B_2, A_1B_3, A_2B_1, A_2B_2, and A_2B_3.

In solving this design, the following three types of hypotheses are tested:

1. Whether loss of sweat differs in two different temperatures irrespective of the exercise machines
2. Whether loss of sweat differs in different exercise machines irrespective of the temperatures
3. Whether interaction between temperature and exercise machine is significant

The first two hypotheses test the main effects of *temperature* and *exercise machine*. Testing these effects is meaningful only when the interaction effect is not significant. But if the interaction effect is significant, then the main effects become meaningless and in that case simple effects of *temperature* and *exercise machine* are evaluated. The simple effect of temperature refers to the effect of *temperature* on sweat loss in each exercise machine and that of simple effect of exercise machine refers to its effect in each temperature condition.

6.4.1   Assumptions in Two-Way Repeated Measures ANOVA

Assumptions of two-way repeated measures ANOVA are similar to that of one-way repeated measures ANOVA. In this analysis, one needs to test the sphericity assumptions for both the independent variables and also for the interaction bet-ween them. Normality assumptions need to be satisfied for the data set in each of the treatment conditions.

6.4.2 Application in Sports Research

Researchers may find this design useful in many situations where less number of subjects is available and individual variation makes a lot of difference in findings. One of the advantages of this design is that it requires less number of subjects. Since each subject is tested in all the treatment conditions, the levels of both the independent variables should not be large say more than three. Otherwise, it may lead to fatigue and boring on the part of the subjects. Some of the specific situations where this design can be used by the researchers are as follows:

1. A sports scientist may like to investigate the effect of warming-up duration (10, 20, and 30 min) and the type of turf (rubberized and cinder) on athlete's performance in an 800-meter event. Here warming-up duration and court types are the two independent within-subjects variables having three and two levels, respectively. A group of randomly selected athletes may be tested for their performance on 800-meter event in each of the six treatment conditions (10 min—rubberized, 20 min—rubberized, and 30 min—rubberized; 10 min—cinder, 20 min—cinder, and 30 min—cinder). In this design, researchers can test whether the two main effects for warming-up duration and turf type affect the 800-meter performance of athletes. Simultaneously, the researcher can also test the significance of interaction between warming-up and turf type on the 800-meter performance.

2. In order to develop an appropriate exercise regimen for the people, an exercise scientist may plan a study to investigate the effect of exercise intensity and the temperature on heart rate. In doing so, he may select three exercise intensities (low, medium, and high) and two temperatures (25° and 30°) for the study. Thus, a random sample of subjects may be asked to undergo all the six treatment conditions (low—25°, medium—25°, and high—25°; low—30°, medium—30°, and high—30°) after that they may be tested for their heart rate. This way the effect of exercise, temperature, and their interaction on heart rate may be tested for their significance.

6.4.3 Steps in Solving Two-Way Repeated Measures ANOVA

The steps in solving two-way repeated measures ANOVA with SPSS are as follows:

1. Check normality assumption for the data in each treatment condition.
2. Formulate all hypotheses concerning main and interaction effects that are required to be tested.

3. Use SPSS to generate the following output:
   (a) Descriptive statistics
   (b) Mauchly's test of sphericity
   (c) F-table for testing within-subjects effects
   (d) Estimates of marginal means of independent variable(s) if F value for the independent variable is significant
   (e) Pair-wise comparison of marginal means of variable(s) if F value for the independent variable is significant
   (f) Estimates of mean recovery time in each cell (*Environment × Intervention*) if F value for the interaction is significant
   (g) Marginal means plots of independent variable(s) if F value for the variable is significant
   (h) Marginal means plots of interaction if F value for the interaction is significant
4. Test sphericity assumption for each of the independent variable and the interaction by means of Mauchly's test. If Mauchly's test is significant ($p < 0.05$) for any effect, sphericity assumption is said to be violated and in that case correction in the degrees of freedom is applied for testing the significance of F; whereas if the sphericity assumption is not violated, no correction is applied.
5. In case sphericity is violated for an effect, look for the value of epsilon (ε). If its value is less than 0.75, apply Greenhouse-Geisser correction. Otherwise, apply Huynh-Feldt correction.
6. If F is significant, do the pair-wise comparisons among group means by applying Bonferroni correction.
7. Report the findings.

6.5 TWO-WAY REPEATED MEASURES ANOVA USING SPSS

Example 6.2

A coach wishes to investigate the effect of intervention program and environment condition on the recovery of the basketball players after treadmill run with the intensity of 75–80% of their maximum heart rate for 30 min. He has taken three intervention therapy (aqua, relaxation, and massage) and two environment levels (hot and cold). Thus, there are six treatment conditions: aqua-hot, relaxation-hot, massage-hot, aqua-cold, relaxation-cold, and massage-cold. In order to have the control in the experiment, he plans a two-way repeated measures design in which all the six subjects in sample are asked to run for 30 min with 75–80% of their maximum heart rate under each of the six treatment conditions. The time taken by each subject to regain their original pulse rate has been noted under each treatment conditions, which are shown in Table 6.8. Let us discuss the procedure used in solving this two-way repeated measures ANOVA with SPSS. We shall use .05 significance level in this study.

Solution

The following three research questions need to be investigated in this design:

1. Does *Environment* significantly affect the recovery time irrespective of intervention?
2. Does *Intervention* significantly affect the recovery time irrespective of environment?
3. Does interaction between *Environment* and Intervention is significant?

The first two questions can be answered by testing the main effects of *Environment* and *Intervention*, whereas the third question can be answered by testing the simple effects of *Environment* and *Intervention*. Thus, the following three sets of hypotheses shall be tested in this experiment:

1. *Main effect of Environment*

$$H_0 : \mu_{Hot} = \mu_{Cold}$$

against $\qquad H_1 : \mu_{Hot} \neq \mu_{Cold}$

2. *Main effect of Intervention*

$$H_0: \mu_{Aqua} = \mu_{Relaxation} = \mu_{Massage}$$

against $\qquad H_1$: At least one group mean differs

3. *Interaction effect (Environment $\times$ Intervention)*

H_0 : There is no interaction between Environment and intervention

against $\qquad H_1$: The interaction effect between Environment and Intervention is significant

TABLE 6.8   Data on Recovery Time in Minutes

	Intervention		
Environment	Aqua	Relaxation	Massage
Hot	5.0	8.0	6.0
	6.0	9.0	5.0
	5.5	7.0	6.5
	6.5	10.0	5.5
	7.0	9.0	6.5
Cold	6.0	12.5	7.5
	6.5	10.5	8.0
	7.5	12.0	6.5
	7.0	11.0	7.5
	7.5	10.0	6.0

6.5.1 Computation in Two-Way Repeated Measures ANOVA

6.5.1.1 Preparation of Data File   A data file needs to be prepared in solving two-way repeated measures ANOVA with SPSS. In preparing data file, six variables need to be defined. Data in each treatment condition is treated as separate variable. The following variables have been defined in preparing the data file:

Hot_Aqua
Hot_Relaxation
Hot_Massage
Cold_Aqua
Cold_Relaxation
Cold_Massage

Readers who are using SPSS for the first time are advised to refer to Chapter 1 for a detailed procedure in preparing the data file. The data file will look like as shown in Figure 6.8.

6.5.1.2 SPSS Commands   It is advisable to save the data file in the desired location before further processing. Do the following steps:

1. *Initiating SPSS commands*: In the data file, click the **Data View** and process the following commands in sequence.

   Analyze → General Linear Model → Repeated Measures

2. *Selecting variables for analysis:* After clicking **Repeated Measures** option, the screen shown in Figure 6.9 shall be obtained where variables can be defined. By default, the within-subject factor name is written as factor 1. Do the following:

   (a) Replace the factor 1 name by the first independent variable *Environment* and write the number of levels as 2 as there are two levels (hot and cold). Click **Add** to move this information into the box.

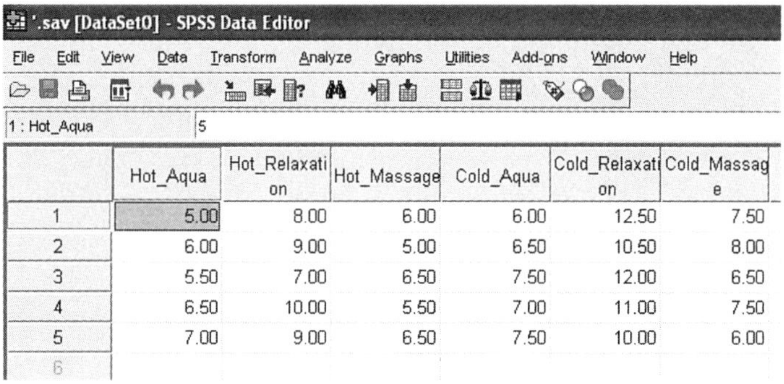

	Hot_Aqua	Hot_Relaxation	Hot_Massage	Cold_Aqua	Cold_Relaxation	Cold_Massage
1	5.00	8.00	6.00	6.00	12.50	7.50
2	6.00	9.00	5.00	6.50	10.50	8.00
3	5.50	7.00	6.50	7.50	12.00	6.50
4	6.50	10.00	5.50	7.00	11.00	7.50
5	7.00	9.00	6.50	7.50	10.00	6.00
6						

FIGURE 6.8   Data file in two-way repeated ANOVA.

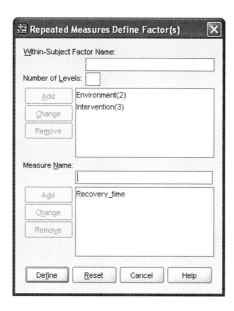

FIGURE 6.9   Defining independent and dependent variables.

(b) Write the name of second independent variable *Intervention* in the "Within-Subject Factor" area and write the number of levels as 3 because *Intervention* has three levels (aqua, relaxation, and massage). Click **Add** to move this information into the box.

(c) In the "Measure Name" section, type *Recovery_time*. Click **Add** to move this information into the box. While writing the name of the independent and dependent variables, the first letter should always be alphabet and no gap should be left in between the two words. However, if the variable name contains two or more words, they must be joined with an underscore.

3. *Selecting options for computation:* Clicking **Define** command in the screen shown in Figure 6.9 shall take you to the screen as shown in Figure 6.10 for selecting the within-subjects variables. Select all six variables from the left panel and bring them to the "Within-Subjects Variables" section of the screen.

After selecting variables, option needs to be defined for generating outputs. Do the following:

(a) Click **Plots** command to get the screen as shown in Figure 6.11.

   (i) Transfer *Environment* variable from the "Factors" section to the "Horizontal Axis" area for generating means plot of the main effect of *Environment* on recovery time. Click **Add.**

   (ii) Transfer *Intervention* variable from the "Factors" section to the "Horizontal Axis" area for generating means plot of the main effect of *Intervention* on recovery time. Click **Add.**

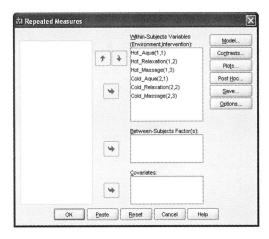

FIGURE 6.10 Selecting variables in two-way repeated ANOVA.

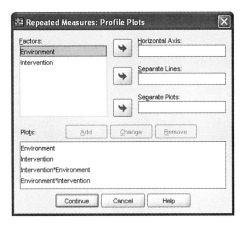

FIGURE 6.11 Selecting options for means plot.

(iii) Transfer *Intervention* and *Environment* variables from the "Factors" section to the "Separate Lines" and "Horizontal Axis" areas, respectively, for generating mean plots to compare simple effects of intervention in each level of the environment. Click **Add** to get the mean plot.

(iv) Transfer *Environment* and *Intervention* variables from the "Factors" section to the "Separate Lines" and "Horizontal Axis" areas, respectively, for generating means plot to compare simple effects of environment in each level of the intervention. Click **Add** and **Continue** to get back to the screen as shown in Figure 6.10.

(b) Click **Options** command to obtain the screen as shown in Figure 6.12 for generating various outputs in the design. Do the following:

(i) Transfer *Environment, Interaction*, and *Environment*Interaction* variables from the "Factor(s) and Factor Interactions" section to the "Display Means for" section. Do the following:

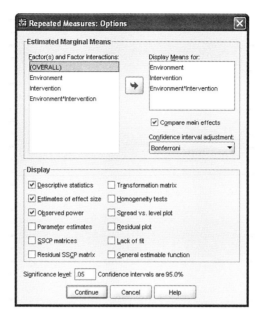

FIGURE 6.12 Selecting options for computing descriptive statistics and pair-wise comparison of means using Bonferroni correction.

(ii) Check 'Compare main effects' option.

(iii) Select Bonferroni correction by clicking on the sign ▼ in "Confidence interval adjustment" drop down menu.

(iv) Check 'Descriptive statistics' option for computing mean and standard deviation in each treatment condition. Ensure that the level of significance is selected as 0.05. In fact by default, it is selected as 0.05. Let all other options remain as it is.

(v) Check 'Estimates of effect size' option

(vi) Click **Continue** and **Add** to get the outputs.

6.5.1.3 SPSS Output   Many outputs are generated in the output panel, but only relevant outputs are selected for discussion. These outputs are shown in the Tables 6.10, 6.11, 6.12, 6.13, 6.14, 6.15, 6.16, and 6.17 and Figures 6.13, 6.14, and 6.15.

6.5.2 Interpretation of Findings

Before interpreting the findings of this design, let us test its assumptions first.

6.5.2.1 Testing Assumptions   Before solving this design, let us see whether its assumptions holds true.

1. Here both the independent variables, that is, *Environment* and *Intervention* are categorical and the dependent variable, *recovery time*, is measured on ratio scale; hence, the assumption about the data type is satisfied.

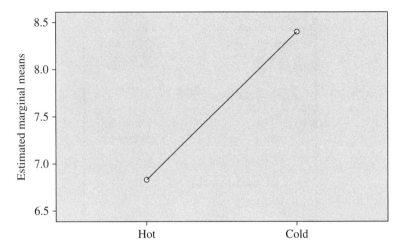

FIGURE 6.13   Means plot of recovery time in different environmental groups.

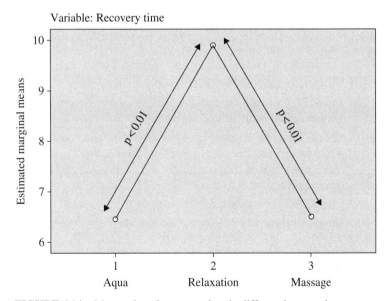

FIGURE 6.14   Means plot of recovery time in different intervention groups.

2. Since all the subjects have been tested independently within each treatment condition, the data can be considered to be independent to each other.

3. Since Shapiro–Wilk statistic is not significant ($p > 0.05$) for all six data sets in different treatment conditions as shown in Table 6.9, the assumption of normality holds true. Readers are advised to test normality of data with SPSS by using the procedure discussed in Chapter 2.

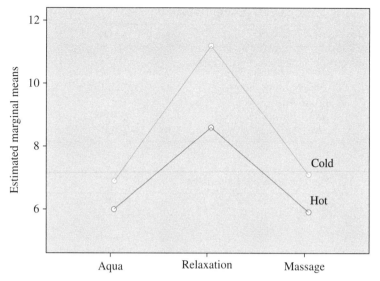

FIGURE 6.15   Means plot in *Intervention × Environment.*

TABLE 6.9   Test of Normality

Treatment Groups	Shapiro–Wilk Statistic	df	Sig.
Hot_Aqua_Score	0.987	5	0.967
Hot_Relaxation_Score	0.961	5	0.814
Hot_Massage_Score	0.902	5	0.421
Cold_Aqua_Score	0.902	5	0.421
Cold_Relaxation_Score	0.952	5	0.754
Cold_Massage_Score	0.914	5	0.490

4. Sphericity assumption shall be tested on the basis of the output generated in the SPSS later in this chapter. If sphericity assumption is violated correction shall be made depending on the severity of the sphericity.

6.5.2.2   Outputs Selected   The following outputs have been selected for the discussion of findings:

- Descriptive statistics (Table 6.10)
- Mauchly's test of sphericity (Table 6.11)
- F-table for testing within-subjects effects (Table 6.12)
- Estimates of marginal means of *Environment* (Table 6.13)
- Pair-wise comparison of marginal means of *Environment* (Table 6.14)
- Estimates of marginal means of *Intervention* (Table 6.15)

TABLE 6.10   Descriptive Statistics

	Mean	SD	N
Hot_Aqua_Score	6.0000	0.79057	5
Hot_Relaxation_Score	8.6000	1.14018	5
Hot_Massage_Score	5.9000	0.65192	5
Cold_Aqua_Score	6.9000	0.65192	5
Cold_Relaxation_Score	11.2000	1.03682	5
Cold_Massage_Score	7.1000	0.82158	5

TABLE 6.11   Mauchly's Test of Sphericity[a]

Measure: Recovery Time

Within-Subjects Effect	Mauchly's W	Approx. Chi-Square	df	Sig. (p Value)	Epsilon[b] Greenhouse-Geisser	Huynh-Feldt	Lower Bound
Environment	1.000	0.000	0	–	1.000	1.000	1.000
Intervention	0.412	2.659	2	0.265	0.630	0.784	0.500
*Environment * Intervention*	0.429	2.542	2	0.281	0.636	0.800	0.500

Tests the null hypothesis that the error covariance matrix of the orthonormalized transformed dependent variables is proportional to an identity matrix.
[a] Design: intercept.
Within-subjects design: *Environment + Intervention + Environment * Intervention*.
[b] May be used to adjust the degrees of freedom for the averaged tests of significance. Corrected tests are displayed in the Tests of Within-Subjects Effects table.

- Pair-wise comparison of marginal means of *Intervention* (Table 6.16)
- Estimates of mean recovery time in each cell (*Environment × Intervention*) (Table 6.17)
- Marginal mean plots of *Environment* (Fig. 6.13)
- Marginal means plots of *Intervention* (Fig. 6.14)
- Marginal means plots of *Intervention × Environment* (Fig. 6.15)
- Marginal means plots of *Environment × Intervention* (Fig. 6.16)

6.5.2.3   Descriptive Statistics   Table 6.10 shows the descriptive statistics for the data on recovery time in each treatment condition. These means are used to draw inferences about the effect of different treatment conditions on the recovery time. In fact, marginal means for *Environment* and *Intervention* are computed on the basis of these means.

6.5.2.4   Testing Sphericity   Since both the independent variables are within-subjects, sphericity of *Environment, Intervention,* and the *Interaction (Environment × Intervention)*

TABLE 6.12 F-Table for Testing Significance of Within-Subjects Effects

Measure: Recovery Time

Source		Type III SS	df	Mean Square	F	Sig. (p Value)	Partial Eta Squared
Environmental	Sphericity assumed	18.408	1.000	18.408	**17.124**	**0.014**	0.811
	Greenhouse-Geisser	18.408	1.000	18.408	17.124	0.014	0.811
	Huynh-Feldt	18.408	1.000	18.408	17.124	0.014	0.811
	Lower bound	18.408	1.000	18.408	17.124	0.014	0.811
Error (Environment)	Sphericity assumed	4.300	4.000	1.075			
	Greenhouse-Geisser	4.300	4.000	1.075			
	Huynh-Feldt	4.300	4.000	1.075			
	Lower bound	4.300	4.000	1.075			
Intervention	Sphericity assumed	78.217	2.000	39.108	**70.307**	**0.000**	0.946
	Greenhouse-Geisser	78.217	1.260	62.096	70.307	0.000	0.946
	Huynh-Feldt	78.217	1.568	49.871	70.307	0.000	0.946
	Lower bound	78.217	1.000	78.217	70.307	0.001	0.946
Error (Intervention)	Sphericity assumed	4.450	8.000	0.556			
	Greenhouse-Geisser	4.450	5.038	0.883			
	Huynh-Feldt	4.450	6.274	0.709			
	Lower bound	4.450	4.000	1.113			
Environment * Intervention	Sphericity assumed	4.117	2.000	2.058	1.926	0.208	0.325
	Greenhouse-Geisser	4.117	1.273	3.235	1.926	0.230	0.325
	Huynh-Feldt	4.117	1.600	2.573	1.926	0.220	0.325
	Lower bound	4.117	1.000	4.117	1.926	0.238	0.325
Error (*Environment * Intervention*)	Sphericity assumed	8.550	8.000	1.069			
	Greenhouse-Geisser	8.550	5.091	1.679			
	Huynh-Feldt	8.550	6.400	1.336			
	Lower bound	8.550	4.000	2.138			

TABLE 6.13 Estimates of Marginal Mean Recovery Time in Different Environment

Measure: Recovery Time

Environment	Mean	Std. Error	95% CI Lower Bound	95% CI Upper Bound
Hot	6.833	0.247	6.147	7.520
Cold	8.400	0.155	7.971	8.829

TABLE 6.14 Pair-Wise Comparison of Marginal Means of Recovery Time in Each Environmental Group

Measure: Recovery Time

(I) Environment	(J) Environment	Mean Difference (I−J)	Std. Error	Sig[a]	95% CI for Difference[a] Lower Bound	95% CI for Difference[a] Upper Bound
Hot	Cold	−1.567*	0.379	0.014	−2.618	−0.516
Cold	Hot	1.567*	0.379	0.014	0.516	2.618

Based on estimated marginal means.
[a] Adjustment for multiple comparisons: Bonferroni.
*The mean difference is significant at the 0.05 level.

TABLE 6.15 Estimates of Marginal Mean Recovery Time in Each Intervention Group

Measure: Recovery Time

Intervention	Mean	Std. Error	95% CI Lower Bound	95% CI Upper Bound
Aqua	6.450	0.289	5.647	7.253
Relaxation	9.900	0.203	9.336	10.464
Massage	6.500	0.079	6.281	6.719

TABLE 6.16 Pair-Wise Comparison of Marginal Mean Recovery Time in Different Intervention Groups

Measure: Recovery Time

(I) Intervention	(J) Intervention	Mean Difference (I−J)	Std. Error	Sig.[a]	95% CI for Difference[a] Lower Bound	95% CI for Difference[a] Upper Bound
Aqua	Relaxation	−3.450*	0.414	0.003	−5.089	−1.811
	Massage	−0.050	0.366	1.000	−1.499	1.399
Relaxation	Aqua	3.450*	0.414	0.003	1.811	5.089
	Massage	3.400*	0.170	0.000	2.728	4.072
Massage	Aqua	0.050	0.366	1.000	−1.399	1.499
	Relaxation	−3.400*	0.170	0.000	−4.072	−2.728

Based on estimated marginal means.
[a] Adjustment for multiple comparisons: Bonferroni.
*The mean difference is significant at the 0.05 level.

TABLE 6.17   Estimates of Mean Recovery Time in Each Cell (Environment × Intervention)

Measure: Recovery Time

Environment	Intervention	Mean	Std. Error	95% CI	
				Lower Bound	Upper Bound
Hot	Aqua	6.000	0.354	5.018	6.982
	Relaxation	8.600	0.510	7.184	10.016
	Massage	5.900	0.292	5.091	6.709
Cold	Aqua	6.900	0.292	6.091	7.709
	Relaxation	11.200	0.464	9.913	12.487
	Massage	7.100	0.367	6.080	8.120

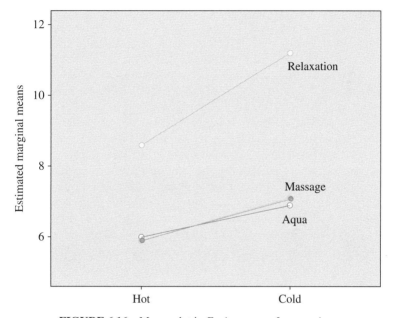

FIGURE 6.16   Means plot in *Environment × Intervention*.

needs to be checked. Table 6.11 shows the Mauchly's test of sphericity for within-subjects effects. It can be seen from the table that Mauchly's test is not significant for *Intervention and Environment × Intervention* because none of the significance value (p value) is less than 0.05. Readers please note that significance value of Mauchly's W statistic for *Environment* has not been computed as there is no question of sphericity if the factor has only two levels. Since sphericity assumption is not violated in any of these effects, no correction is required in the degrees of freedom for any of the effect.

6.5.2.5   F-Table for Testing Within-Subjects Effects
Since sphericity assumption is not violated in any of the three effects, F value for each effect would be tested for their significance without making any correction. From Table 6.12, it can be seen that the F values for the two main effects, *Environment* and *Interaction*, are significant as p values associated with them are 0.014 and 0.000, respectively, which are less than 0.05.

On the other hand, F value for the Interaction effect is not significant because its associated p value is 0.208 which is more than 0.05.

Since the main effects of *Environment* and *Intervention* are significant, pair-wise comparison of means shall be made for these effects to get the clear picture about the group difference. Readers should note that in case of repeated measures design, no post hoc test is applicable because the data is obtained by repeated measures. It is because of this reason that SPSS does not show the option for post hoc when variable is within-subjects. Thus, in case of within-subjects variables pair-wise comparison of means is done by applying the paired t-test and using the Bonferroni correction. Due to multiple comparisons of paired group means, the value of α gets inflated and to correct this error the Bonferroni correction is applied. By choosing the option for Bonferroni as shown in Figure 6.12, the SPSS automatically makes the correction and enhances the value of p associated with each pair mean difference. Since SPSS does this correction automatically, you need not worry and test the significance of the mean difference as usual at 0.05 level if that is the level of significance at which you want to test the results.

Since *Interaction* effect is not significant, no action is taken further in testing the simple effects.

6.5.2.6 Main Effect of Environment
Since main effect of *Environment* is significant, it may be concluded that *Environment* affects the recovery time. To further know as to which environment is better for recovery, the marginal means must be compared. Since environment has only two levels (hot and cold), only one pair of marginal means is required to be compared. Table 6.13 shows the descriptive statistics.

Table 6.14 shows that the mean difference is significant for hot and cold groups as the p value for the difference is 0.014 which is less than 0.05. Since there are only two levels of environment, once the F value is significant you can directly draw the conclusion as to which marginal mean is higher by looking to the magnitude. Since marginal mean for hot environmental group is less than that of Cold group, it may be concluded that the recovery time is less in hot climate in comparison to that of cold. Comparison of marginal means for *Environment* is shown graphically in Figure 6.13.

6.5.2.7 Main Effect for Intervention
Like *Environment*, the *Intervention* is also a within-subjects variable; hence, no post hoc comparison is possible in SPSS. Therefore, comparison of paired marginal means is done by means of paired t-test using the Bonferroni correction. Table 6.15 shows the descriptive means for *Intervention*. These marginal means are used to obtain the mean plots for the main effect of *Intervention*.

Table 6.16 shows that the mean difference between aqua and relaxation groups and that of relaxation and massage groups are significant as their associated p values are 0.003 and 0.000, respectively, which are less than 0.05. However, no difference exists between aqua and massage groups. The means plot for the main effect of *Intervention* has been shown in Figure 6.14.

From Figure 6.14, it may be concluded that the recovery time in aqua and massage is significantly lower in comparison to that of relaxation *Intervention.*

6.5.2.8   Interaction   If *Interaction* effect is not significant, then simple effects are not tested and in that case no outputs related to it should be reported in the findings. However, just for the sake of understanding, the outputs in Table 6.17 and two plots for simple effects have been shown in Figures 6.15 and 6.16. No conclusion should be drawn based on these plots because *Intervention* effect is not significant. The mean recovery time in each cell shown in Table 6.17 is used to obtain the means plots in *Intervention × Environment* as well as *Environment × Intervention* plot.

6.5.2.8.1   Intervention × Environment   It can be seen from Figure 6.15 that in the Aqua group, the recovery time for the basketball players is high in cold group in comparison to that of hot group. Similar trend exists in relaxation and massage groups. The most interesting feature is that the largest difference in the recovery time exists in the relaxation group in comparison to that of other two intervention groups.

6.5.2.8.2   Environment × Intervention Plot   Figure 6.16 shows the means plots for the simple effects of intervention in each of the environment group. In hot environment, the recovery time for the relaxation group is higher than that of massage and aqua groups. Similar trend is observed in cold climate. However, massage and aqua intervention have an equal effect on the recovery time of the basketballers both in hot and in cold environment.

6.5.3   Findings of the Study

Since Mauchly's test is not significant for *Intervention*, and the *Interaction* (*Environment × Intervention*) in Table 6.11, sphericity assumption is not violated for any of these effects; hence, no correction in the degrees of freedom has been made for investigating the significance of F values. The main effects of *Environment* and *Interaction* are significant as shown in Table 6.12, whereas *Interaction* effect is not significant.

While investigating marginal means plot of the main effect of *Environment*, it may be concluded that the recovery is fast in *hot* climate in comparison to that of *cold* (Fig. 6.13).

Means plot for the main effect *Intervention* shows that the recovery in *aqua* and *massage* groups is fast in comparison to that of *relaxation* group.

6.5.4   Inference

On the basis of the sampled data, it may be concluded that the recovery of basketballers is fast in hot climate in comparison to that of cold climate irrespective of the intervention. Further, the aqua and massage intervention are more effective in recovery of the basketballers after the treadmill run irrespective of the climatic conditions.

6.6 SUMMARY OF THE SPSS COMMANDS FOR ONE-WAY REPEATED MEASURES ANOVA

1. After preparing the data file, change the within-subject factor name as *Time* and write the number of levels as 4. Write the Measure Name as 'VO$_2$ max'. Click **Add**.
2. Click **Define** command and select all the four variables from the left panel and bring them to the "Within-Subjects Variables" section of the screen.
3. Click **Plots** command and transfer *Time* variable from the "Factor" section into the "Horizontal Axis" area. Click **Add** command and **Continue**.
4. Click **Option** command and transfer the *Time* variable from left panel to the "Display Means for" section. Check 'Compare main effects' option.
5. Select Bonferroni correction and check 'Descriptive statistics' option and click **Continue** and **OK** commands for generating outputs.

6.7 SUMMARY OF THE SPSS COMMANDS FOR TWO-WAY REPEATED MEASURES ANOVA

1. Prepare the data file by defining six variables: *Hot_Aqua, Hot_Relaxation, Hot_Massage, Cold_Aqua, Cold_Relaxation*, and *Cold_Massage*
2. After preparing the data file, in the **Data View** click the following commands in sequence.

Analyze → General Linear Model → Repeated Measures

3. Change "Within-Subject Factor" name by the first independent variable *Environment* and write the number of levels as 2. Click **Add** to move this information into the box. In the same box again, write the name of the second independent variable *Intervention* and write the number of levels as 3. Click **Add**.
4. In the "Measure Name" area, type 'Recovery_time' and click **Add**.
5. Click **Define** command and select all six variables from the left panel to the "Within-Subjects Variables" section of the screen.
6. Click **Plots** command and do the following:
   (a) Transfer the *Environment* variable from the "Factors" section to the "Horizontal Axis" and click **Add**.
   (b) Transfer *Intervention* variable from the "Factors" section to the "Horizontal Axis" area and click **Add**.
   (c) Transfer *Intervention* and *Environment* variables from the "Factors" section to the "Separate Lines" and "Horizontal Axis" areas, respectively, for generating mean plots to compare simple effects of intervention in each level of the environment and click **Add**.

(d) Transfer *Environment* and *Intervention* variables from the "Factors" section to the "Separate Lines" and "Horizontal Axis" areas, respectively, for generating mean plots to compare simple effects of environment in each level of the intervention. Click **Add** and **Continue**.

7. Click **Options** command and transfer the variables *Environment, Interaction*, and *Environment*Interaction* from the "Factor(s) and Factor Interactions" section to the "Display Means for" section.

8. Check 'Compare main effects' option and select Bonferroni correction.

9. Check 'Descriptive statistics' and 'Estimates of effect size' options. Click **Continue** and **OK** commands to generate outputs.

6.8   EXERCISE

6.8.1   Short Answer Questions

Note: Write answer to each of the following questions in not more than 200 words.

Q.1   What assumptions are required for repeated measures design? Explain the method for testing them.

Q.2   Explain the procedure of solving one-way repeated measures ANOVA design.

Q.3   What do you mean by the main effects and simple effects? Explain by means of an example.

Q.4   Discuss an example where two-way repeated measures design can be applied. Explain the hypotheses which you would like to test in the design.

Q.5   Discuss the method used in solving one-way repeated measures ANOVA design.

Q.6   What do you mean by Bonferroni correction? In what situation it is used and why.

Q.7   What is sphericity? What correction is made if sphericity assumption is violated?

6.8.2   Multiple Choice Questions

Note: Questions 1–10 have four alternative answers for each question. Tick mark the one that you consider the closest to the correct answer.

1   Choose the correct sequence of SPSS commands for two-way repeated measures ANOVA
  (a) Analyze → Linear Model → Repeated Measures
  (b) Analyze → Repeated Measures → Linear Model
  (c) Analyze → General Linear Model → Repeated Measures
  (d) Analyze → Repeated Measures → General Linear Model

2   In repeated measures design,
    (a) Data in each treatment conditions are independent
    (b) Data in each treatment condition come from same population
    (c) Data in each treatment condition are highly related
    (d) Data in each treatment conditions are dependent

3   Main effects are interpreted when
    (a) *Interaction* effect is not significant
    (b) Main effect is significant
    (c) *Interaction* effect is significant
    (d) Main effect is not significant

4   Choose the correct statement
    (a) Between-subjects factor refers to the same subjects being tested in all the treatment conditions.
    (b) Between-subjects factor is a dependent variable.
    (c) Within-subjects factor refers to the same subjects being tested in all the treatment conditions.
    (d) Within-subjects factor is a dependent variable.

5   Mauchly's test is significant
    (a) If $p \leq 0.05$
    (b) If $p < 0.05$
    (c) If $p > 0.05$
    (d) If $p \geq 0.05$

6   If sphericity is violated, then apply
    (a) Greenhouse-Geisser correction if $\varepsilon < 0.75$ and Huynh-Feldt correction if $\varepsilon \geq 0.75$
    (b) Huynh-Feldt correction if $\varepsilon < 0.75$ and Greenhouse-Geisser correction if $\varepsilon \geq 0.75$
    (c) Greenhouse-Geisser correction if $\varepsilon > 0.75$ and Huynh-Feldt correction if $\varepsilon \leq 0.75$
    (d) Huynh-Feldt correction if $\varepsilon > 0.75$ and Greenhouse-Geisser correction if $\varepsilon \leq 0.75$

7   Bonferroni correction is used when
    (a) Factor is a between-subjects
    (b) Factor is a within-subjects
    (c) Post hoc test is applied
    (d) Post hoc test is not possible

8   If *interaction* effect is significant, then
    (a) Both the factors are not correlated
    (b) Trends in all the levels of one factor is same in all the levels of the other factor

(c) Both the factors are correlated

(d) None of the above is true

9   If ε is 0.7 and degrees of freedom attached to F are (3,15), then corrected values
    of the degrees of freedom would be

(a) (3.7,15.7)

(b) (2.3,14.3)

(c) (4.3,21.4)

(d) (2.1,10.5)

10   In $A \times B$ factorial design marginal mean of factor A denotes

(a) Mean of the dependent variable in each level of the factor A across the
    level B

(b) Mean of the dependent variable in each level of the factor B across the
    level A

(c) Mean of the dependent variable in each cell

(d) None of the above is true

6.8.3 Assignment

A sport scientist was interested in investigating the effect of different types of
drinks used by tennis players on their body weight in a set of five matches. Three
teams were randomly made with equal-level tennis players and they were asked
to consume three different types of drinks (mineral water, lemon water, and
vitamin water) in equal amount during three different matches played against
their opponents. Before and after the match, their body weights were measured
and the loss of weight in lbs was recorded (see Table 6.18). Apply one-way
repeated measures ANOVA to investigate the effect of drinks on the reduction of
weights during play.

**TABLE 6.18   Data on Weight Reduction (in lb) During Tennis
Match While Consuming Different Types of Drinks**

Mineral Water	Lemon Water	Vitamin Water
8.8	7.1	7.9
6.7	6.0	6.4
6.0	5.6	6.4
7.8	6.7	7.1
9.2	9.5	8.5
8.1	7.4	7.1

6.9   CASE STUDY ON REPEATED MEASURES DESIGN

Objective

A sports psychologist was interested to investigate the effect of cognitive therapy on the stress level of sports persons during competition. He conducted a study on randomly selected six male sports persons. All subjects were tested for their stress level under each of the three treatment conditions (individual counseling, group counseling, and audiovisual counseling) before the tournament. The data so obtained is shown in Table 6.19.

Research Questions

Following research questions were investigated:

1. Whether cognitive therapy affects stress of the sports persons?
2. Whether stress score differs if therapy is given individually, in group, or by using audiovisual method.
3. Which therapy is better in improving the stress of the sports persons?

Data Format

The format used for preparing data file in SPSS is shown in the Table 6.19.

Analyzing Data

Since in this study subjects were repeatedly measured and there is only one within-subject factor, one-way repeated measures ANOVA design was used. Before analyzing the data, it is required to test the assumptions of normality and sphericity.

Testing Assumption

1. Normality assumption can be tested in SPSS by using the commands **Analyze, Descriptive Statistics,** and **Explore** in sequence. By selecting variables and checking the option 'Normality plots with test'; output for testing normality

TABLE 6.19   **Data on Stress Under All the Treatment Conditions**

Cognitive Therapy		
Individual	Group	Audiovisual
35	36	38
32	28	41
29	31	40
28	34	42
30	33	39

TABLE 6.20   Test of Normality

Treatment Groups	Shapiro–Wilk Statistic	df	Sig.
Individual	0.939	5	0.656
Group	0.981	5	0.940
Audiovisual	0.987	5	0.967

TABLE 6.21   Descriptive Statistics

	Mean	Std. Deviation	N
Individual	30.8000	2.77489	5
Group	32.4000	3.04959	5
Audiovisual	40.0000	1.58114	5

can be generated. Table 6.20 shows the Shapiro–Wilk statistic which tests the normality of data for each group. In this table, it can be seen that the Shapiro–Wilk statistic is not significant for any of the group data, hence the assumption of normality holds.

2. Assumption about the sphericity shall be tested on the basis of the output generated in the SPSS later.

Testing the Significance of Effect

For investigating research questions, one-way repeated measures ANOVA was carried out by using SPSS. Before testing the significance of F value assumption of sphericity was tested. Looking to the status of sphericity, the corrections were made in the degrees of freedom and accordingly the significance of F value was tested. By using the sequence of commands **Analyze, General Linear Model,** and **Repeated measures** in SPSS, defining the variables, selecting the Bonferroni correction, and checking the options 'Descriptive statistics' and 'Estimates of effect size' the outputs were generated, which are shown in Tables 6.21, 6.22, 6.23, and 6.24 and Figure 6.17.

Since Mauchly's test of sphericity in Table 6.22 is not significant ($p=0.138$), the assumption of sphericity is not violated; hence, no correction was required in the degrees freedom

Table 6.23 shows that the F ratio for the cognitive therapy is significant ($p=0.002$); hence, it may be concluded that the cognitive therapy effects stress level of the sports persons. In order to know as to which therapy is more useful, a post hoc test was carried out by using the Bonferroni correction.

Marginal Means Plot

The means plot is shown in Figure 6.17. This plot indicates that the individual counseling is the best in reducing stress level of the sports person. However,

TABLE 6.22 Mauchly's Test of Sphericity[a]

Measure: Stress score

Within-Subjects Effect	Mauchly's W	Approx. Chi-Square	df	Sig.	Epsilon[b] Greenhouse-Geisser	Huynh-Feldt	Lower Bound
Factor 1	0.983	0.050	2	0.975	0.984	1.000	0.500

Tests the null hypothesis that the error covariance matrix of the orthonormalized transformed dependent variables is proportional to an identity matrix.
[a] Design: Intercept.
Within Subjects Design: Counseling.
[b] May be used to adjust the degrees of freedom for the averaged tests of significance. Corrected tests are displayed in the Tests of Within-Subjects Effects table.

TABLE 6.23 Tests of within-subjects effects

Measure: Stress score

Source		Type III Sum of Squares	df	Mean Square	F	Sig.	Partial Eta Squared
Cognitive_Therapy	Sphericity assumed	241.600	2.000	120.800	15.825	**0.002**	0.798
	Greenhouse-Geisser	241.600	1.967	122.806	15.825	0.002	0.798
	Huynh-Feldt	241.600	2.000	120.800	15.825	0.002	0.798
	Lower bound	241.600	1.000	241.600	15.825	0.016	0.798
Error (Cognitive_Therapy)	Sphericity assumed	61.067	8.000	7.633			
	Greenhouse-Geisser	61.067	7.869	7.760			
	Huynh-Feldt	61.067	8.000	7.633			
	Lower bound	61.067	4.000	15.267			

TABLE 6.24 Pairwise Comparisons

Measure: Stress score

(I) Cognitive Therapy	(J) Cognitive Therapy	Mean Difference (I−J)	Std. Error	Sig.[a]	95% CI for Difference[a] Lower Bound	Upper Bound
Individual	Group	−1.600	1.631	1.000	−8.060	4.860
	Audiovisual	−9.200*	1.800	0.021	−16.329	−2.071
Group	Individual	1.600	1.631	1.000	−4.860	8.060
	Audiovisual	−7.600*	1.806	0.041	−14.751	−0.449
Audiovisual	Individual	9.200*	1.800	0.021	2.071	16.329
	Group	7.600*	1.806	0.041	0.449	14.751

Based on estimated marginal means.
[a] Adjustment for multiple comparisons: Bonferroni.
*The mean difference is significant at the 0.05 level.

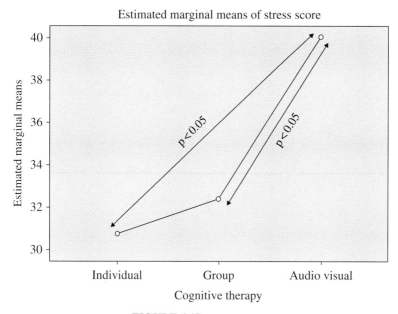

FIGURE 6.17 Means plot.

pair-wise comparison shown in Table 6.24 also suggests that on the basis of the sampled data, individual and group counseling is equally effective.

Reporting

- Since Mauchly's test was not significant, sphericity assumption was not violated; hence, no correction was required in the degrees of freedom.
- Since F ratio was significant, it may be concluded on the basis of the sampled data that the cognitive therapy affects stress level of sports persons.
- Paired mean comparison revealed that a significant difference existed between individual therapy and audiovisual therapy ($p = 0.021$) and that of between group therapy and audiovisual therapy ($p = 0.041$).
- Means plot indicated that the individual counseling is most effective in reducing stress among sports persons.

7

ANALYSIS OF COVARIANCE

LEARNING OBJECTIVES

After completing this chapter, you should be able to do the following:

- Understand the use of analysis of covariance in analyzing comparative effectiveness of treatments
- Know the importance of controlling covariate
- Formulate the hypotheses in analysis of covariance
- Describe the situations where analysis of covariance should be used
- Prepare data file in SPSS
- Understand the steps involved in using SPSS for analysis of covariance
- Interpret the output obtained in analysis of covariance
- Learn to write the results of analysis in a model way

7.1   INTRODUCTION

In homogeneous population, treatments are randomly allocated to the subjects in an experimental research. If we know that a particular variable influences the effectiveness of treatments, experimental groups may be formed by matching the subjects on that variable. On many occasions using randomization and

Sports Research with Analytical Solution using SPSS®, First Edition. J. P. Verma.
© 2016 John Wiley & Sons, Inc. Published 2016 by John Wiley & Sons, Inc.
Companion website: www.wiley.com/go/Verma/Sportsresearch

matching methods may not be feasible for the researchers. Sometimes, a researcher may not have a choice to assign treatments randomly and may be compelled to administer treatments to intact groups that are not homogeneous. The subjects in these intact groups may differ initially on many parameters, and therefore statistical control is necessary to reduce the experimental error due to such initial differences in groups.

Thus, in experimental research, the individual variations that appear within the measures on the dependent variable (DV) are potentially correlated with something else. If the dependent variable is a measure of how well the subjects learn swimming under one or the other of the two methods of instructions, the potential correlates are likely to include such parameters as prior relevant learning, endurance, strength, motivation, self-discipline, intelligence, etc. These potential correlates are known as covariates. Analysis of covariance (ANCOVA) can be used to compare the effectiveness of these instructional methods on learning swimming after removing the effect of the identified covariates.

7.2 CONCEPTUAL FRAMEWORK OF ANALYSIS OF COVARIANCE

In analysis of covariance, the aim of the analysis is to compare the post-treatment means of different groups by adjusting initial variations in the groups. The statistical control is achieved by including measures on concomitant variable (X) in addition to the variable of primary interest (Y) after implementing the treatments. The concomitant variable that may not be of experimental interest is called "covariate" and is denoted by X. Let us denote the variable which is of interest in the experiment by Y, also known as dependent variable. Thus, in ANCOVA design, two observations (X and Y) are obtained on each subject. Measurements on X (covariate) are obtained prior to the administration of treatments and is mainly used to adjust the measurements on Y (DV). Covariate is the variable that is assumed to be associated with the dependent variable. When X and Y are associated, a part of the variability of Y is due to the variation in X. If the value of covariate X is constant over the experimental units, there would be corresponding reduction in the variance of Y.

Let us consider an example in which the ANCOVA can be applied to reduce the experimental error. Suppose an experiment is conducted to study the effect of two different types of pranayama, that is, Bhastrika and Ujjayi on the cardiovascular efficiency of the subjects. Further, an experimenter is forced to use three intact groups of subjects from three different colleges. However, there is a freedom to assign treatments (types of pranayama) randomly to the groups. Out of the three groups, one may serve as control. Since the treatments cannot be randomly assigned to the subjects, the possibility of initial differences (before administration of treatment) among the groups on their cardiovascular efficiency exists. Thus, one may decide to have initial measurement (X) of cardiovascular efficiency on each subject before applying treatment. This measure of covariate, to be measured before implementing the pranayama, is used to adjust measurements on the cardiovascular efficiency (Y) obtained after the treatment.

Thus, the variables X and Y can be defined as follows:

X = Pre-treatment scores of the cardiovascular efficiency in each of the three treatment groups

Y = Post-treatment scores of the cardiovascular efficiency in each of the three treatment groups

In ANCOVA, the means of the dependent variable Y in different treatment groups are adjusted to compensate the variation in the covariate X in the treatment groups. For mathematical details on covariance analysis, readers are advised to read the book titled *Statistics for Exercise Science and Health with Microsoft Office Excel* (Verma, 2014).

Thus, in ANCOVA the following null hypothesis is tested:

$$H_0 : \mu_{Adj\_Po\_Bastrika} = \mu_{Adj\_Po\_Ujjai} = \mu_{Adj\_Po\_Control}$$

Against the alternative hypothesis that at least one adjusted post-treatment group mean differs.

ANCOVA table generated in SPSS output contains the value of F-statistic along with significance value. Thus, if F is significant, the null hypothesis is rejected and in that case post hoc test is used to compare the adjusted post-treatment means of different groups in pairs.

7.3   APPLICATION OF ANCOVA

Consider a situation where it is decided to start a conditioning program for the students to improve their physical efficiency. Three conditioning programs (C1, C2, and C3) having different intensities and durations have been suggested by the experts. A researcher needs to decide as to which program should be implemented. For this, he conducts an experiment on college students in which he allocates C1 treatment on the undergraduate, C2 on the graduate, and C3 on the research students. Since these groups differ in their age, variation in their post-treatment performance on the physical efficiency may be partly due to variation in their age. Here age (X) is a covariate and post-treatment data on PFI (Y) is a dependent variable. The ANCOVA design may be used to compare the effectiveness of these conditioning programs by compensating the variation in age.

Note of Caution

Applying one-way ANOVA on the data obtained by taking the difference of post- and pre-testing in all the treatment groups results in wrong conclusion. This is because treatment effect is not compensated due to initial variations among the groups.

7.4 ANCOVA WITH SPSS

Example 7.1

An experiment was conducted to study the effect of 4-week Bhastrika and Ujjayi pranayama on resting pulse rate. Three groups of subjects were selected for the study. Each group consisted of 15 subjects. The first group was given Bhastrika pranayama, the second, the Ujjayi pranayama, and the third served as Control group. Resting pulse rate was measured before and after the treatment in all the three groups. The data so obtained are shown in Table 7.1.

Solution: Here it is required to compare the adjusted post-treatment means of resting pulse rate among Bhastrika, Ujjayi, and Control groups. Thus, the following null hypothesis needs to be tested against the alternative hypothesis that at least one post treatment adjusted group mean differs.

$$H_0 : \mu_{\text{Adj\_Po\_Bhastrika}} = \mu_{\text{Adj\_Po\_Ujjai}} = \mu_{\text{Adj\_Po\_Control}}.$$

where

$\mu_{\text{Adj\_Po\_Bhastrika}}$: Adjusted post-treatment mean of resting pulse rate in Bhastrika group

$\mu_{\text{Adj\_Po\_Ujjai}}$: Adjusted post-treatment mean of resting pulse rate in Ujjayi group

$\mu_{\text{Adj\_Po\_Control}}$: Adjusted post-treatment mean of resting pulse rate in Control group

TABLE 7.1   Data on Resting Pulse Rate (Beat/min) Before and After the Treatment

	Bhastrika Pranayama		Ujjayi Pranayama		Control Group	
S.N.	Pre	Post	Pre	Post	Pre	Post
1	70	68	69	67	71	71
2	73	72	72	71	72	73
3	69	67	70	70	80	79
4	71	70	68	66	78	78
5	80	78	82	81	69	70
6	69	69	68	67	68	66
7	78	77	72	69	75	73
8	73	73	76	74	73	74
9	68	67	69	68	79	78
10	80	77	80	78	68	68
11	74	73	72	72	74	75
12	69	68	75	74	87	85
13	67	67	67	67	69	68
14	72	71	74	73	73	73
15	70	69	76	75	82	81

The SPSS output provides ANCOVA table along with pair-wise comparison of adjusted post-treatment means of different treatment groups. The pair-wise comparison of means provided in the output should be used only when the F-ratio is significant.

The ANCOVA table generated in the SPSS output looks similar to that of one-way ANOVA table as only the adjusted post-treatment group means are compared here. The F value is shown along with its significance value (p value). The F value would be significant at 5% level. If the value of p associated with it is less than 0.05. Once the F value is found to be significant, a pair-wise comparison of means is done by using the Bonferroni correction. The SPSS output provides the significance value for each pair of group means difference. Thus, by looking at the values of means, the best treatment may be identified.

7.4.1 Computation in ANCOVA

7.4.1.1 Preparation of Data File After preparing the data file, the SPSS commands can be used for getting the output in ANCOVA. After starting the SPSS as discussed in Chapter 1, select the option 'Type in data.' The sequence of commands for starting SPSS on your computer is as follows:

Start → All Programs → SPSS Inc → SPSS 20.0 → Type in Data

7.4.1.2 Defining Variables Here three variables, namely *Pre_Resting*, *Post_Resting*, and *Treatment*, need to be defined along with their properties. *Pre_Resting* and *Post_ Resting* are the scale variables, whereas *Treatment* is a nominal variable. These variables along with their characteristics can be defined in the **Variable View** as follows:

- Click **Variable View** on the left corner at the bottom of the screen as shown in Figure 7.1 to define variables and their properties.
- Write short name of the variables as *Pre_Resting*, *Post_Resting*, and *Treatment* under the column heading "Name."
- Under the column heading "Label," define full name of these variables as *Pre_ resting pulse rate*, *Post_resting pulse rate*, and *Treatment*. Other names may also be chosen for describing these variables.
- Under the column heading "Measure," select the 'Scale' option for the *Pre_ Resting* and *Post_Resting* variables and 'Nominal' for the *Treatment* variable.
- For the variable *Treatment*, double click the cell under the column "Values" and add the following values to different labels:

Value	Label
1	Bhastrika
2	Ujjayi
3	Control

- Use default entries in rest of the columns.

After defining variables in **Variable View**, the screen shall look like as shown in Figure 7.1.

	Name	Type	Width	Decimals	Label	Values	Missing	Columns	Align	Measure
1	Pre_Resting	Numeric	8	2	Pre resting pu...	None	None	8	Right	Scale
2	Post_Resting	Numeric	8	2	Post resting p...	None	None	8	Right	Scale
3	Treatment	Numeric	8	2	Treatment	{1.00, Bhas...	None	8	Right	Nominal

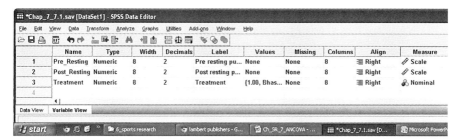

FIGURE 7.1 Defining variables along with their characteristics.

	Pre_Resting	Post_Resting	Treatment
1	70.00	68.00	1.00
2	73.00	72.00	1.00
3	69.00	67.00	1.00
4	71.00	70.00	1.00
5	80.00	78.00	1.00
6	69.00	69.00	1.00
7	78.00	77.00	1.00
8	73.00	73.00	1.00
9	68.00	67.00	1.00
10	80.00	77.00	1.00
11	74.00	73.00	1.00
12	69.00	68.00	1.00
13	67.00	67.00	1.00
14	72.00	71.00	1.00
15	70.00	69.00	1.00
16	69.00	67.00	2.00
17	72.00	71.00	2.00
18	70.00	70.00	2.00
19	68.00	66.00	2.00
20	82.00	81.00	2.00
21	68.00	67.00	2.00
22	72.00	69.00	2.00
23	76.00	74.00	2.00
24	69.00	68.00	2.00
25	80.00	78.00	2.00
26	72.00	72.00	2.00
27	75.00	74.00	2.00
28	67.00	67.00	2.00
29	74.00	73.00	2.00
30	76.00	75.00	2.00
31	71.00	71.00	3.00
32	72.00	73.00	3.00
33	80.00	79.00	3.00
34	78.00	78.00	3.00
35	69.00	70.00	3.00
36	68.00	66.00	3.00
37	75.00	73.00	3.00
38	73.00	74.00	3.00
39	79.00	78.00	3.00
40	68.00	68.00	3.00
41	74.00	75.00	3.00
42	87.00	85.00	3.00
43	69.00	68.00	3.00
44	73.00	73.00	3.00
45	82.00	81.00	3.00

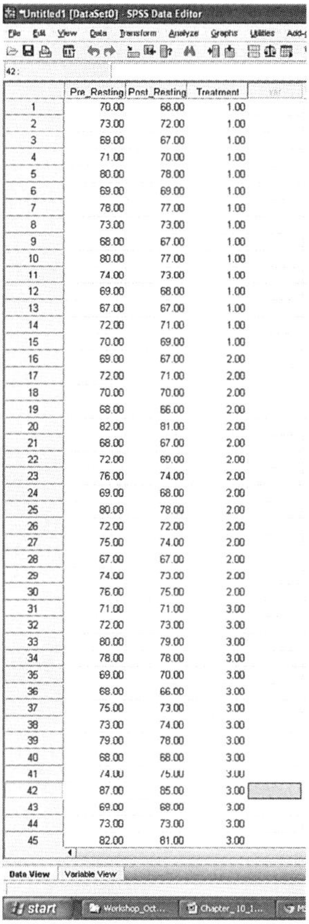

FIGURE 7.2 Data file of resting pulse rate for analysis of covariance.

7.4.1.3 Entering Data After defining the variables in the **Variable View**, click on **Data View** on the screen shown in Figure 7.1 to open the format for entering the data column-wise. After entering data, the screen will look like as shown in Figure 7.2. Save the data file in the desired location before further processing.

7.4.1.4 SPSS Commands While being in the **Data View**, follow the below mentioned steps for generating outputs in the ANCOVA:

1. *Initiating SPSS:* In **Data View**, click on the following commands in sequence:

   Analyze → General Linear Model → Univariate

   The screen shall look like as shown in Figure 7.3.

2. *Selecting variables:* After clicking the **Univariate** option, you will be directed to the next screen for selecting variables. Do the following:
   (a) Select *Post_Resting* variable from left panel and bring it to the "Dependent variable" section in the right panel.
   (b) Select *Treatment* variable from left panel and bring it to the "Fixed Factor(s)" section in the right panel.
   (c) Select *Pre_Resting* variable from the left panel and bring it to the "Covariate(s)" section in the right panel.

   The screen will look like as shown in Figure 7.4 as shown below.

3. *Selecting options for computation:* After selecting variables, option needs to be defined for generating the output in ANCOVA. Do the following:
   (a) Click **Model** command in the screen shown in Figure 7.4 and select the 'Sum of squares' option as "Type I." The screen will look like as shown in Figure 7.5. Click **Continue** to go back to the screen shown in Figure 7.4.
   (b) Click **Options** command to get the screen as shown in Figure 7.6. Do the following:
      (i) Select *Treatment* variable from the left panel and bring it to the "Display Means for" section in the right panel.
      (ii) Check 'Compare main effects' option and select 'Bonferroni' correction.
      (iii) Check 'Descriptive statistics' and 'Estimates of effect size' options.
      (iv) Ensure 'Significance level' as 0.05. This value is written by default.
   (c) Click **Continue** and **OK** for generating outputs.

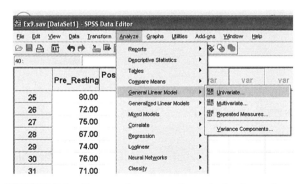

FIGURE 7.3   Command sequence for analysis of covariance.

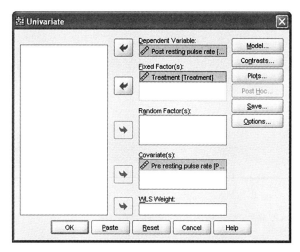

FIGURE 7.4 Selection of variables for ANCOVA.

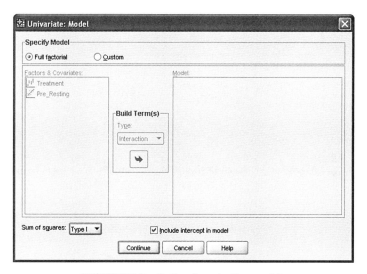

FIGURE 7.5 Option for selecting model.

4. *Getting the output:* After clicking **OK** in the screen shown in Figure 7.4, various results shall be generated in the output window. The following relevant outputs shall be selected for discussion:

   (a) Descriptive statistics

   (b) ANCOVA table

   (c) Post hoc comparison table

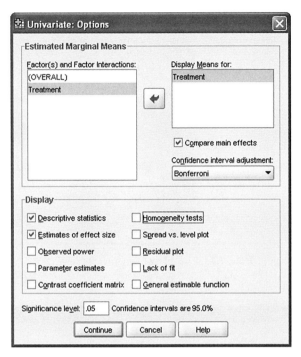

FIGURE 7.6   Options for various outputs in ANCOVA.

7.4.1.5   Interpretation of Findings   The outputs of the ANCOVA produced by the SPSS are shown in Tables 7.2, 7.3, 7.4, 7.5, and 7.6.

TABLE 7.2   Mean and Standard Deviation of Different Post-treatment Groups

Treatment	Mean	Std. Deviation	N
Bhastrika	71.0667	3.82598	15
Ujjayi	71.4667	4.40562	15
Control	74.1333	5.28970	15
Total	72.2222	4.65095	45

TABLE 7.3   Adjusted Mean and Standard Error of Different Post-treatment Groups

			95% Confidence Interval	
Treatment	Mean	Std. Error	Lower Bound	Upper Bound
Bhastrika	71.932[a]	0.232	71.464	72.401
Ujjayi	71.900[a]	0.231	71.434	72.365
Control	72.835[a]	0.234	72.363	73.307

[a] Covariates appearing in the model are evaluated at the following values: Pre-treatment score of resting pulse rate = 73.1333.

TABLE 7.4   Tests "Between-Subjects" Effects

Dependent Variable: Post-treatment Score of Resting Pulse Rate

Source	Type I Sum of Squares	df	Mean Square	F	Sig.	Partial Eta Square
Corrected model	919.146[a]	3	306.382	384.954	0.000	0.966
Intercept	234722.222	1	234722.222	2.949E5	0.000	1.000
Pre_Resting	911.057	1	911.057	1.145E3	0.000	0.965
Treatment	8.089	2	4.045	5.082	0.011	0.199
Error	32.632	41	0.796			
Total	235674.000	45				
Corrected total	951.778	44				

[a] $R^2 = 0.966$ (Adjusted $R^2 = 0.963$).

TABLE 7.5   ANCOVA Table for the Post-treatment Data on Resting Pulse Rate

Source	Type I Sum of Squares	df	Mean Square	F	Sig.	Partial Eta Square
Pre_Resting	911.057	1	911.057	1.145E3	0.000	0.965
Treatment	8.089	2	4.045	5.082	**0.011**	0.199
Error	32.632	41	0.796			
Corrected total	951.778	44				

TABLE 7.6   Pair-Wise Comparisons

Dependent Variable: Post-treatment Resting Pulse Rate

(I) Treatment Group	(J) Treatment Group	Mean Diff. (I−J)	SE	Sig.[a]	95% Confidence Interval for Difference[a]	
					Lower Bound	Upper Bound
Bhastrika	Ujjayi	0.033	0.326	1.000	−0.781	0.847
	Control	−0.902*	0.333	**0.029**	−1.732	−0.072
Ujjayi	Bhastrika	−0.033	0.326	1.000	−0.847	0.781
	Control	−0.935*	0.330	**0.021**	−1.759	−0.111
Control	Bhastrika	0.902*	0.333	**0.029**	0.072	1.732
	Ujjayi	0.935*	0.330	**0.021**	0.111	1.759

Based on estimated marginal means.
[a] Adjustment for multiple comparisons: Bonferroni.
* The mean difference is significant at the 0.05 level.

7.4.1.5.1 Descriptive Statistics of the Post-treatment Group   The value of mean and standard deviation for the data on resting pulse rate in different post-treatment groups are shown in Table 7.2. If readers are interested to compute different descriptive statistics for pre-treatment measurements on resting pulse rate in different groups, the procedure discussed in Chapter 2 may be used. The SPSS does not generate these statistics during ANCOVA analysis.

7.4.1.5.2 Descriptive Statistics of the Post-treatment Groups after Adjustment   Further, post-treatment adjusted means and standard deviation for the data on resting pulse rate of different groups have been shown in Table 7.3. Readers may note that these values are different from that of the unadjusted values shown in Table 7.2. The advantage of using the ANCOVA is that the differences in the post-treatment means are compensated for the initial differences in the scores. In other words, it may be said that the effect of covariate is eliminated in comparing the effectiveness of the treatment in post-treatment testing.

7.4.1.5.3 ANCOVA Table for the Post-treatment Data on Resting Pulse Rate   Table 7.4 is the main result of the ANCOVA analysis. By deleting some of the contents that are not required, the final table can be obtained as shown in Table 7.5 for discussing the findings.

Table 7.5 shows the F value for comparing the post-treatment adjusted means of the three groups (Bhastrika, Ujjayi, and Control). Since p value associated with F is 0.011 which is less than 0.05; hence, F is significant. Thus, the null hypothesis of no difference among the adjusted post-treatment group means for the data on resting pulse rate may be rejected at 5% level.

7.4.1.5.4 Pair-wise Comparison of Post-treatment Adjusted Group Means   Since the F value in Table 7.5 is significant, a pair-wise comparison has been made in Table 7.6. The post hoc comparison of means for the post-treatment measurements can be shown graphically by using the values of different adjusted post-group means in Table 7.3 and using p values of mean differences in Table 7.6. These comparisons are shown in Table 7.7.

Since F value is significant, pair-wise comparison of means has been made by using the Bonferroni correction which is shown in Table 7.6. It may be noted that the p value associated with the mean difference between Bhastrika and Control is 0.029 and between Ujjayi and Control is 0.021. Both these p values are less than 0.05 and the differences are significant at 5% level. Thus, the following conclusions can be drawn:

1. There is a significant difference in the adjusted means resting pulse rate of the Bhastrika and Control groups.
2. There is a significant difference in the adjusted means resting pulse rate of the Ujjayi and Control groups.
3. There is no significant difference in the adjusted means resting pulse rate of the Bhastrika and Ujjayi groups.

TABLE 7.7   Pair-Wise Comparisons of Post-treatment Group Means of the Data on Resting Pulse Rate Shown with Graphics

Control	Bhastrika	Ujjayi
72.835	**71.932**	**71.900**

"└─────────┘" represents no significant difference between the means at 5% level.

In order to find as to which treatment is the best, one can see the adjusted mean values of different treatment groups during post-treatment testing given in Table 7.3. Clubbing these adjusted means with the three results of the Table 7.6, one may get the answer. However, this task becomes much easier if Table 7.7 is created. In this table, the adjusted post-means of different groups have been shown in descending order. If the difference between any two group means is significant (which can be seen from Table 7.6), nothing is done and if the mean difference is not significant, a line is drawn covering the two groups. Thus, it may be concluded that the resting pulse rate of the Bhastrika and Ujjayi groups are equal and is significantly less than that of the Control group.

Hence, it may be inferred that Bhastrika and Ujjayi pranayamas are equally effective in reducing the resting pulse rate among the subjects in comparison to that of the Control group.

7.5   SUMMARY OF THE SPSS COMMANDS

1. Start SPSS by using the following sequence of commands

   Start → All Programs → SPSS Inc → SPSS 20.0

2. Click **Variable View** and define *Pre_Resting* and *Post_Resting* as a scale variables and *Treatment* as nominal.

3. Under the column heading "Values" define '1' for Bhastrika; '2' for Ujjayi, and '3' for Control.

4. Type data for these variables by clicking **Data View**.

5. In the **Data View**, follow the below-mentioned command sequence:

   Analyze → General Linear Model → Univariate

6. Select *Post_Resting*, *Treatment*, and *Pre_Resting* variables from left panel and bring them to the "Dependent variable" section, "Fixed Factor(s)" section, and "Covariate(s)" section, respectively, in the right panel.

7. Click **Model** command and select the 'Type I' as an option in 'Sum of Squares.' Click **Continue**.

8. Click **Options** command and select *Treatment* variable from the left panel and bring it into the "Display Means for" section of the right panel. Check 'Compare main effects' and select 'Bonferroni' correction.

9. Check 'Descriptive statistics' and 'Estimates of effect size' options. Keep significance value as 0.05 or 0.01 as the case may be. Click **Continue** and **OK** for getting outputs.

7.6   EXERCISE

7.6.1   Short Answer Questions

Note: Write answers to each of the following questions in not more than 200 words.

Q.1   What do you mean by covariate? How is it controlled in ANCOVA? Give a specific example.

Q.2   Describe an experimental situation where ANCOVA can be applied. Construct null hypothesis and all alternative hypotheses.

Q.3   Thirty boys in the age category of 7–9 years were selected for swimming classes. They did not have any prior exposure in swimming. In order to compare the effectiveness of three swimming techniques, namely Breast stroke, Butterfly stroke, and Freestyle stroke in learning swimming which statistical analysis would you suggest and why?

Q.4   How ANOVA and ANCOVA differs from one another? Discuss briefly.

7.6.2   Multiple Choice Questions

Note: Questions 1–10 have four alternative answers for each question. Tick mark the one that you consider the closest to the correct answer.

1   One of the methods of having control in an experiment is to match the groups initially. This matching is done on the variable which is
  (a) Independent
  (b) Extraneous
  (c) Dependent
  (d) Any variable found suitable

2   Covariate is a variable which is supposed to be correlated with
  (a) Independent variable
  (b) Moderating variable
  (c) Dependent variable
  (d) None of the above

3   In ANCOVA while doing post hoc analysis, which group means are compared?
   (a) Pre-treatment group means
   (b) Post-treatment group means
   (c) Pre-treatment adjusted group means
   (d) Post-treatment adjusted group means

4   In order to compare the effectiveness of three training programs on dribbling accuracy in basketball, an experiment was planned. Three treatment groups were tested for their performance in pre- and post-training. While using SPSS for ANCOVA, three variables, namely Pre_Drib, Post_Drib, and Treatment_Group need to be defined. Choose the correct statement.
   (a) Pre_Drib and Post_Drib are Scale and Treatment_Group is Ordinal.
   (b) Pre_Drib and Post_Drib are Nominal and Treatment_Group is Scale.
   (c) Pre_Drib and Treatment_Group are Scale and Post_Drib is Nominal.
   (d) Pre_Drib and Post_Drib are Scale and Treatment_Group is Nominal.

5   While using SPSS for ANCOVA, the three variables, namely Pre_Test, Post_Test, and Treatment_Group are classified as
   (a) Post_Test as Dependent variable, whereas Pre_Test and Treatment_Group as Fixed Factors
   (b) Post_Test as Dependent variable, Pre_Test as Covariate and Treatment_Group as Fixed Factors
   (c) Treatment_Group as Dependent variable, Pre_Test and Post_Test as Fixed Factors
   (d) Treatment_Group as Dependent variable, Post_Test as Covariate, and Pre_Test as Fixed Factor.

6   Choose the correct sequence of commands in SPSS for starting ANCOVA
   (a) Analyze → Univariate → General Linear Model
   (b) Analyze → General Linear Model → Multivariate
   (c) Analyze → General Linear Model → Univariate
   (d) Analyze → General Linear Model → Repeated Measures

7.6.3   Assignment

In an experiment, three groups of basketballers were given three different heights of depth jump training for 6 weeks to see their effectiveness on vertical jump performance. Three depth jump heights were 30, 25, and 20 inches. A control group was also taken in the study on which no training was imparted. The vertical jump performance was measured before and after the treatment for 6 weeks, and the data so obtained is shown in Table 7.8. Apply ANCOVA to find as to which depth jump height is the best in improving vertical jump performance among the basketballers. Test your hypothesis at 0.05 and 0.01 level of significance.

TABLE 7.8   Data on Vertical Jump Performance (in Inches) in Different Depth Jump Height Group During Pre- and Post-treatment Testing

	Depth Jump 30 Inches		Depth Jump 25 Inches		Depth Jump 20 Inches		Control	
S.N.	Pre	Post	Pre	Post	Pre	Post	Pre	Post
1	45	47	45	47	53	56	53	52
2	38	40	43	45	52	55	45	44
3	60	63	44	48	36	40	47	48
4	41	43	47	49	43	48	54	54
5	46	48	43	46	49	53	40	40
6	49	51	40	41	51	54	39	43
7	40	41	49	52	45	50	45	48
8	44	46	46	48	54	57	54	55
9	61	64	44	46	53	56	46	48
10	47	49	41	44	48	52	40	44

7.7   CASE STUDY ON ANCOVA DESIGN

Objective

A sports scientist conducted a study to test the effectiveness of Uchikomi, Randori, and Kata practices of Judo on strength index. These Judo practices were administered on the three intact groups of athletes for 4 weeks and their strength was measured before and after treatments. A control group was also taken in the study. The data so obtained from the study is shown in Table 7.9.

TABLE 7.9   Data on Strength Index in Different Judo Practice Groups Before and After Treatment

	Uchikomi		Randori		Kata		Control	
S.N.	Pre	Post	Pre	Post	Pre	Post	Pre	Post
1	211	240	211	244	208	236	207	210
2	209	241	208	249	210	241	209	221
3	202	220	205	258	198	222	210	213
4	208	221	212	227	195	230	202	205
5	201	239	221	243	202	232	219	217
6	200	237	210	242	208	235	215	218
7	207	221	209	247	212	242	206	208
8	210	219	205	256	195	220	209	215
9	210	240	210	226	195	128	215	220
10	212	242	221	245	201	230	217	215

Research Questions

The following research questions were investigated:

1. Does Judo training affect the strength index?
2. Whether any one technique is more effective than others?

Data Format

The format used for preparing data file in SPSS is shown in Table 7.10.

TABLE 7.10   Data Format Used in SPSS for Strength Index

Pre_Testing	Post_Testing	Group
211	240	1
209	241	1
202	220	1
208	221	1
201	239	1
200	237	1
207	221	1
210	219	1
210	240	1
212	242	1
211	244	2
208	249	2
205	258	2
212	227	2
221	243	2
210	242	2
209	247	2
205	256	2
210	226	2
221	245	2
208	236	3
210	241	3
198	222	3
195	230	3
202	232	3
208	235	3
212	242	3
195	220	3
195	128	3
201	230	3
207	210	4

(continued)

TABLE 7.10   (continued)

Pre_Testing	Post_Testing	Group
209	221	4
210	213	4
202	205	4
219	217	4
215	218	4
206	208	4
209	215	4
215	220	4
217	215	4

Group code: 1, Uchikomi; 2, Randori; 3, Kata; 4, Control.

TABLE 7.11   Tests of Between-Subjects Effects

Dependent Variable: Post_Testing

Source	Type I Sum of Squares	df	Mean Square	F	Sig.
Corrected model	6198.113[a]	4	1549.528	4.882	0.003
Intercept	2077080.625	1	2077080.625	6.544E3	0.000
Pre_testing	1586.699	1	1586.699	4.999	0.032
Group	4611.414	3	1537.138	**4.843**	**0.006**
Error	11108.262	35	317.379		
Total	2094387.000	40			
Corrected total	17306.375	39			

[a] $R^2 = 0.358$ (Adjusted $R^2 = 0.285$).

Analyzing Data

Since the experimental groups were intact and were not drawn randomly, there is a possibility that their initial conditions might have been different. Thus, to control the effect of extraneous variance, ANCOVA was used in this study to address the research issues. The researcher was interested to test the null hypothesis that all the three judo techniques are equally effective in increasing the strength index against the alternative hypothesis that at least one technique is more effective than others. The F value obtained in the ANCOVA design was tested for its significance and the pair-wise comparison was done by using the Bonferroni test.

The one-way ANCOVA design was applied in SPSS by using the following commands in sequence: **Analyze, General Linear Model,** and **Univariate.** The dependent variable, group variable, and covariate were placed in the appropriate locations in the dialogue box. The output in the analysis was obtained by selecting 'mean plot', 'comparing mean effect', and 'descriptive statistics' options that are shown in Tables 7.11, 7.12, and 7.13 and in Figure 7.7

TABLE 7.12   Pair-Wise Comparisons

Dependent Variable: Post_Testing

(I) Group	(J) Group	Mean Difference (I–J)	Std. Error	Sig.[a]	95% Confidence Interval for Difference[a] Lower Bound	Upper Bound
Uchikomi	Randori	−7.251	8.274	1.000	−30.391	15.888
	Kata	5.528	8.334	1.000	−17.779	28.835
	Control	21.931	8.233	0.070	−1.092	44.954
Randori	Uchikomi	7.251	8.274	1.000	−15.888	30.391
	Kata	12.779	9.239	1.000	−13.060	38.617
	Control	29.182*	7.969	**0.005**	6.897	51.468
Kata	Uchikomi	−5.528	8.334	1.000	−28.835	17.779
	Randori	−12.779	9.239	1.000	−38.617	13.060
	Control	16.403	9.160	0.492	−9.212	42.019
Control	Uchikomi	−21.931	8.233	0.070	−44.954	1.092
	Randori	−29.182*	7.969	0.005	−51.468	−6.897
	Kata	−16.403	9.160	0.492	−42.019	9.212

Based on estimated marginal means.
[a] Adjustment for multiple comparisons: Bonferroni.
* The mean difference is significant at the 0.05 level.

TABLE 7.13   Estimates: Adjusted Mean and Standard Error of Different Groups After Post-treatment

Dependent Variable: Post_Testing

Group	Mean	Std. Error	95% Confidence Interval Lower Bound	Upper Bound
Uchikomi	2.329E2	5.653	221.451	244.403
Randori	2.402E2	5.904	228.191	252.165
Kata	2.274E2	6.341	214.526	240.272
Control	2.110E2	5.859	199.102	222.890

E2 means 10^2.

Interpreting Findings

Table 7.11 shows that the F value is significant ($p = 0.006$) beyond 0.05 level; hence, the null hypothesis was rejected. Since null hypothesis was rejected, pair-wise comparisons of mean were done by using the Bonferroni test on the adjusted post means among all the four treatment groups. Table 7.12 shows the pair-wise comparisons of mean. The table reveals that only Randori technique is significantly different than the Control group.

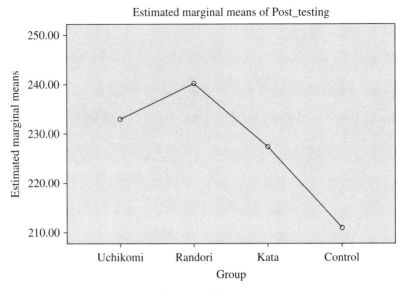

FIGURE 7.7   Means plot.

Means Plot

Figure 7.7 shows the means plot of the adjusted mean of all the four treatment groups. Based on the sampled data mean plot reveals that mean strength index of the Randori group was significantly higher than that of the Control group.

Reporting

- Since the F ratio (=4.843) was significant (p=0.006), the null hypothesis that all the three techniques are equally effective in improving the strength index was rejected. Thus, based on the sampled data, it can be concluded that the Judo training was effective in improving the strength index.
- Pair-wise comparison of means suggests that the Randori treatment was significantly better in improving the strength in comparison to those where no training was given.
- The means plot suggested that the Randori treatment was the best in improving the strength index.

8

NONPARAMETRIC TESTS IN SPORTS RESEARCH

LEARNING OBJECTIVES

After completing this chapter, you should be able to do the following:

- Understand the research situations in which the nonparametric tests can be used
- Learn to construct hypothesis in using each test
- Understand the procedure of making data file in applying different nonparametric tests in SPSS
- Know the procedure of testing goodness of fit and association between two attributes
- Interpret the outputs generated in SPSS for hypothesis testing in different nonparametric tests

8.1 INTRODUCTION

Nonparametric tests are used in a situation when data is measured on nonmetric scale. In other words if the measurements are categorical in nature, these tests are used in hypothesis testing experiment. Nonparametric tests can also be used for metric data if assumptions of parametric tests are severely violated. This makes

Sports Research with Analytical Solution using SPSS®, First Edition. J. P. Verma.
© 2016 John Wiley & Sons, Inc. Published 2016 by John Wiley & Sons, Inc.
Companion website: www.wiley.com/go/Verma/Sportsresearch

these tests even more useful. In research studies, quite often distribution of the population from which the sample is drawn is unknown, and therefore in such situations nonparametric tests are the best option. In using nonparametric tests, no assumption is made about the distribution of the population from which the samples are obtained; hence, these tests are also known as distribution-free test. Not many assumptions are required for using nonparametric tests; hence, it can be easily used by the researchers. On the other hand, all parametric tests are based on the assumption that the distribution of the population from which the samples are drawn is normal. Besides this, each parametric test requires certain assumptions to be made. Thus, in all those situations where normality assumption violated, required assumptions of the parametric test breaks down, or if the data is measured on nominal or ordinal scales, nonparametric tests are used in hypothesis testing.

In parametric tests, hypothesis concerning proportion, mean, or variance is usually tested; whereas in nonparametric tests, hypothesis concerning median is tested for its significance. In parametric tests, parent population is assumed to be normally distributed. All tests that we have read so far in this book like z, t, and F are known as parametric tests. Since these tests investigate the hypothesis concerning parameters, they are known as parametric tests. On the other hand in nonparametric tests distribution of the population need not to be normally distributed. Since hypothesis testing does not involve any parameter, these tests are known as nonparametric tests. Nonparametric tests are simple to understand and easy to use.

In nonparametric tests, a test statistic is computed on the basis of ranks, signs, order relations or category frequencies. Because of this reason, these tests are useful if subjectivity in the measurement is an issue.

Many situations arise in sports research where the data is obtained either on ordinal or nominal scale. For example, assessment of playing ability, quality of cricket shot, and performance in soccer produce data on ordinal scale. On the other hand performance on minimum muscular fitness test and match result in hockey results in nominal data as these performances are assessed on pass/fail or winning/ loosing format, respectively. In all such situations, nonparametric tests are well suited for hypothesis testing.

The procedure of testing hypothesis is similar in nonparametric and parametric tests. The only difference is in terms of constructing hypothesis and computing test statistic. In most of the commonly used parametric tests, there is an alternative test available in nonparametric. For example, chi-square and Mann–Whitney U tests are alternative tests to the two sample t-test, and Wilcoxon signed-rank test is an alternative to the paired t-test. Similarly, nonparametric tests such as Kruskal– Wallis and Friedman can be used as an alternative to the one-way ANOVA and repeated measures ANOVA, respectively. In this chapter, some of the most widely used nonparametric tests including chi-square shall be discussed in detail. The readers will learn to use SPSS in solving their problems based on these tests discussed in this chapter.

8.2 CHI-SQUARE TEST

Chi-square test is used in investigating nature of categorical data in many of the inferential studies. This test is widely used by the researchers in survey studies. It can be used to investigate whether a sample has been drawn from a population having specific distribution. For example if preferences toward specialization like sports biomechanics, sports psychology, and exercise physiology had been in the proportion of $2:4:5$ in a college, the authority may wish to know whether this distribution still holds true on the basis of the response obtained from the sample of students selected randomly.

The chi-square is pronounced as "Kye" square and is denoted by the Greek letter χ^2. It is computed by the following formula:

$$\chi^2 = \Sigma \frac{\left(f_o - f_e\right)^2}{f_e}$$

Where f_o and f_e represent observed and expected frequencies, respectively. This χ^2 statistic follows a chi-square distribution with $(r-1)$ degrees of freedom, where r is the number of categories. The chi-square statistic requires data to be measured on nominal scale and is computed on the basis of frequencies instead of scores. The chi-square test is easy to apply and requires fewer assumptions. It is not affected by the outliers. One of the essential conditions in computing the chi-square is that none of the cell frequency should be less than 5, otherwise Yates' correction needs to be applied.

Chi-square test is mainly used for the two applications given in the following text. These applications shall be discussed in detail by using the SPSS software.

1. Testing goodness of fit
2. Testing independence of attributes

8.2.1 Testing Goodness of Fit

In testing goodness of fit, we intend to test whether the sample has been obtained from a population that follows a particular frequency distribution. For instance, to know whether all three shoe brands like Nike, Adidas, and Reebok are equally popular among athletes, an equal occurrence hypothesis can be tested. Here, null and alternative hypothesis can be written as follows:

H_0: All three sports shoe brands are equally popular.

H_1: All three sports shoe brands differ in their popularity.

To test the null hypothesis, degree of freedom is taken as $r-1$, where r is the number of groups.

If calculated $\chi^2 >$ tabulated $\chi^2_{0.05}$ $(r-1)$, H_0 is rejected at the significance level 0.05 and if calculated $\chi^2 \leq$ tabulated $\chi^2_{0.05}$ $(r-1\ df)$, we fail to reject H_0

If null hypothesis is not rejected, it is interpreted that the fit is good and all three brands of sports shoes are equally popular. Thus, in testing goodness of fit, an experimenter's interest is not to reject the null hypothesis so as to say that the fit is good. Another useful application of goodness of fit is to test the normality of data, which is one of the main assumptions in using parametric test for testing a hypothesis.

8.2.2 Yates' Correction

If any of the cell frequency is 5 or less, then Yates' correction needs to be applied while calculating chi-square. This correction was suggested by F. Yates (1934) and is known as Yates' correction for continuity. Normally in such situations, the cell having frequency 5 or less is merged with the nearby cell so as to make the expected frequency more than 5 and then the analysis is done as usual. But if the cells are merged in a 2×2 contingency table, then the chi-square will have zero degree of freedom which is meaningless. In applying this correction, 0.5 is subtracted from each difference of the observed and expected cell frequencies. Thus, the formula for chi-square (χ^2) with Yates' correction is given by

$$\chi^2 = \Sigma\Sigma\frac{\left(f_o - f_e - 0.5\right)^2}{f_e}$$

8.2.3 Contingency Coefficient

Contingency coefficient (C) provides magnitude of association between any two attributes. Its value can range from 0 (no association) to 1 (the theoretical maximum possible association). Chi-square simply tests whether an association between the two attributes is significant or not. But it does not give the magnitude of association. Thus, if χ^2 is significant, one must compute the contingency coefficient (C) to know the extent of association between the two attributes. It is computed using the following formula:

$$C = \sqrt{\frac{\chi^2}{\chi^2 + N}}$$

Where, "N" is the sum of all frequencies in the contingency table.

8.3   GOODNESS OF FIT WITH SPSS

Example 8.1

Consider a study in which response of 110 students were taken to compare the popularity of three different brands of tracksuits among them. The responses of the students so obtained are shown in Table 8.1. Let us compute chi-square for investigating the issue.

Solution: Here, the hypotheses that are required to be tested are as follows:

H_0: All three brands are equally popular.

H_1: All three brands are not equally popular.

We shall use SPSS to compute chi-square for testing the null hypothesis.

TABLE 8.1 Summary of Student's Response About Their Preferences

	Brand A	Brand B	Brand C
Q. Which brand of tracksuits do you like?	50	20	40

8.3.1 Computation in Goodness of Fit

8.3.1.1 Preparation of Data File After starting SPSS, select the option 'Type in data' to define variables. There are two variables, *Brand* and *Frequency*, which need to be defined. Do the following:

1. Click on **Variable View** to define variables and their properties.
2. Write *Brand*, short name of the variable under the column heading "Name."
3. For this variable, define full name, that is, *Brand of Track Suit* under the column heading "Label."
4. Under the column heading "Values" define '1' for Brand A, '2' for Brand B, and '3' for Brand C.
5. Under the column heading "Measure," select the 'Nominal' option because *Brand* is a nominal variable.
6. Similarly, define another variable *Frequency* in the next row as scale variable.
7. Use default entries in rest of the columns.

After defining variables in the **Variable View**, the screen shall look like as shown in Figure 8.1.

8.3.1.2 Entering Data Once the variable *Brand* and *Frequency* have been defined, click **Data View** on the left bottom of the screen to open the format for data entry column-wise as shown in Figure 8.2.

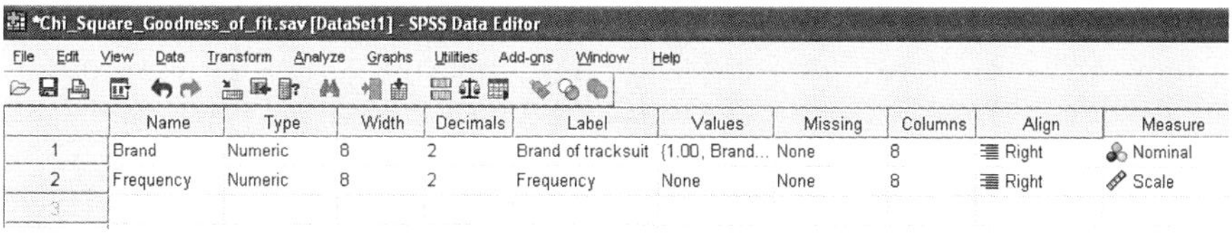

	Name	Type	Width	Decimals	Label	Values	Missing	Columns	Align	Measure
1	Brand	Numeric	8	2	Brand of tracksuit	(1.00, Brand...	None	8	Right	Nominal
2	Frequency	Numeric	8	2	Frequency	None	None	8	Right	Scale
3										

FIGURE 8.1 Defining variable along with their characteristics.

8.3.1.3 Define Weights After entering the data, identify the variable for 'Weight cases by' option by doing the following:

1. Click on **Data** command in the header of the data file and click on **Weight Cases ...** option to get the screen as shown in Figure 8.3.
2. Select the option *Weight cases by*
3. Select variable *Frequency* from the left panel and bring it into "Frequency Variable" section in the right panel.
4. Click on **OK** and go back to the data file.

8.3.1.4 SPSS Commands After entering data and defining 'Weight cases by' option, follow the steps for computing chi-square as follows:

1. In **Data View**, click on the following commands in sequence:

   Analyze → Nonparametric Tests → Chi-Square

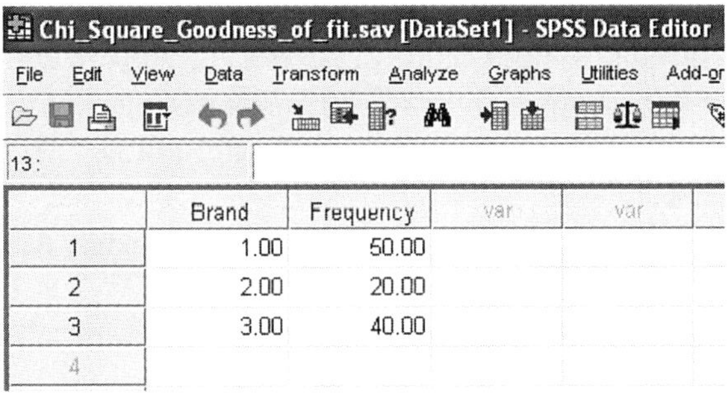

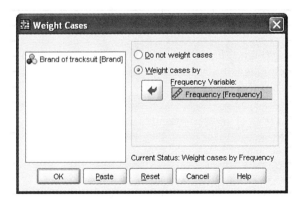

FIGURE 8.2 Data file of brand response for goodness of fit.

FIGURE 8.3 Selecting variable for 'Weight cases by' option.

2. After clicking 'Chi-Square' option, you will be taken to the next screen for selecting variable. Select *Brand* variable from the left panel and bring it to the "Test Variable List" section in the right panel. The screen shall look like as shown in Figure 8.4.

3. Click on **Option** command and check 'Descriptive' option to generate descriptive statistics as shown in Figure 8.5.

4. Click on **Continue** and **OK** to get the output.

5. The output panel shall have two results that are shown in Tables 8.2 and 8.3. These outputs can be selected by using the right click of the mouse and may be pasted in the word file.

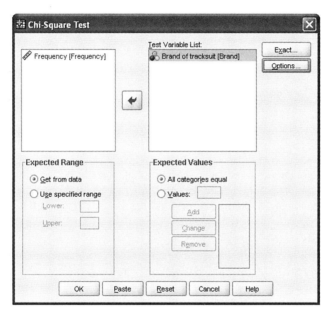

FIGURE 8.4   Option for selecting variable.

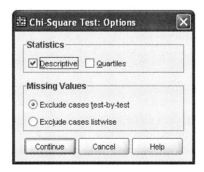

FIGURE 8.5   Option for descriptive statistics.

TABLE 8.2   Observed and Expected Frequencies of the Response for Different Track Suit Brands

	Frequencies of the Response		
	Observed N	Expected N	Residual
Brand A	50	36.7	13.3
Brand B	20	36.7	−16.7
Brand C	40	36.7	3.3
Total	110		

TABLE 8.3   Chi-Square for the Data On Brand Option

	Brand of Track Suit
Chi-square	12.727[a]
df	2
Asymp. sig.	0.002

The minimum expected cell frequency is 36.7.
[a] 0 cells (0%) have expected frequencies less than 5.

8.3.2   Interpretation of Findings

Table 8.2 shows the observed and expected frequencies of different brands. No cell frequency is less than 5; and therefore, no correction has been made by the SPSS in computing chi-square. In Table 8.3, the value of χ^2 is 12.727 which is significant at 5% level, as the p value is 0.002 which is less than 0.05. Thus, we may reject the null hypothesis.

In other words, it can be interpreted that all the three responses are not equally distributed and the fit is not good. So long the value of p is less than 0.05, the value of chi-square is significant at 5% level; and if it exceeds 0.05, the chi-square becomes insignificant.

8.4   TESTING INDEPENDENCE OF TWO ATTRIBUTES

Chi-square is used for testing the independence of two attributes. For instance, it may be interesting to test whether there is any association between IQ and minimum muscular fitness test. A subject may be categorized into high or low IQ as well as into pass or fail category based on minimum muscular fitness test. Thus, all subjects in the sample can be classified into 2×2 table, known as contingency table. The chi-square test can also be applied if frequencies are classified into $m \times n$ table as well, where m and n are integers, but it is more efficient in a 2×2 contingency table.

Let us consider that the two attributes A and B represent IQ and performance (on minimum muscular fitness test), respectively, and are dichotomous in nature. Frequencies of the subjects possessing these attributes can be shown in a 2×2

TABLE 8.4 Observed Frequencies (f_o)

		Minimum Muscular Fitness Test (B)		
		Pass	Fail	Total
IQ (A)	High	a	b	a+b
	Low	c	d	c+d
	Total	a+c	b+d	N

contingency table (Table 8.4). The symbol "a" represents the frequency of subjects having high IQ and has passed the minimum muscular fitness test, whereas "d" represents the frequency of subjects having low IQ and fail to qualify the minimum muscular fitness test. On the other hand, the symbol "b" represents the frequency of those subjects having high IQ but fail to qualify the test, whereas symbol "c" represents the frequency of those who qualify the test and has low IQ. Here, the null hypothesis of no association between the two attributes A and B is tested.

Under the null hypothesis that the attributes are independent, the expected cell frequency for each cell is calculated as follows:

$$a_e = \frac{(a+b) \times (a+c)}{N}, \quad b_e = \frac{(a+b) \times (b+d)}{N}$$

$$c_e = \frac{(c+d) \times (a+c)}{N}, \quad d_e = \frac{(c+d) \times (b+d)}{N}$$

The chi-square (χ^2) statistic can be calculated using the following formula:

$$\chi^2 = \sum\sum \frac{(f_o - f_e)^2}{f_e}$$

Where f_o and f_e are the observed and expected frequencies as shown in Tables 8.4 and 8.5, respectively. The distribution of this statistic follows chi-square distribution with $(r-1) \times (c-1)$ degrees of freedom.

The chi-square statistic can also be computed directly without computing the expected frequencies using the following formula:

$$\chi^2 = \frac{N(ad - bc)^2}{(a+b)(c+d)(a+c)(b+d)}$$

The critical value of chi-square with $(r-1) \times (c-1)$ degrees of freedom and at α significance level can be seen in Table A.5. The procedure in testing the independence of attributes has been shown by using SPSS in the following example.

Let us understand the procedure used in testing the independence of attributes by using the chi-square test through an example. Consider a situation in which we wish to test the independence of gender and smoking knowledge. Responses in Table 8.6

TABLE 8.5 Expected Frequencies (f_e)

		Minimum Muscular Fitness Test (B)	
		Pass	Fail
IQ (A)	High	a_e	b_e
	Low	c_e	d_e

TABLE 8.6 Statement: Cigarette Contains Nicotine

		Response		
		Correct	Do not Know	Incorrect
Gender	Male	30	4	10
	Female	10	5	25

have been obtained from the subjects on the statement "Cigarette contains nicotine." Subjects were asked to respond by choosing any one of the following options: correct, do not know, and incorrect.

To test the independence of Gender and Response, the hypotheses may be written as follows:

$$H_0: \text{ Gender and Response are independent.}$$

$$H_1: \text{ Gender and Response are associated.}$$

After computing chi-square, it needs to be tested for its significance at certain level of significance and $(r-1)(c-1)$ degrees of freedom. Significance of χ^2 is tested by using the following criteria:

If calculated χ^2 > tabulated $\chi^2_{0.05}$ $((r-1)(c-1))$, H_0 is rejected at the significance level 0.05 (r is the number of row and c is the number column. Here r = 2 and c = 2)

and if, calculated $\chi^2 \leq$ tabulated $\chi^2_{0.05}$ $((r-1)(c-1))$, we fail to reject H_0.

8.4.1 Interpretation

If H_0 is rejected, we interpret that there is a significant association between the gender and their response toward the knowledge about smoking. Here significant association simply means that the response pattern of male and female differs. Thus, readers may note that chi-square statistic is used to test the significance of association, but ultimately we get the comparison between the levels of one attribute across the levels of other attribute.

8.5   TESTING ASSOCIATION WITH SPSS

Example 8.2

A survey was conducted in which college men and women were asked to give their opinion on drinking coffee for relaxation. The responses so obtained are shown in Table 8.7.

Let us compute chi-square to test the significance of association between Gender and Response.

Solution: Here, the hypotheses that are required to be tested are as follows:

H_0: Gender and Response are independent.

H_1: There is an association between Gender and Response.

Chi-square for two samples shall be computed by using SPSS software. The chi-square so obtained shall be used for testing the null hypothesis.

TABLE 8.7   Response on Drinking Coffee for Relaxation

Q. Drinking Coffee Is a Healthy Way of Relieving Fatigue		Response		
		Never	Sometimes	Always
Gender	Men	10	6	20
	Women	18	6	7

8.5.1   Computation in Chi-Square

8.5.1.1   Preparation of Data File   After starting SPSS, select the option 'Type in data' to define variables for computing chi-square. There are three variables, *Gender, Response*, and *Frequency*, which need to be defined. Do the following:

1. Click on **Variable View** to define all three variables and their properties.
2. Write short name of the variables *Gender, Response*, and *Frequency* under the column heading "Name."
3. Under the column heading "Label," full name of the variables *Gender, Response*, and *Frequency* may be defined.
4. For the variable *Gender*, double click the cell under the column "Values" and add the following values to different labels:

Value	Label
1	Men
2	Women

5. Similarly for the variable *Response*, double click the cell under the column "Values" and add the following values to different labels:

Value	Label
1	Never
2	Sometimes
3	Always

There is no specific rule of defining the code of these variables. Even "Never," "Sometimes," and "Always" may be defined as 3, 4, and 5, respectively.

6. Under the column "Measure," select the option 'Nominal' for the variables *Gender* and *Response* and scale for *Frequency*.

7. Use default entries in rest of the columns.

After defining variables in the **Variable View**, the screen shall look like as shown in Figure 8.6.

8.5.1.2 Entering Data   Once the variables *Gender, Response*, and *Frequency* are defined, click **Data View** to open the format for entering data column-wise as shown in Figure 8.7.

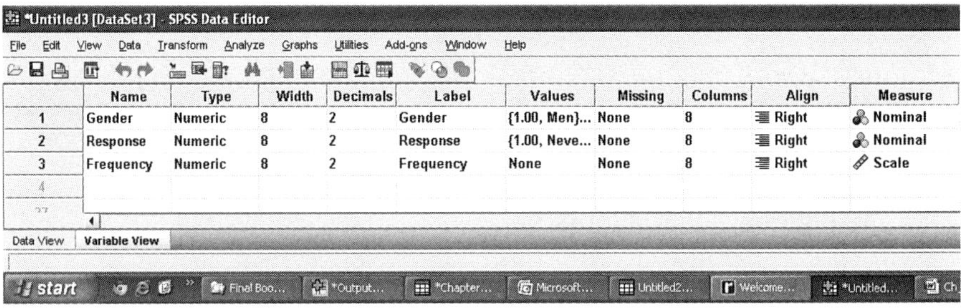

FIGURE 8.6   Defining variables along with their characteristics.

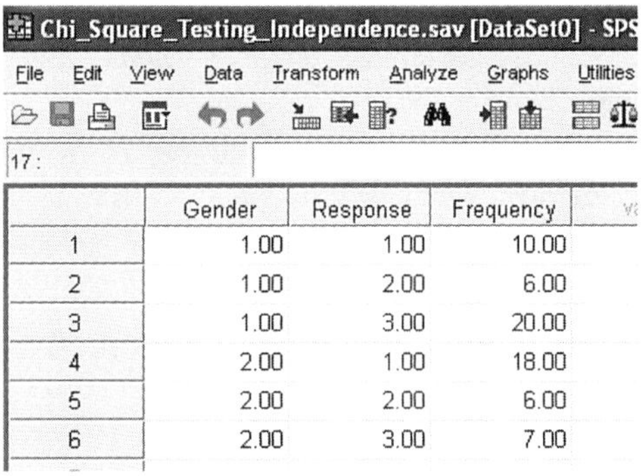

FIGURE 8.7   Data file of coffee data for chi-square.

8.5.1.3 Define Weights   After entering data, identify the variable for 'Weight cases by' option by doing the following:

1. Click on **Data** command in the header of the data file and select **Weight Cases ...** option to get the screen as shown in Figure 8.8.
2. Select the option *Weight cases by*.
3. Select variable *Frequency* from the left panel and bring it into "Frequency Variable" section in the right panel.
4. Click on **OK** and go back to the data file.

8.5.1.4 SPSS Commands   After entering data and defining 'Weight cases by' option, follow the steps listed down for computing chi-square:

1. In **Data View**, click on the following commands in sequence:

   Analyze → Descriptive Statistics → Crosstabs

2. After clicking 'Crosstabs' option, you shall be directed to the next screen for selecting variables. Select variables *Gender* and *Response* from the left panel and bring them into the "Row(s)" and "Column(s)" sections in the right panel. The screen shall look like as shown in Figure 8.9.
3. *Selecting options for computation:* After selecting variables, option need to be defined for generating outputs. Do the following:
   (a) Click on **Statistics** command and check the options 'Chi-Square' and 'Contingency Coefficient' as shown in Figure 8.10. Click **Continue**.
   (b) Click on **Cell** command and check 'Expected,' 'Row,' 'Column,' and 'Total' options as shown in Figure 8.11.
   (c) Click on **Continue** and **OK** options to get the output.
   (d) Select outputs from the output window of SPSS as shown in Tables 8.8, 8.9, and 8.10 for discussion.

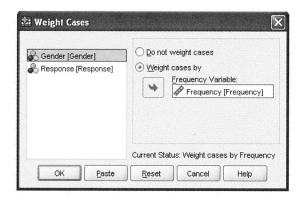

FIGURE 8.8   Selecting variable for 'Weight cases by' option.

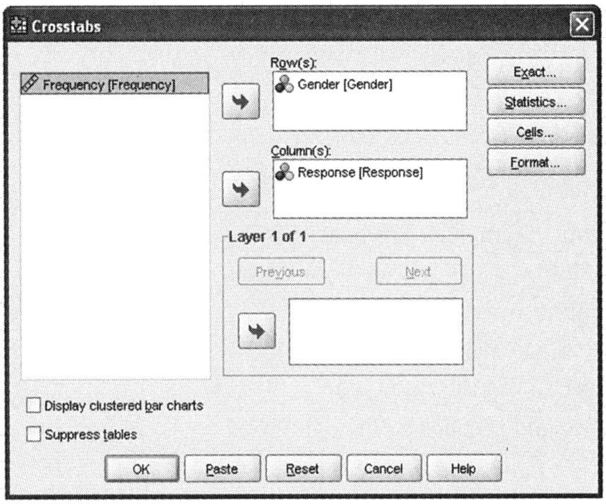

FIGURE 8.9 Option for selecting variables for chi-square.

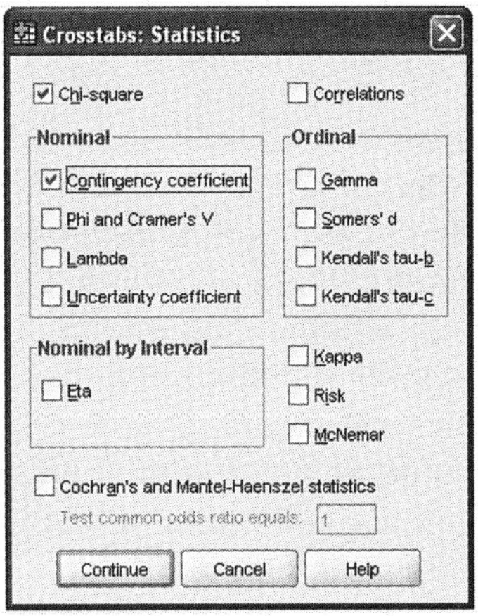

FIGURE 8.10 Option for computing chi-square and contingency coefficient.

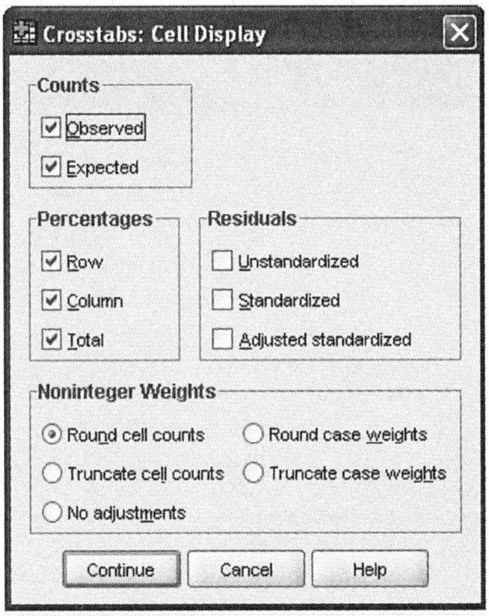

FIGURE 8.11 Option for computing observed and expected frequencies.

TABLE 8.8   Gender * Response Cross Tabulation

			Never	Sometimes	Always	Total
			Response			
Gender	Men	Count	10	6	20	36
		Expected count	15.0	6.4	14.5	36.0
		% within-gender	27.8	16.7	55.6	100.0
		% within-response	35.7	50.0	74.1	53.7
		% of total	14.9	9.0	29.9	53.7
	Women	Count	18	6	7	31
		Expected count	13.0	5.6	12.5	31.0
		% within-gender	58.1	19.4	22.6	100.0
		% within-response	64.3	50.0	25.9	46.3
		% of total	26.9	9.0	10.4	46.3
	Total	Count	28	12	27	67
		Expected count	28.0	12.0	27.0	67.0
		% within gender	41.8	17.9	40.3	100.0
		% within LOC	100.0	100.0	100.0	100.0
		% of total	41.8	17.9	40.3	100.0

TABLE 8.9   Chi-Square for the Data On Gender * Options

	Value	df	Asymp. Sig. (Two-Sided)
Pearson chi-square	8.218[a]	2	0.016
Likelihood ratio	8.471	2	0.014
Linear-by-linear association	8.001	1	0.005
Number of valid cases		67	

The minimum expected count is 5.55.

[a] 0 cells (0.0%) have expected count less than 5.

TABLE 8.10   Contingency Coefficient for the Data On Gender * Options

		Value	Approx. Sig. (p Value)
Nominal by nominal	Contingency coefficient	0.331	0.016
Number of valid cases			67

8.5.2   Interpretation of Findings

Table 8.8 shows the observed and expected frequencies of the *Gender × Response*. No cell frequency is less than 5; hence, no correction was made by the SPSS while computing chi-square. If any of the cell frequency had value 5 or less, then SPSS would have computed the chi-square after applying Yates' correction.

In Table 8.9, the value of chi-square (χ^2) is 8.218, which is significant ($p < 0.05$). Thus, we may reject the null hypothesis that the gender and response are independent. It may be concluded that there is a significant association between gender and their responses on the issue of "Drinking coffee is a healthy way of relieving fatigue."

In other words, it may be interpreted that the response pattern of the male and female on the issue differs significantly.

In Table 8.10, the value of contingency coefficient is 0.331. This is a measure of association between gender and response. Further, the value of contingency coefficient is significant as its p value is 0.016 which is less than 0.05.

8.6   MANN–WHITNEY U TEST: COMPARING TWO INDEPENDENT SAMPLES

If assumptions of t-test are seriously violated, then the Mann–Whitney U test may be used to compare two independent groups. In this test, no assumption is required about the distribution of population from which the samples have been drawn. In using Mann–Whitney U test we intend to test whether the two samples come from the same population or not. Since this test can be used both for parametric and nonparametric data, it is considered to be the most powerful nonparametric test. The Mann–Whitney U test can be used more efficiently as an alternative to the t-test if we wish to avoid the assumptions like equality of variance and normality of the population distribution. The only assumption in using this test is that the data must be measured at least on the ordinal scale and samples must be randomly drawn.

Example 8.3

In physical education colleges postgraduate students are considered to be less active than the undergraduates due to the nature of their curriculum. To investigate this fact, a study was planned in which 10 students were randomly chosen from the undergraduate as well as from the postgraduate classes. These subjects were tested for their cardio-respiratory endurance by means of VO_2 max. The data so obtained are shown in Table 8.11. The assumptions of t-test are seriously violated; hence, let us see how to apply Mann–Whitney U test to investigate the research question.

Solution: We need to test the following hypotheses:

H_0: VO_2 max is similar in both the groups.

H_1: VO_2 max is not similar in both the groups.

8.6.1   Computation in Mann–Whitney U Statistic Using SPSS

8.6.1.1   Preparation of Data File   To prepare data file, define *Course* as a nominal and *VO₂ max* as scale variables in the **Variable View**. For *Course* variable, give code 1 to undergraduate and code 2 to postgraduate by clicking the cell under the column heading "Values." After defining variables, the screen shall look like as shown in Figure 8.12.

8.6.1.2 Entering Data After defining variables, click on **Data View** to open the format for entering data column-wise. Enter the data as shown in Figure 8.13.

8.6.1.3 SPSS Commands After entering data in the **Data View**, do the following steps:

1. *Initiating SPSS commands:* In **Data View**, click on the following commands in sequence:

   Analyze → Nonparametric Tests → 2 Independent Samples....

2. *Selecting variable*: After clicking **2 Independent Samples** option, you will be taken to the screen as shown in Figure 8.14 for selecting variables and defining other options. Do the following:

   (a) Select *VO₂ max* and *Course* variables from the left panel and bring them into the "Test Variable List" and "Grouping Variable" sections in the right panel.

   (b) Enter 1 and 2 in Group 1 and Group 2, respectively, as shown in Figure 8.14.

   (c) Ensure that the 'Mann–Whitney U' option is checked.

   (d) Click on **Options** command and check 'Descriptive' (Fig. 8.15).

   (e) Click on **Continue** and **OK** options to get the outputs.

3. *Getting the output*: The outputs generated by the SPSS are shown in Tables 8.12 and 8.13.

TABLE 8.11   Data On VO_2 Max (in Ml.kg.min⁻¹)

Undergraduate	Postgraduate
66	60
68	60
62	58
64	65
60	62
63	55
54	53
55	57
59	48
65	49
59	55
69	61

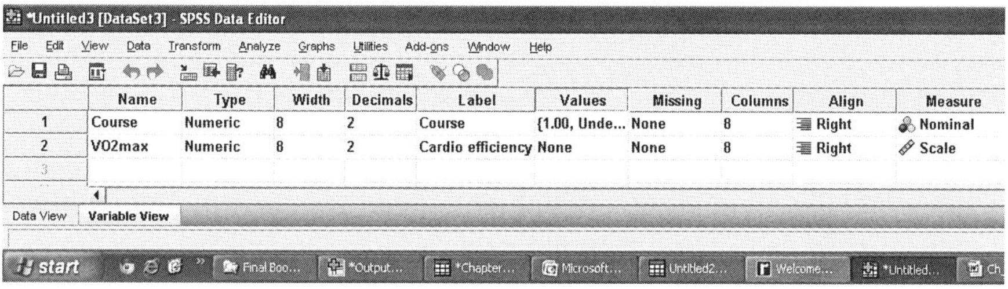

FIGURE 8.12   Defining independent and dependent variables.

	Course	VO2max	var
1	1.00	66.00	
2	1.00	68.00	
3	1.00	62.00	
4	1.00	64.00	
5	1.00	60.00	
6	1.00	63.00	
7	1.00	54.00	
8	1.00	55.00	
9	1.00	59.00	
10	1.00	65.00	
11	1.00	59.00	
12	1.00	69.00	
13	2.00	60.00	
14	2.00	60.00	
15	2.00	58.00	
16	2.00	65.00	
17	2.00	62.00	
18	2.00	55.00	
19	2.00	53.00	
20	2.00	57.00	
21	2.00	48.00	
22	2.00	49.00	
23	2.00	55.00	
24	2.00	61.00	

FIGURE 8.13   Data file of VO$_2$ max for Mann–Whitney U test.

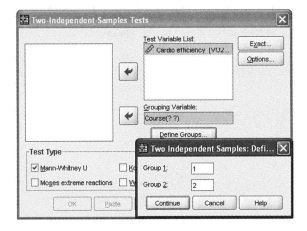

FIGURE 8.14   Selecting independent and dependent variables.

8.6.2   Interpretation of Findings

Table 8.12 shows the mean rank in both the groups, whereas Table 8.13 shows the Mann–Whitney U statistic and other results. To interpret the findings, we need to consider the z statistic and two tailed p value, corrected for ties.

The output indicates that the z statistic is significant, $|z| = 2.141$, $p < 0.05$; hence, significant differences in cardio-respiratory endurance exists between undergraduate and postgraduate students.

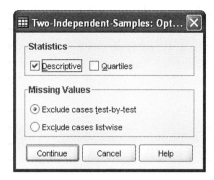

FIGURE 8.15   Selecting option for descriptive statistics.

TABLE 8.12   Ranks

	Course	N	Mean Rank	Sum of Ranks
Cardio efficiency	Undergraduate	12	15.58	187.00
	Postgraduate	12	9.42	113.00
	Total	24		

TABLE 8.13   Test Statistics[a]

	Cardio Efficiency
Mann–Whitney U	35.000
Wilcoxon W	113.000
Z	−2.141
Asymp. sig. (two-tailed)	0.032
Exact sig. [2*(one-tailed sig.)]	0.033[b]

[a] Grouping variable: Course.
[b] Not corrected for ties.

8.7   WILCOXON SIGNED-RANK TEST: FOR COMPARING TWO RELATED GROUPS

The Wilcoxon signed-rank test is a nonparametric alternative to the paired t-test. This test is used to compare two groups when the data in both groups is related in some sense and we wish to test whether the members of a pair differ. For large sample, this test is almost as sensitive as the paired t-test, and for small sample with unknown distributions this test is even more sensitive. Mostly researchers are not sure that the scores are normally distributed hence this test may be preferred over the paired t-test.

Example 8.4

A 4-week health awareness program was launched in which 12 housewives participated. Their weights were measured before and after the program. The data obtained in the study is shown in Table 8.14. The data violates the assumption of paired t-test. Let us investigate whether the program was effective in reducing participant's weight at 5% level.

Solution: In this example, we need to test the following hypotheses:

H_0: No difference between pre- and post-program testing data on weight exists.

H_1: Significant difference exists between pre- and post-program testing data on weight.

8.7.1 Computation in Wilcoxon Signed-Rank Test Using SPSS

8.7.1.1 Preparation of Data File   Before applying Wilcoxon signed-rank test, a data file needs to be prepared. This can be done by defining the variables *Pre_test* and *Post_test* as Scale in **Variable View**. Under the heading "Label," expanded name of the variables can be defined. Leave other entries as selected by default. After defining the variables, the screen shall look like as shown in Figure 8.16.

8.7.1.2 Entering Data   After defining variables, click on **Data View** to open the format for entering the data column-wise. Kindly note the difference of data feeding layout which is different than the one we used in case of Mann–Whitney U test. After data entry, the screen shall look like as shown in Figure 8.17.

8.7.1.3 SPSS Commands   After entering data in the **Data View**, do the following steps:

TABLE 8.14   Data On Weight Obtained On Housewives

Pre Test	Post Test
87	85
85	80
94	88
65	64
56	57
72	70
70	69
68	68
57	58
90	79
61	59
74	72

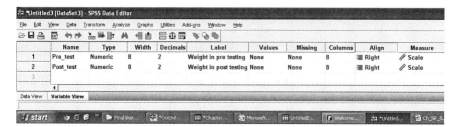

FIGURE 8.16   Defining variables.

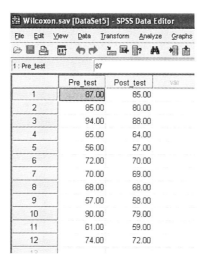

FIGURE 8.17   Data file for Wilcoxon signed-rank test.

1. *Initiating SPSS commands:* In **Data View**, click on the following commands in sequence:

    Analyze → Nonparametric Tests → 2 Related Samples….

2. *Selecting variable*: After clicking **2 Related Samples** option, you will be taken to the screen as shown in Figure 8.18 for selecting variables and selecting option. Do the following:

    (a) Select *Pre_test* and *Post_test* variables from the left panel and bring them into the "Test Pairs" section in the right panel.

    (b) Ensure that the 'Wilcoxon' option is checked.

    (c) Click on **Options** command and check 'Descriptive' (Fig. 8.19).

    (d) Click on **Continue** and **OK** options to get the outputs.

3. *Getting the output:* The outputs generated by the SPSS are shown in Tables 8.15, 8.16, and 8.17.

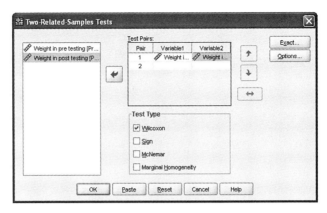

FIGURE 8.18   Selecting pre- and post-test variables.

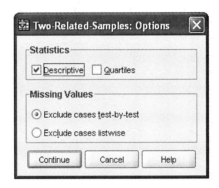

FIGURE 8.19   Selecting option for descriptive statistics.

TABLE 8.15   Descriptive Statistics

	N	Mean	Std. Deviation	Minimum	Maximum
Weight in pre testing	12	73.2500	12.99738	56.00	94.00
Weight in post testing	12	70.7500	10.45445	57.00	88.00

8.7.2   Interpretation of Findings

Table 8.16 shows the summary of negative and positive ranks in both the groups, whereas Table 8.17 shows z statistic and p value. To interpret the Wilcoxon signed-rank test, z statistic needs to be examined for testing two-tailed hypothesis.

The output indicates that the z statistic is significant, $|z| = 2.514$, $p < 0.05$; hence, health awareness program was effective in reducing weight of the participants.

TABLE 8.16 Ranks

		N	Mean Rank	Sum of Ranks
Weight in post testing –	Negative ranks	9[a]	6.78	61.00
Weight in pre testing	Positive ranks	2[b]	2.50	5.00
	Ties	1[c]		
	Total	12		

[a] Weight in post testing < Weight in pre testing.
[b] Weight in post testing > Weight in pre testing.
[c] Weight in post testing = Weight in pre testing.

TABLE 8.17 Test Statistics[a]

	Weight in Post Testing – Weight in Pre Testing
Z	−2.514[b]
Asymp. sig. (2-tailed)	0.012

[a] Wilcoxon signed-rank test.
[b] Based on positive ranks.

8.8 KRUSKAL–WALLIS TEST

The Kruskal–Wallis test is a nonparametric alternative to the one-way ANOVA. It is used to compare three or more samples simultaneously and decide whether they belong to the same population or not. This test is used when the data obtained are measured at least on ordinal scale. The Kruskal–Wallis test can be used for parametric data if the assumption of normality does not hold or other assumptions required for one-way ANOVA violates.

Example 8.5

A gymnastic coach wanted to improve flexibility for her gymnasts. She was offered three circuit training programs with different intensities to choose from. In order to take decision, she conducted a study in which these programs were randomly allocated to the subjects in the sample for 6 weeks. After the treatment was over, flexibility of the subjects was measured in three groups, which are shown in Table 8.18.

Solution: We need to test the following hypotheses:

H_0: All three groups are equal.

H_1: All three groups differ.

TABLE 8.18 Data On Flexibility (in Inches)

Program Intensity		
Low	Medium	High
11	12	10
9	10	8
8	7	9
10	11	9
8	10	9
9	10	11
10	12	9
12	10	11
7	9	10
8	10	9

8.8.1 Computation in Kruskal–Wallis Test Using SPSS

8.8.1.1 Preparation of Data File   To prepare data file, define *Circuit_training* as a nominal and *Flexibility* as scale variables in the **Variable View**. For *Circuit_training* variable, define code 1 for Low intensity, 2 for Medium intensity, and 3 for High intensity by clicking cell under the column heading "Values." After defining variables, the screen shall look like as shown in Figure 8.20.

8.8.1.2 Entering Data   After defining variables, click on **Data View** to open the format for entering data column-wise. Enter the data as shown in Figure 8.21.

8.8.1.3 SPSS Commands   After entering data in the **Data View**, do the following steps:

1. *Initiating SPSS commands*: In **Data View**, go to the following commands in sequence:

   Analyze → Nonparametric Tests → K Independent Samples….

2. *Selecting variables*: After clicking **K Independent Samples** option, you will be directed to the screen as shown in Figure 8.22 for selecting variables and defining other options. Do the following:

   (a) Select *Flexibility* and *Circuit_training* variables from the left panel and bring them into the "Test Variable List" and "Grouping Variable" sections in the right panel.

   (b) Enter 1 in the box labeled "Minimum" and 3 in the "Maximum" as shown in Figure 8.22.

   (c) Ensure that the 'Kruskal–Wallis H' option is checked.

   (d) Click on **Options** command and check 'Descriptive' (Fig. 8.23).

   (e) Click on **Continue** and **OK** options to get the output.

3. *Getting the output*: The outputs generated by the SPSS are shown in Tables 8.19 and 8.20.

	Name	Type	Width	Decimals	Label	Values	Missing	Columns	Align	Measure
1	Circuit_training	Numeric	8	2	Circuit training intensity	{1.00, Low ...	None	8	Right	Nominal
2	Flexibility	Numeric	8	2	Flexibility	None	None	8	Right	Scale

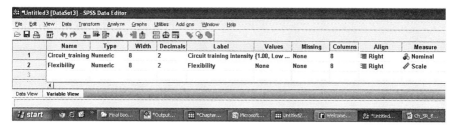

FIGURE 8.20 Defining variables.

	Circuit_training	Flexibility
1	1.00	11.00
2	1.00	9.00
3	1.00	8.00
4	1.00	10.00
5	1.00	8.00
6	1.00	9.00
7	1.00	10.00
8	1.00	12.00
9	1.00	7.00
10	1.00	8.00
11	2.00	12.00
12	2.00	10.00
13	2.00	7.00
14	2.00	11.00
15	2.00	10.00
16	2.00	10.00
17	2.00	12.00
18	2.00	10.00
19	2.00	9.00
20	2.00	10.00
21	3.00	10.00
22	3.00	8.00
23	3.00	9.00
24	3.00	9.00
25	3.00	9.00

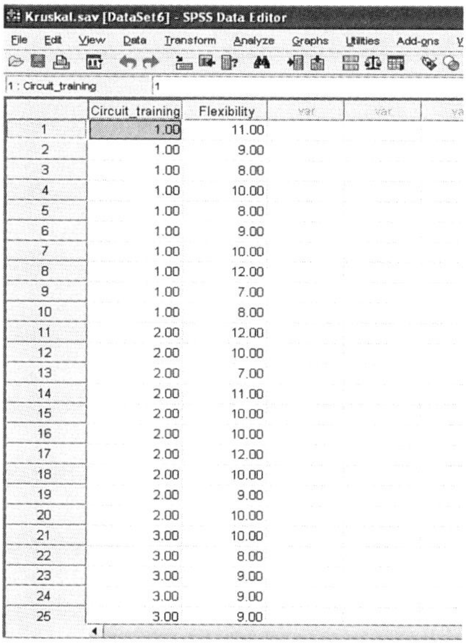

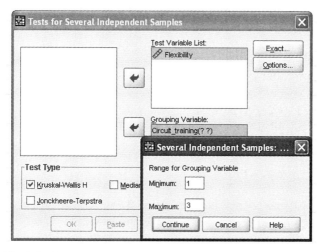

FIGURE 8.21 Data file of flexibility for Kruskal–Wallis test.

FIGURE 8.22 Selecting independent and dependent variables and option for descriptive statistics.

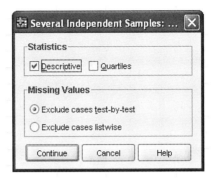

FIGURE 8.23   Option for descriptive statistics.

TABLE 8.19   Ranks of Different Groups

	Circuit Training Intensity	N	Mean Rank
Flexibility	Low intensity	10	12.85
	Medium intensity	10	19.05
	High intensity	10	14.60
	Total	30	

TABLE 8.20   Test Statistics[a,b]

	Flexibility
Chi-square	2.778
df	2
Asymp. sig.	0.249

[a] Kruskal–Wallis test.
[b] Grouping variable: circuit training intensity.

8.8.2   Interpretation of Findings

The results of the Kruskal–Wallis test can be interpreted by looking to the value of chi-square, degrees of freedom, and significance value (p), which has been corrected for ties. Since $\chi^2 (= 2.778)$ is not significant (p>0.05), it may be concluded that the flexibility did not differ in the three treatment groups.

8.9   FRIEDMAN TEST

The Friedman test is a nonparametric test and can be used in place of one-way ANOVA with repeated measures if its assumptions violate. This test is used in a situation when repeated measures are obtained on the same set of subjects. In using this test, we try to detect differences in treatments across multiple test attempts. This test can be used if the following assumptions are satisfied:

1. Sample is randomly drawn
2. Three or more repeated measures have been obtained on the same subjects
3. Dependent variable is measured at least on ordinal scale.

Example 8.6

A sports scientist wanted to investigate the progress of his athlete on muscular strength during his 4-week weight training program. Eight athletes participated in the program. These athletes were tested for their strength before starting the training and after 2 and 4 weeks in the experiment. The data so obtained is shown in Table 8.21. Since data violated the stringent assumptions of repeated measures ANOVA, it was decided to apply Friedman test.

Solution: We need to test the following hypotheses:

H_0: All three samples are from the same population or from populations with equal medians.

H_1: All three samples are not from the same populations. They differ in their median values.

TABLE 8.21   Data On Strength (in Lb)

	Time	
0 Day	2 Weeks	4 Weeks
150	145	165
180	210	265
220	210	280
140	150	190
150	190	195
160	165	180
170	175	170
180	190	195

8.9.1   Computation in Friedman Test Using SPSS

8.9.1.1   Preparation of Data File   To prepare data file, define *Zero_day, Two_week*, and *Four_week* as scale variables in the **Variable View** as shown in Figure 8.24.

8.9.1.2   Entering Data   After defining variables, click on **Data View** to open the format for entering the data column-wise. Enter the data as shown in Figure 8.25.

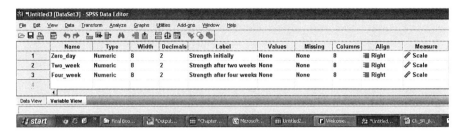

FIGURE 8.24   Defining variables.

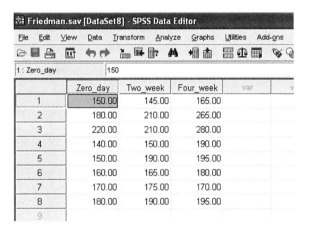

FIGURE 8.25   Data file of strength scores for Friedman test.

8.9.1.3   SPSS Commands   After entering data in the **Data View**, do the following steps:

1. *Initiating SPSS commands:* In **Data View**, go to the following commands in sequence:

   Analyze → Nonparametric Tests → K Related Samples….

2. *Selecting variable:* After clicking **K Related Samples** option, you will be taken to the screen as shown in Figure 8.26 for selecting variables and defining other options. Do the following:

   (a) Select *Zero_day, Two_week* and *Four_week* variables from the left panel and bring them into the "Test Variables" section in the right panel.

   (b) Ensure that the 'Friedman' option is checked.

   (c) Click on **Statistics** command and check 'Descriptive.'

   (d) Click on **Continue** and **OK** options to get the outputs.

3. *Getting the output:* The outputs generated by the SPSS are shown in Tables 8.22 and 8.23.

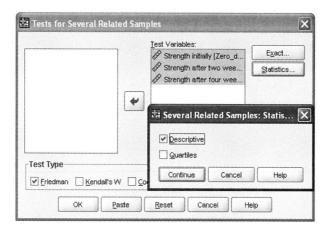

FIGURE 8.26   Selecting variables and defining option for descriptive statistics.

TABLE 8.22   Descriptive Statistic

	N	Mean	Std. Deviation	Minimum	Maximum
Strength initially	8	1.6875E2	25.31939	140.00	220.00
Strength after 2 weeks	8	1.7938E2	24.99107	145.00	210.00
Strength after 4 weeks	8	2.0500E2	43.26001	165.00	280.00

TABLE 8.23   Test Statistics[a]

N	8
Chi-square	9.484
df	2
Asymp. sig.	0.009

[a] Friedman test.

8.9.2   Interpretation of Findings

In Friedman test, hypothesis is tested by using the chi-square statistic. Table 8.23 indicates that $\chi^2(2, n = 8) = 9.484$ is significant ($p < 0.05$); hence, it may be concluded that the significant differences do exist in strength across duration and that duration appears to increase strength of the subjects considerably.

8.10   SUMMARY OF THE SPSS COMMANDS

8.10.1   Computing Chi-Square Statistic (for Testing Goodness of Fit)

1. Create data file by choosing the option 'Type in data.'
2. In **Variable View**, define *Brand* as a nominal and *Frequency* as a scale variable.

3. For the variable *Brand*, define "1" for Brand A, "2" for Brand B, and "3" for Brand C under the column heading "Values."

4. Enter the data column-wise for all three categories of Brand.

5. Click on **Data** command in the header of the data file and select the *Frequency* variable for the **Weight Cases …** option. Click **OK**.

6. Click on the following commands in sequence:

Analyze → Nonparametric Tests → Chi-Square

7. After selecting variable, click the **Option** command and check the 'Descriptive' option.

8. Click on **Continue** and **OK** options to get the outputs.

8.10.2   Computing Chi-Square Statistic (for Testing Independence)

1. Prepare data file by defining *Gender* and *Response* variables as nominal and *Frequency* as scale.

2. For *Gender* variable, define "1" for Male and "2" for Female under the column heading "Values."

3. Similarly, define the code for *Response* variable as "1" for Never, "2" for Sometimes, and "3" for Always.

4. Enter the data column-wise.

5. Click on **Data** command in the header of the data file and select the *Frequency* variable for the **Weight Cases …** option. Click **OK**.

6. Click on the following commands in sequence:

Analyze → Descriptive Statistics → Crosstabs

7. Click on **Statistics** command and check the options 'Chi-Square' and 'Contingency Coefficient'. Click on **Continue** button.

8. Click on **Cell** command and check the options 'Expected,' 'Row,' 'Column,' and 'Total.'

9. Click on **Continue** and then **OK** to get the outputs.

8.10.3   Computation in Mann–Whitney U Test

1. Create data file by defining *Course* as nominal and VO_2 *max* as scale variable.

2. For *Course* variable, define "1" for Undergraduate and "2" for Postgraduate under the column heading "Values."

3. Enter the data column-wise.

4. Click on the following commands in sequence:

Analyze → Nonparametric Tests → 2 Independent Samples….

5. Select VO_2 *max* and *Course* variables from the left panel and bring them in the "Test Variable List" and "Grouping Variable" sections in the right panel.

6. Enter 1 and 2 in Group 1 and Group 2, respectively.
7. Ensure that the 'Mann–Whitney U' option is checked.
8. Click on **Options** command and check 'Descriptive' option.
9. Click on **Continue** and **OK** options to get the outputs.

8.10.4   Computation in Wilcoxon Signed-Rank Test

1. Create data file by defining *Pre_test* and *Post_test* as scale variables.
2. For *Course* variable, define "1" for Undergraduate and "2" for Postgraduate under the column heading "Values."
3. Enter the data column-wise for both the variables.
4. Click on the following commands in sequence:

        Analyze → Nonparametric Tests → 2 Related Samples….

5. Select *Pre_test* and *Post_test* variables from the left panel and bring them in the "Test Pairs" section in the right panel.
6. Ensure that the 'Wilcoxon' option is checked.
7. Click on **Options** command and check 'Descriptive' option.
8. Click on **Continue** and **OK** options to get the outputs.

8.10.5   Computation in Kruskal–Wallis Test

1. Create data file by defining *Circuit_training* as a nominal and *Flexibility* as scale variables.
2. For *Circuit_training* variable, define "1" for Low intensity, "2" for Medium intensity, and "3" for High intensity.
3. Enter the data column-wise.
4. Click on the following commands in sequence:

        Analyze → Nonparametric Tests → K Independent Samples….

5. Select *Flexibility* and *Circuit_training* variables from the left panel and bring them into the "Test Variable List" and "Grouping Variable" sections in the right panel.
6. Enter 1 in the box labeled "Minimum" and 3 in the "Maximum."
7. Ensure that the 'Kruskal–Wallis H' option is checked.
8. Click on **Options** command and check 'Descriptive' option.
9. Click on **Continue** and **OK** options to get the outputs.

8.10.6   Computation in Friedman Test

1. Create data file by defining *Zero_day, Two_week* and *Four_week* as scale variables.
2. Enter the data column wise.
3. Click on the following commands in sequence:

        Analyze → Nonparametric Tests → K Related Samples….

4. Select *Zero_day*, *Two_week* and *Four_week* variables from the left panel and bring them in the "Test Variables" section in the right panel.

5. Ensure that the 'Friedman option' is checked.

6. Click on **Statistics** command and check 'Descriptive' option.

7. Click on **Continue** and **OK** options to get the outputs.

8.11   EXERCISE

8.11.1   Short Answer Questions

Note: Write answer to each question in not more than 200 words.

Q.1   Responses were obtained from male and female on different questions related to their knowledge about smoking. There were three possible responses for each question: Agree, Undecided, and Disagree. How will you compare the knowledge of male and female about smoking?

Q.2   Explain two important applications of chi-square.

Q.3   Discuss the assumptions of nonparametric tests.

Q.4   Explain a situation where Friedman test can be applied.

Q.5   Is there any similarity between z-test and chi-square test? Explain in detail by means of an example.

Q.6   How will you frame a null hypothesis in testing the significance of an association between gender and IQ where IQ is classified into high and low category? Write decision criteria in testing this hypothesis.

Q.7   Can the chi-square be used for comparing the attitude of men and women on the issue of "Coach uses innovative practices," if the 2×5 frequencies are given in Table 8.24. Under what situation chi-square becomes the most robust test?

Q.8   If chi-square comes out to be significant, then it indicates that the association between the two attributes exists. How would you find the magnitude of an association?

Q.9   What is Phi coefficient? In what situation it is used? Explain by means of an example.

TABLE 8.24   Responses On "Coach Uses Innovative Practices"

		Strongly Agree	Agree	Undecided	Disagree	Strongly Disagree
Gender	Men	30	15	10	10	15
	Women	40	10	5	15	10

8.11.2   Multiple Choice Questions

Note: Questions 1–10 have four alternative answers for each question. Tick marks the one that you consider the closest to the correct answer.

1   In computing chi-square with SPSS, the sequence of commands is
    (a) Analyze → Nonparametric Tests → Chi-Square
    (b) Analyze → Descriptive → Crosstabs
    (c) Analyze → Chi-Square → Nonparametric Tests
    (d) Analyze → Crosstabs → Chi-Square

2   Choose the most appropriate statement about the null hypothesis in chi-square
    (a) There is an association between gender and response.
    (b) There is no association between gender and response.
    (c) There are 50–50% chances of significant and insignificant association.
    (d) None of the above is correct.

3   Student's response on their preference toward optional paper is as follows:

	Response of the Students		
Subjects	Psychology	Biomechanics	Exercise Physiology
No. of students	15	20	25

The value of chi-square is
(a) 2
(b) 2.5
(c) 50
(d) 25

4   The value of chi-square for the given data is

		Gender	
		Male	Female
Level	State	15	5
	National	15	25

(a) 7.5
(b) 75
(c) 12.5
(d) 750

5   Chi-square is used for
    (a) Finding magnitude of an association between two attributes.
    (b) Finding significance of an association between two attributes.
    (c) Comparing the variation between two attributes.
    (d) Comparing median of two attributes.

6   Chi-Square is the most robust test if the frequency table is
    (a) 2×2
    (b) 2×3
    (c) 3×3
    (d) $m \times n$

7   While using chi-square for testing an association between two attributes, SPSS
    provides Crosstabs option. Choose the most appropriate statement.
    (a) Crosstabs treat all data as nominal.
    (b) Crosstabs treat all data as ordinal.
    (c) Crosstabs treat some data as nominal and some data as ordinal.
    (d) Crosstabs treat data as per the problem.

8   If responses are obtained in the form of the frequency on a five-point scale and
    it is required to compare the responses of male and female on a specific issue
    "Yoga is good for children," then which statistical test you would prefer?
    (a) Two sample t-test
    (b) Paired t-test
    (c) One-way ANOVA
    (d) Chi-square test

9   If p value for a chi-square is 0.02, what conclusion can you draw?
    (a) Chi-square is significant at 99% confidence interval.
    (b) Chi-square is not significant at 95% confidence interval.
    (c) Chi-square is significant at 0.01 levels.
    (d) Chi-square is significant at 0.05 levels.

10 The degrees of freedom of chi-square in an $r \times c$ table can be calculated by the
    formula
    (a) $r + c$
    (b) $r + c - 1$
    (c) rc
    (d) $(r - 1)(c - 1)$

11 In Mann–Whitney U test, hypothesis is tested by using
    (a) z-test
    (b) Chi-square test
    (c) F-test
    (d) t-test

12 In Kruskal–Wallis test, null hypothesis is tested by using
    (a) t-test
    (b) F-test
    (c) Chi-square test
    (d) z-test

13 In a 6-week fitness program if 15 subjects are tested for their cardio-respiratory
    endurance before starting the program and after 2, 4, and 6 weeks during the

TABLE 8.25   Responses of the Students About Their Subject Preferences

Subjects	Biomechanics	Sports Psychology	Sport Physiology
Frequency	20	40	30

program and if the assumption of normality is seriously violated, which test would you prefer to compare the three groups?
(a) t-test
(b) Mann–Whitney U test
(c) Chi-square test
(d) Friedman test

14   In testing the effectiveness of an exercise program, which test should be used if the assumption of parametric test fails?
(a) Chi-square test
(b) Wilcoxon signed-rank test
(c) Mann–Whitney U test
(d) Friedman test

8.11.3   Assignment

1. In a study, 90 students were asked to give their preference about one of the three specialization papers namely biomechanics, sports psychology, and sports physiology in their master's program. Compute chi-square using SPSS for testing whether all the three subjects are equally popular on the basis of the data given in Table 8.25.

8.12   CASE STUDY ON TESTING INDEPENDENCE OF ATTRIBUTES

Objective

A coach wanted to investigate whether minimum muscular fitness is gender specific. He conducted a study on a randomly selected sample of the university students including both male and female. These subjects were tested for their performance on minimum muscular fitness test, and the results so obtained are shown in Table 8.26.

Research Questions

The following research questions were investigated:

1. Is there any association between minimum muscular fitness and gender?
2. Does minimum muscular fitness for male and female differ?

Analyzing Data

The two research questions were investigated in this study. First, whether association between gender and minimum muscular fitness exists and second, whether performance of the male and female differs on this test. In fact, the second research question can be derived using the result obtained from the first. For addressing these two issues, chi-square and contingency coefficient were computed by using SPSS, which are shown in Tables 8.28 and 8.29, respectively.

The chi-square and contingency coefficient were obtained by using the commands **Analyze, Descriptive Statistics,** and **Crosstabs** in sequence. *Frequency* variable was selected for 'Weight cases by' option. After clicking on **Statistics** option, 'Chi-square' and 'Contingency coefficient' were selected. Further, after selecting options for 'Expected,' 'Row,' 'Column,' and 'Total' by clicking on the **Cell** command, results were obtained as shown in Tables 8.27, 8.28, and 8.29.

TABLE 8.26 Performance of the Students On Fitness Test

		Minimum Muscular Test	
		Pass	Fail
Gender	Male	15	5
	Female	7	18

TABLE 8.27 Gender * Min_Mus_Fit Cross Tabulation

			Min_Mus_Fit		
			Pass	Fail	Total
Gender	Male	Count	15	5	20
		Expected count	9.8	10.2	20.0
	Female	Count	7	18	25
		Expected count	12.2	12.8	25.0
	Total	Count	22	23	45
		Expected count	22.0	23.0	45.0

TABLE 8.28 Chi-Square for the Data On Gender * Min_Mus_Fit

	Value	df	Asymp. Sig. (Two-Sided)
Pearson chi-square	9.823 [a]	1	0.002
Continuity correction [b]	8.032	1	0.005
Likelihood ratio	10.220	1	0.001
Fisher's exact test			
Linear-by-linear association	9.604	1	0.002
Number of valid cases [b]	45		

[a] Significant at 5% level.
[b] Computed only for a 2×2 table.

TABLE 8.29   Contingency Coefficient for the Data On Gender * Min_Mus_Fit

		Value	Approx. Sig. (p Value)
Nominal by nominal	Contingency coefficient	0.423	0.002
Number of valid cases		45	

Testing Association

Table 8.28 shows that the chi-square value is 9.823 which is significant as its associated p value is 0.002 which is less than 0.05. Thus, on the basis of the sample observation, it may be inferred that the association between gender and minimum muscular fitness is significant. Table 8.29 shows that the contingency coefficient is 0.423. This shows the strength of the association between the two attribute gender and minimum muscular fitness test.

Since the association between gender and minimum muscular fitness is significantly associated, it may be concluded that the performance of male and female on this test differs significantly.

Reporting

- Since chi-square was significant ($p < 0.01$), it may be inferred that the association between gender and minimum muscular fitness was significant. The strength of the association was 0.423
- Significance of association between gender and minimum muscular fitness indicates that the performance of male and female differs on this test.

9

REGRESSION ANALYSIS AND MULTIPLE CORRELATIONS

LEARNING OBJECTIVES

After completing this chapter, you should be able to do the following:

- Explain the use of regression analysis and multiple correlation in research
- Interpret various terms involved in regression analysis
- Learn to use SPSS for doing regression analysis
- Understand the procedure of identifying the most efficient regression model
- Know the method of constructing the regression equation based on the SPSS output.

9.1 INTRODUCTION

The purpose of regression analysis is to explain the variation in a dependent variable on the basis of variation in one or more independent variables. A dependent variable is also termed "criterion variable." Correlation coefficient may be used to know as to how an athlete's performance on 400-meter event is affected by the variation in his height, leg length, leg strength, stride length, etc. If variability in a dependent variable is explained by only one independent variable, the model is known as simple regression. If it is explained by more than one independent variable, it is known as multiple regression. The regression equation can either be linear or curvilinear, but our discussion shall be limited to linear regression only.

Sports Research with Analytical Solution using SPSS®, First Edition. J. P. Verma.
© 2016 John Wiley & Sons, Inc. Published 2016 by John Wiley & Sons, Inc.
Companion website: www.wiley.com/go/Verma/Sportsresearch

A lot of studies have been conducted on regression analysis in forecasting human performance in the area of sports. Besides regression analysis, there are other quantitative and qualitative methods used in performance forecasting. But the regression analysis is one of the most popularly used quantitative techniques.

Higher multiple correlation ensures greater accuracy in estimating the value of dependent variable on the basis of predictor variables in the regression model variables. Due to this reason multiple correlation is computed in regression analysis to indicate the efficiency of regression model. It is customary to show the value of multiple correlation along with regression equation. One can see that many researchers, while suggesting a regression model for estimating fat% on the basis of skin fold measurement, do show the value of multiple correlation. Any regression model having higher multiple correlation gives better estimate in comparison to that of other models. We will see an explanation of multiple correlation while discussing a solved example later in this chapter.

9.2 UNDERSTANDING REGRESSION EQUATION

Regression equation is a linear equation developed for estimating the value of dependent variable on the basis of some independent variables. The regression equation is of the form

$$Y = a + b_1 X_1 + b_2 X_2 + b_3 X_3 + b_4 X_4$$

where

Y is a dependent variable
X_1, X_2, X_3, and X_4 are the independent variables, and
a, b_1, b_2, b_3, and b_4 are the regression coefficients

While doing regression analysis using SPSS, regression coefficients are generated along with other statistics in the output. Significance of these regression coefficients is tested by means of t-test. A regression coefficient is significant at 5% level if its significance value (p value) provided in the output is less than 0.05. Significance of regression coefficient indicates that the corresponding variable significantly explains variation in the dependent variable and contributes to the regression model.

9.2.1 Methods of Regression Analysis

In a study based on regression analysis, independent variables are selected on the basis of either literature or some known information. In doing so, a large number of independent variables are studied; and therefore, there is a need to identify only those independent variables that explain maximum variation in the dependent variable. This can be done by using any of the following two methods: "stepwise regression" or "backward regression."

9.2.1.1 Stepwise Regression In stepwise regression analysis, independent variables are selected one by one depending upon relative importance in the regression model. In other words, the first entered variable in the model is the one that has largest contribution in explaining variation in the dependent variable. A variable is included in the model only if its regression coefficient is significant at 5% level. Thus, if the stepwise regression method is used for regression analysis, the variables are selected one by one, and finally the regression coefficients of the retained variables are generated in the output. These regression coefficients are used in developing the required regression equation.

9.2.1.2 Backward Regression In this method, a regression model is developed by including all the independent variables taken in the study, and then these variables are dropped one by one on the basis of their least contribution in the model. A variable is dropped if its regression coefficient is not significant at 10% level. Thus, we get several models having different number of independent variables. Robustness of these models is determined on the basis of R^2, where R is the multiple correlation.

9.2.2 Multiple Correlation

Multiple correlation determines the strength of relationship between dependent variable and a group of independent variables. Thus, it is an indicator of robustness of a regression model. The multiple correlation is represented by "R," and the generalized formula is given as follows:

$$R_{12.345...n} = \sqrt{1 - \left(1 - r_{12}^2\right)\left(1 - r_{13.2}^2\right)\left(1 - r_{14.23}^2\right)\cdots\left(1 - r_{1n.23...(n-1)}^2\right)}$$

The limits of multiple correlation are 0 to +1. It is computed with the help of product moment correlation coefficients; and therefore, it also measures linear relationship only.

In regression analysis, another statistic R^2 is also computed for assessing the validity of a model. R^2 can be defined as the variance explained in the dependent variable by the independent variables in a model. If in the regression model R^2 is 0.6, it means that all independent variables together in the model explain 60% of the variability in the dependent variable.

9.3 APPLICATION OF REGRESSION ANALYSIS

Researchers are constantly engaged in finding ways and means to improve performance in sports. This is done by conducting an exploratory study where the performance is estimated on the basis of certain independent parameters. For instance, to identify parameters that are required in estimating high jump performance of an athlete, a regression study may be planned. Similarly, in estimating fat% on the basis of body girths, one may opt for regression analysis.

Regression analysis may provide knowledge about the independent variables, which may be used for developing training schedule. Further, it may be used to estimate the value of dependent variable at some point of time if the values of independent variables are known. This is more relevant in a situation where the dependent variable is difficult to measure. For instance, fat% of the subjects in field situation cannot be assessed by underwater weighing, and therefore regression analysis may be useful in this situation in developing an appropriate model for estimating fat% on the basis of some parameters of body girths and skin fold measurements.

9.4 MULTIPLE REGRESSION ANALYSIS WITH SPSS

Example 9.1

Consider a study on badminton players in which a regression model was developed for estimating playing ability on the basis of physical and anthropometric variables. The data on 25 badminton players were recorded, which is shown in Table 9.1. Let us see how the regression equation can be developed for estimating the playing ability.

Solution: In order to get the solution, the following needs to be done:

1. Use "stepwise regression" method in SPSS to get the regression coefficients of the retained independent variables in the model for developing regression equation.
2. Test the significance of regression coefficients using t-test and significance value (p) in the output.
3. Test the regression model for its significance through the F-test using its significance value (p) in the output.
4. Use the value of R^2 in output for testing robustness of the model.

The steps involved in regression analysis with SPSS have been explained in the sections that follow.

9.4.1 Computation in Regression Analysis

9.4.1.1 Preparations of Data File Data file needs to be prepared before using SPSS commands for the computation of regression coefficients. After starting the SPSS as discussed in Chapter 1, select the 'Type in data' option.

9.4.1.2 Defining Variables There are 14 variables in this example which need to be defined along with their properties. Since all the variables are quantitative in

TABLE 9.1 Data on Physical and Anthropometric Variables Along with Playing Ability of Badminton Players

S.N.	Playing Ability (X_1)	Age (years) (X_2)	Height (cm) (X_3)	Weight (kg) (X_4)	Arm Length (cm) (X_5)	Leg Length (cm) (X_6)	Trunk Length (cm) (X_7)	Hand Girth (cm) (X_8)	Thigh Girth (cm) (X_9)	Calf Girth (cm) (X_{10})	Shoulder Width (s) (X_{11})	Hip Width (kg) (X_{12})	50 Meter Sprint (X_{13})	Explosive Strength (X_{14})
1	83	32	180	68.5	72	91	83	31	52	36	43	36	7.30	41
2	87	30	184	64.5	76	94	90	27	54	36	43	31	6.90	50
3	87	26	176	66.6	78	95	85	31	53	34	44	31	6.82	45
4	79	20	168	76.8	78	89	80	28	53	35	42	35	7.14	36
5	86	23	177	76.5	79	90	87	30	55	40	45	33	6.75	53
6	87	36	180	97.0	77	89	91	37	54	41	48	35	6.90	50
7	73	19	171	65.3	76	85	86	27	54	34	42	34	7.10	33
8	72	18	163	61.0	76	84	79	28	56	36	42	32	7.18	33
9	75	22	168	65.5	81	88	78	33	52	37	43	30	7.01	35
10	66	21	163	74.0	70	85	79	28	57	39	42	36	7.29	33
11	60	20	162	74.2	72	84	78	27	50	36	43	34	7.32	34
12	72	22	167	59.7	75	84	83	28	51	35	43	32	7.08	33
13	79	24	173	69.5	80	85	87	29	54	36	38	31	7.00	33
14	85	23	177	67.3	84	88	89	25	52	35	35	35	6.92	38
15	75	27	172	78.2	73	91	80	32	53	36	42	36	7.00	42
16	86	19	180	67.8	86	88	92	27	50	34	43	35	6.90	33
17	87	31	188	78.8	81	95	92	28	54	36	48	36	6.80	45
18	76	18	181	52.0	74	96	86	24	46	33	38	31	7.90	47
19	88	25	176	72.8	82	88	88	28	51	34	44	37	6.76	38
20	91	24	187	73.5	85	94	92	29	50	34	43	35	6.90	55
21	79	23	181	68.7	73	96	84	26	54	33	41	34	7.20	59
22	81	24	175	67.3	77	88	86	27	53	34	42	33	7.10	38
23	93	19	180	61.5	80	90	91	24	47	33	39	32	6.09	40
24	68	22	175	65.5	72	91	84	33	52	38	43	30	7.30	33
25	60	24	166	67.0	71	88	77	26	53	36	44	34	7.30	29

nature, they are treated as scale variables. The procedure of defining the variables and their characteristics in SPSS is as follows:

1. Click on **Variable View** to define variables and their properties.
2. Write short name of the variables as *PlaAbl, Age, Ht, Wt, ArmLength, LegLength, TrunkLength, HandGirth, ThighGirth, CalfGirth, ShoulderWidth, HipWidth, FiftyMt* and *ExploStren* under the column heading "Name."
3. Under the column heading "Label," full name of these variables may be defined as Playing Ability, Age, Height, Weight, Arm Length, Leg Length, Trunk Length, Hand Girth, Thigh Girth, Calf Girth, Shoulder Width, Hip Width, 50 meter, and Explosive Strength, respectively. Readers have the liberty to choose some other names of these variables as well.
4. Under the column heading "Measure," select the 'Scale' option for all the variables as all these variables are quantitative in nature.
5. Use default entries in rest of the columns.

After defining variables in the **Variable View**, the screen shall look like as shown in Figure 9.1.

9.4.1.3 Entering Data Once all the 14 variables are defined in the **Variable View**, click on **Data View** on the left corner at the bottom of the screen, shown in Figure 9.1, to open the format for entering data. For each variable, data can be entered column-wise. After data entry the screen will look like as shown in Figure 9.2. Save this data file in the desired location before further processing.

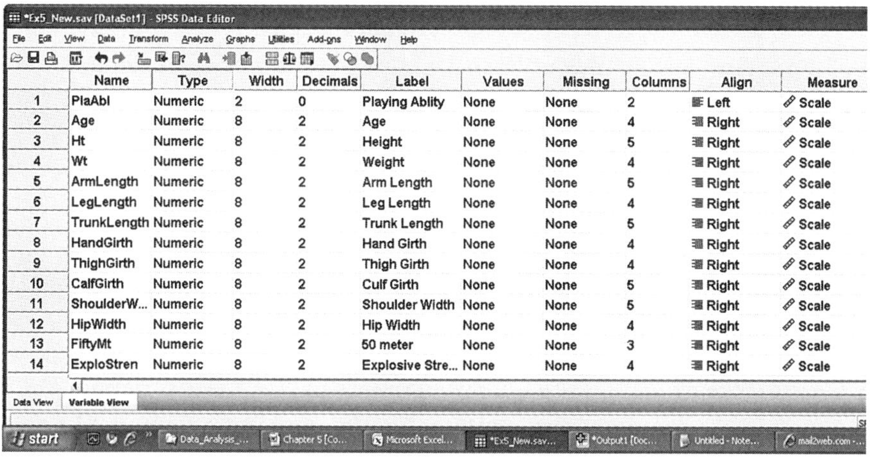

	Name	Type	Width	Decimals	Label	Values	Missing	Columns	Align	Measure
1	PlaAbl	Numeric	2	0	Playing Ability	None	None	2	Left	Scale
2	Age	Numeric	8	2	Age	None	None	4	Right	Scale
3	Ht	Numeric	8	2	Height	None	None	5	Right	Scale
4	Wt	Numeric	8	2	Weight	None	None	4	Right	Scale
5	ArmLength	Numeric	8	2	Arm Length	None	None	5	Right	Scale
6	LegLength	Numeric	8	2	Leg Length	None	None	4	Right	Scale
7	TrunkLength	Numeric	8	2	Trunk Length	None	None	5	Right	Scale
8	HandGirth	Numeric	8	2	Hand Girth	None	None	4	Right	Scale
9	ThighGirth	Numeric	8	2	Thigh Girth	None	None	4	Right	Scale
10	CalfGirth	Numeric	8	2	Culf Girth	None	None	5	Right	Scale
11	ShoulderW...	Numeric	8	2	Shoulder Width	None	None	5	Right	Scale
12	HipWidth	Numeric	8	2	Hip Width	None	None	4	Right	Scale
13	FiftyMt	Numeric	8	2	50 meter	None	None	3	Right	Scale
14	ExploStren	Numeric	8	2	Explosive Stre...	None	None	4	Right	Scale

FIGURE 9.1 Defining variables along with their characteristics.

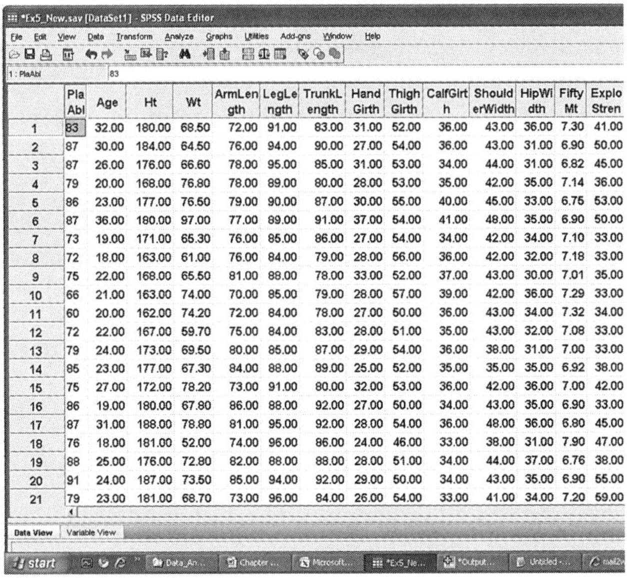

	Pla Abl	Age	Ht	Wt	ArmLen gth	LegLe ngth	TrunkL ength	Hand Girth	Thigh Girth	CalfGirt h	Should erWidth	HipWi dth	Fifty Mt	Explo Stren
1	83	32.00	180.00	68.50	72.00	91.00	83.00	31.00	52.00	36.00	43.00	36.00	7.30	41.00
2	87	30.00	184.00	64.50	76.00	94.00	90.00	27.00	54.00	36.00	43.00	31.00	6.90	50.00
3	87	26.00	176.00	66.60	78.00	95.00	85.00	31.00	53.00	34.00	44.00	31.00	6.82	45.00
4	79	20.00	168.00	76.80	78.00	89.00	80.00	28.00	53.00	35.00	42.00	35.00	7.14	36.00
5	86	23.00	177.00	76.50	79.00	90.00	87.00	30.00	55.00	40.00	45.00	33.00	6.75	53.00
6	87	36.00	180.00	97.00	77.00	89.00	91.00	37.00	54.00	41.00	48.00	35.00	6.90	50.00
7	73	19.00	171.00	65.30	76.00	85.00	86.00	27.00	54.00	34.00	42.00	34.00	7.10	33.00
8	72	18.00	163.00	61.00	76.00	84.00	79.00	28.00	56.00	36.00	42.00	32.00	7.18	33.00
9	75	22.00	168.00	65.50	81.00	88.00	78.00	33.00	52.00	37.00	43.00	30.00	7.01	35.00
10	66	21.00	163.00	74.00	70.00	85.00	79.00	28.00	57.00	39.00	42.00	36.00	7.29	33.00
11	60	20.00	162.00	74.20	72.00	84.00	78.00	27.00	50.00	36.00	43.00	34.00	7.32	34.00
12	72	22.00	167.00	59.70	75.00	84.00	83.00	28.00	51.00	35.00	43.00	32.00	7.08	33.00
13	79	24.00	173.00	69.50	80.00	85.00	87.00	29.00	54.00	36.00	38.00	31.00	7.00	33.00
14	85	23.00	177.00	67.30	84.00	88.00	89.00	25.00	52.00	35.00	35.00	35.00	6.92	38.00
15	75	27.00	172.00	78.20	73.00	91.00	80.00	32.00	53.00	36.00	42.00	36.00	7.00	42.00
16	86	19.00	180.00	67.80	86.00	88.00	92.00	27.00	50.00	34.00	43.00	35.00	6.90	33.00
17	87	31.00	188.00	78.80	81.00	95.00	92.00	28.00	54.00	36.00	48.00	36.00	6.80	45.00
18	76	18.00	181.00	52.00	74.00	96.00	86.00	24.00	46.00	33.00	38.00	31.00	7.90	47.00
19	88	25.00	176.00	72.80	82.00	88.00	88.00	28.00	51.00	34.00	44.00	37.00	6.76	38.00
20	91	24.00	187.00	73.50	85.00	94.00	92.00	29.00	50.00	34.00	43.00	35.00	6.90	55.00
21	79	23.00	181.00	68.70	73.00	96.00	84.00	26.00	54.00	33.00	41.00	34.00	7.20	59.00

FIGURE 9.2   Screen showing data entered for all the variables in the data view.

9.4.1.4   SPSS Commands   After entering all data in the **Data View**, do the following steps for regression analysis:

1. *Initiating SPSS commands for regression analysis*: In **Data View**, click on the following commands in sequence:

   Analyze → Regression → Linear

   The screen shall look like as shown in Figure 9.3.

2. *Selecting variables*: After clicking on **Linear** option, you will be directed to the next screen as shown in Figure 9.4 for selecting variables for the regression analysis. Select *Playing Ability* (dependent variable) from left panel and bring it to the "Dependent" section in the right panel. Select all independent variables from left panel and bring them to the "Independent(s)" section on the right panel.

   Either the variable selection is made one by one or all at once. The arrow tag is used to transfer the variable from left to right panel. After selection of variables, the screen shall *look like as sh*own in Figure 9.4.

3. *Selecting options for computation*: After selecting the variables, option needs to be defined for the regression analysis. Do the following on the screen shown in Figure 9.4:

   (a) Click on **Statistics** command for getting the screen shown in Figure 9.5. Check 'R squared change,' 'Descriptive,' and 'Part and partial correlations' options.

   (b) By default, the options "Estimates" and "Model fit" are checked. Ensure that they remain checked.

(c) Click on **Continue**, you will be taken back to the screen shown in Figure 9.4. *Checking 'R squared change' option shall provide the values of R^2 and adjusted R^2 in the output. Similarly, checking the option 'Descriptive' shall provide the values of mean and standard deviations along with correlation matrix of all the variables. Whereas checking the option 'Part and partial correlations' shall provide partial correlations of various orders between*

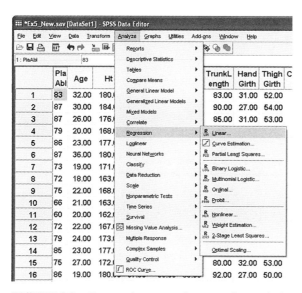

FIGURE 9.3 Command sequence for regression analysis.

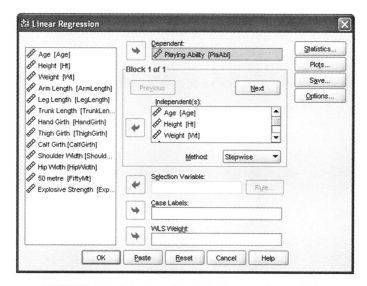

FIGURE 9.4 Selection of variables in regression analysis.

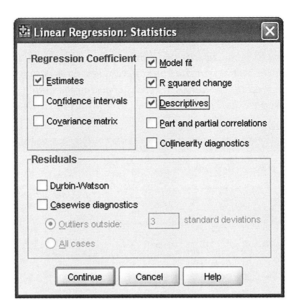

FIGURE 9.5   Selection of options in computing different outputs in regression analysis.

playing ability and other variables. Readers are advised to try other options and see what changes they get in their output.

(d) In the option "Method" shown in Figure 9.4, select 'Stepwise' and click on **OK**. This will generate the required results.

4. *Getting output*: Results will be generated in a separate window of the SPSS from which the relevant output can be copied by using right click of the mouse and pasted in the word file. The output panel shall have the following results:

(a) Descriptive statistics

(b) Correlation matrix along with significance level

(c) Model summary along with the values of R and R^2

(d) ANOVA table showing F values for all the models

(e) Regression coefficients of selected variables in different models along with their t values and partial correlations

In this example, all the outputs so generated by the SPSS have been shown in Tables 9.2, 9.3, 9.4, 9.5, and 9.6.

9.4.2   Interpretation of Findings

From the outputs obtained, the following conclusions can be drawn:

1. The values of mean and standard deviation for all the variables are shown in Table 9.2. These values can be used for further analysis in the study.

2. In Table 9.3, correlation matrix including significance level (p value) for each correlation coefficient at 0.05 level has been shown. Significance has been

TABLE 9.2 Descriptive Statistics for Different Variables of Badminton Players

Variables	Mean	SD	N
Playing ability	79.00	9.170	25
Age	23.68	4.598	25
Height	174.80	7.371	25
Weight	69.58	8.495	25
Arm length	77.12	4.484	25
Leg length	89.44	3.863	25
Trunk length	85.08	4.890	25
Hand girth	28.52	3.016	25
Thigh girth	52.40	2.500	25
Calf girth	35.64	2.099	25
Shoulder width	42.40	2.799	25
Hip width	33.52	2.104	25
50 meter	7.04	0.3172	25
Explosive strength	40.24	8.192	25

tested for one-tailed test. Correlation coefficient with asterisk mark (*) indicates that it is significant at 5% level.

For one-tail test, value of correlation coefficient required for its significance at 0.01 level and 23 (N − 2) df is 0.462 and at 0.05 level is 0.337. These values can be obtained by using Table A.6. Thus, all those correlation coefficients having values more than 0.462 are significant at 1% level. Such correlation coefficients have been shown with two asterisks (**). Readers may also show the correlation matrix by writing the upper diagonal values only.

3. It can be seen in Table 9.3 that playing ability is significantly related with height, arm length, leg length, trunk length, and 50-meter at 1% level, whereas with age and explosive strength at 5% level.

4. Five regression models have been presented in Table 9.4. For the fifth model, the value of R^2 is 0.859, which is maximum; hence, this model shall be used to develop the regression equation. It can be seen from Table 9.6 that in the fifth model, three independent variables, namely, 50-meter distance, height, and arm length have been identified; and therefore, the regression equation shall be developed by using these three variables only. Since R^2 for this model is 0.859, these three independent variables explain 85.9% variability in the playing ability of badminton players. Thus, this model is quite appropriate to estimate playing ability.

5. In Table 9.5, F values for all the models have been shown. Since F value for the fifth model is quite high and significant, it may be concluded that the model selected is highly efficient.

6. Regression coefficients in all the models have been shown in Table 9.6. In the fifth model, t values for all the three regression coefficients are significant as the significance value (p value) associated with them is less than 0.05. Thus, it

TABLE 9.3 Correlation Matrix

	Playing Ability	Age	Height	Weight	Arm Length	Leg Length	Trunk Length	Hand Girth	Thigh Girth	Calf Girth	Shoulder Width	Hip Width	50 Meter	Explosive Strength
Pearson correlation														
Playing ability	1	0.372*	0.794**	0.184	0.714**	0.487**	0.826**	0.041	−0.187	−0.201	0.050	0.134	−0.663**	0.585*
Age		1	0.466**	0.615**	−0.030	0.351*	0.305	0.568**	0.291	0.411*	0.538**	0.294	−0.182	0.418*
Height			1	0.109	0.457*	0.777**	0.849**	−0.016	−0.285	−0.215	0.109	0.101	−0.314	0.716**
Weight				1	0.084	−0.017	0.150	0.604**	0.408*	0.605**	0.579**	0.571**	−0.252	0.266
Arm length					1	0.079	0.665**	−0.070	−0.239	−0.248	−0.074	0.086	−0.582**	0.143
Leg length						1	0.397*	−0.003	−0.235	−0.247	0.114	−0.055	−0.014	0.767**
Trunk length							1	−0.082	−0.262	−0.168	0.049	0.105	−0.520*	0.474**
Hand girth								1	0.347*	0.682**	0.567*	−0.025	−0.049	0.103
Thigh girth									1	0.553**	0.328	0.157	0.014	−0.027
Calf girth										1	0.472**	0.035	0.029	−0.012
Shoulder width											1	0.239	−0.140	0.181
Hip width												1	−0.085	0.075
50 meter													1	−0.157
Explosive strength														1

* Correlation is significant at the level 0.05 (one-tailed). Significance value of the correlation coefficient at 0.05 level with 23 df (one-tailed)=0.337.

** Correlation is significant at the level 0.01 (one-tailed). Significance value of the correlation coefficient at 0.01 level with 23 df (one-tailed)=0.462.

TABLE 9.4   Model Summary Along with the Values of R and R²

Model	R	R²	Adjusted R²	Std. Error of the Estimate	Change Statistics				
					R Square Change	F Change	df1	df2	Sig. F Change
1	0.826[a]	0.682	0.669	5.278	0.682	49.437	1	23	0.000
2	0.870[b]	0.757	0.735	4.721	0.075	6.748	1	22	0.016
3	0.909[c]	0.826	0.801	4.086	0.069	8.372	1	21	0.009
4	0.906[d]	0.820	0.804	4.062	−0.006	0.742	1	21	0.399
5	0.927[e]	0.859	0.839	3.678	0.039	5.829	1	21	0.025

[a] Predictors: (Constant), Trunk length.
[b] Predictors: (Constant), Trunk length, 50 meter.
[c] Predictors: (Constant), Trunk length, 50 meter, height.
[d] Predictors: (Constant), 50 meter, height.
[e] Predictors: (Constant), 50 meter, height, arm length.

TABLE 9.5   ANOVA Table Showing F Values for All the Models

Model		Sum of Squares	df	Mean Square	F	Sig.
1	Regression	1377.250	1	1377.250	49.437	0.000[a]
	Residual	640.750	23	27.859		
	Total	2018.000	24			
2	Regression	1527.649	2	763.825	34.270	0.000[b]
	Residual	490.351	22	22.289		
	Total	2018.000	24			
3	Regression	1667.419	3	555.806	33.293	0.000[c]
	Residual	350.581	21	16.694		
	Total	2018.000	24			
4	Regression	1655.036	2	827.518	50.158	0.000[d]
	Residual	362.964	22	16.498		
	Total	2018.000	24			
5	Regression	1733.891	3	577.964	42.720	0.000[e]
	Residual	284.109	21	13.529		
	Total	2018.000	24			

[a] Predictors: (Constant), Trunk length.
[b] Predictors: (Constant), Trunk length, 50 meter.
[c] Predictors: (Constant), Trunk length, 50 meter, height.
[d] Predictors: (Constant), 50 meter, height.
[e] Predictors: (Constant), 50 meter, height, arm length.

may be concluded that the variables 50-meter, height, and arm length significantly explain the variations in the playing ability. In order to know which is the most contributing predictor in the model out of these three variables one should look for the Beta coefficients in Table 9.6. Larger the absolute value of Beta coefficient more is the contribution of that variable in the model. Thus, height is the most contributory predictor and 50 meter performance is the second most important predictor in the model.

TABLE 9.6 Regression Coefficients of Selected Variables in Different Models Along with Their t Values and Partial Correlations

Model		Unstandardized Coefficients		Standardized Coefficients			Correlations		
		B	Std. Error	Beta	t	Sig. (p Value)	Zero-Order	Partial	Part
1	(Constant)	−52.807	18.776		−2.812	0.010			
	Trunk length	1.549	0.220	0.826	7.031	0.000	0.826	0.826	0.826
2	(Constant)	38.761	39.047		0.993	0.332			
	Trunk length	1.237	0.231	0.660	5.362	0.000	0.826	0.753	0.564
	50 meter	−9.240	3.557	−0.320	−2.598	0.016	−0.663	−0.484	−0.273
3	(Constant)	22.195	34.274		0.648	0.524			
	Trunk length	0.322	0.374	0.172	0.861	0.399	0.826	0.185	0.078
	50 meter	−11.865	3.209	−0.410	−3.697	0.001	−0.663	−0.628	−0.336
	Height	0.646	0.223	0.519	2.893	0.009	0.794	0.534	0.263
4	(Constant)	31.023	32.514		0.954	0.350			
	50 meter	−13.262	2.753	−0.459	−4.817	0.000	−0.663	−0.716	−0.436
	Height	0.808	0.118	0.650	6.824	0.000	0.794	0.824	0.617
5	(Constant)	−18.532	35.891		−0.516	0.611			
	50 meter	−9.604	2.917	−0.332	−3.292	0.003	−0.663	−0.583	−0.270
	Height	0.710	0.115	0.571	6.186	0.000	0.794	0.804	0.507
	Arm length	0.532	0.220	0.260	2.414	0.025	0.714	0.466	0.198

Regression equation: Using regression coefficients (B) of the fifth model shown in the Table 9.6, the regression equation can be developed which is as follows:

Playing ability $= -18.532 - 9.604 \times$ (50-meter timing) $+ 0.710 \times$ (Height) $+ 0.532 \times$ (Arm length)

To conclude, it may be interpreted that the above regression equation is quite reliable as the value of R^2 is 0.859. In other words, the three variables selected in the regression equation explain 85.9% of the total variability in the playing ability which is quite good. Since F value for this regression model is highly significant, the model is reliable. At the same time, all the regression coefficients in this model are highly significant; and therefore, it may be interpreted that all the three variables selected in the model, namely, 50 meter timing, height, and arm length are quite appropriate in estimating the playing ability of a badminton player.

9.5   SUMMARY OF SPSS COMMANDS FOR REGRESSION ANALYSIS

1. Start SPSS by using the following commands:

   Start → All Programs → SPSS Inc → SPSS 20.0

2. Create data file by choosing the 'Type in data' option. Define variables and their characteristics by clicking on the **Variable View**. Once the variables are defined, type data for these variables by clicking on **Data View**.

3. Use the following command sequence for selecting variables from left panel and bring them to the right panel by clicking the arrow.

   Analyze → Regression → Linear

4. Select the dependent variable from left panel and bring it to the "Dependent" section of the right panel. Select all other independent variables from left panel to the "Independent(s)" section of the right panel.

5. After selecting variables for regression analysis click on the **Statistics** option. Check 'R squared change,' 'Descriptive,' and 'Part and partial correlations' options. Click on **Continue**.

6. In the "Method" option, select 'Stepwise' and then click on **OK** to get the different outputs for regression analysis.

9.6   EXERCISE

9.6.1   Short Answer Questions

Note: Write answer to each question in not more than 200 words.

Q.1   What do you mean by regression analysis? Explain the difference between simple regression and multiple regression models.

Q.2   Differentiate between stepwise regression and backward regression.

Q.3   What is the role of R^2 in regression analysis? Explain multiple correlation and its order.

Q.4   Explain a situation where regression analysis can be used.

Q.5   How will you know that the variables that are selected in the regression analysis are valid?

Q.6   What strategy is adopted in dropping variables in backward regression method?

9.6.2   Multiple Choice Questions

Note: Questions 1–10 have four alternative answers for each question. Tick mark the one that you consider the closest to the correct answer.

1   The range of multiple correlation, R is
   (a) −1 to +1
   (b) −1 to 0
   (c) 0 to +1
   (d) None of the above

2   SPSS commands for multiple regression analysis is
   (a) Analyze → Linear → Regression
   (b) Analyze → Regression → Linear
   (c) Analyze → Linear
   (d) Analyze → Regression

3   Choose the most appropriate statement
   (a) R^2 is a measure of multiple correlation.
   (b) R^2 is used for selecting variables in the regression model.
   (c) R^2 indicates the amount of variability explained in the dependent variable by the independent variables.
   (d) All of the above are correct.

4   If p value for the correlation between playing ability and explosive strength is 0.019, what conclusion can be drawn?
   (a) Correlation is significant at 1% level.
   (b) Correlation is significant at 5% level.
   (c) Correlation is not significant at 5% level.
   (d) All above statements are wrong.

5   Regression analysis
   (a) Measures improvement
   (b) Establishes cause and effect

(c) Estimates any independent variable

(d) Establishes a relationship between two variables

6   In regression analysis, four models have been developed. Which model in your opinion is the most appropriate?

Models	No. of Independent Variables	R^2
(a) Model I	5	0.88
(b) Model II	4	0.87
(c) Model III	3	0.86
(d) Model IV	2	0.65

7   In a regression analysis, the following results were obtained:

Independent Variables	B Coefficient	p Value
Agility	1.5	0.04
Reaction time	0.2	0.10
Heart rate	3.1	0.41
Fat%	1.2	0.03

Choose the most appropriate statement

(a) Both Agility and Reaction time are significant at 0.05 level in the model.

(b) Both Agility and Heart rate are significant at 0.05 level in the model.

(c) Both Reaction time and Heart rate are significant at 0.05 level in the model.

(d) Both Agility and Fat% are significant at 0.05 level in the model.

8   Choose the correct statement about B and β coefficients

(a) "B" is a unstandardized coefficient and "β" is a standardized coefficient.

(b) "β" is a unstandardized coefficient and "B" is a standardized coefficient.

(c) Both "B" and "β" are standardized coefficients.

(d) Both "B" and "β" are unstandardized coefficients.

9.6.3 Assignment

1. The data in Table 9.7 shows the measurements on physical and physiological parameters along with the playing ability of badminton players. Develop a regression equation and explain its significance and validity.

TABLE 9.7 Data of Badminton Players on Their Physical and Physiological Parameters and Playing Ability

S.N.	Playing Ability	Agility (sec)	Flexibility (cm)	Reaction Time (sec)	Heart Rate (beat/min)	Excretion of Sweat (kg)	Hb (g/dl)	Fat% (%)	LBW (kg)	VO_2 max (ml/kg)
1	84	11.9	17	0.11	66	0.8	15.0	9.59	61.65	35
2	87	12.0	17	0.12	58	1.1	14.7	8.53	58.81	36
3	87	12.0	18	0.11	60	0.8	14.0	7.96	55.86	35
4	78	12.0	18	0.11	58	0.8	13.9	11.03	68.14	37
5	86	11.9	19	0.11	60	0.9	14.2	10.09	65.30	38
6	87	12.1	19	0.11	62	0.7	14.3	13.11	64.00	35
7	72	12.5	17	0.13	59	1.2	14.5	10.30	58.97	35
8	72	11.5	16	0.12	61	1.1	13.9	10.09	55.29	34
9	75	12.0	17	0.13	56	1.0	13.9	10.57	58.75	35
10	67	12.3	15	0.13	58	1.1	14.2	11.32	68.27	28
12	60	12.0	16	0.14	61	0.7	15.0	11.90	58.60	25
13	72	13.0	18	0.13	68	0.8	14.6	8.53	54.60	33
14	79	12.0	15	0.13	60	0.8	13.8	11.50	61.80	35
15	86	11.1	16	0.11	62	1.1	14.7	9.07	61.15	31
16	75	11.0	15	0.13	64	1.3	13.4	11.30	69.83	33
17	86	11.3	16	0.11	62	0.9	14.4	7.96	62.40	30
18	87	12.1	17	0.11	57	1.1	13.7	10.20	62.20	34
19	76	12.2	16	0.13	59	1.2	15.0	7.90	48.12	46
20	87	11.9	20	0.11	60	1.5	14.2	9.60	61.40	50
21	91	11.2	21	0.11	58	1.4	14.9	7.95	59.20	35
22	79	12.0	18	0.13	62	0.9	14.2	9.52	62.19	38
23	81	12.0	19	0.13	60	0.8	14.3	10.10	60.50	39
24	93	11.2	20	0.13	56	1.1	14.8	10.50	58.56	30
25	68	12.5	17	0.13	58	1.0	13.5	9.20	48.15	27
26	61	12.3	15	0.12	61	0.9	14.7	8.50	61.15	29

9.7 CASE STUDY ON REGRESSION ANALYSIS

Objective

A sport scientist was interested to develop a model through which playing ability of basketball players could be estimated on the basis of some skill parameters. A sample of 30 national basketball players was chosen and the data on five skill tests was collected on them. Their playing ability was measured during a tournament. The data so obtained is shown in Table 9.8. Let us see how this analysis can be carried out.

Research Questions

The following research questions were investigated:

1. Whether regression model developed for estimating the playing ability would be significant.
2. Whether independent variables selected in the model significantly contribute to the model.
3. Whether any particular skill could be identified which is the most contributing predictor in the model.

Data Format

The format used for preparing data file in SPSS is shown in the Table 9.8.

Analyzing Data

In order to investigate the three research issues, regression analysis was done in SPSS. A regression model was developed by using the unstandardized regression coefficients obtained in the output. The developed model was tested for its significance. The regression coefficients were tested for its significance in order to ensure the contribution of the independent variables in the model. Since this was the exploratory study, 'Stepwise' method was chosen for identifying the independent variables in the model. The outputs are shown in Tables 9.9 and 9.11. Finally, adjusted R^2 was reported to explain the worth of the developed regression model.

The regression analysis was done by using the commands; **Analyze, Regression**, and **Linear** in sequence in SPSS. By selecting the dependent and independent variables and choosing the Stepwise procedure the output of the regression analysis was generated. Further by checking the option 'R Squared Changed' in **Statistics** command the value of R^2 as generated is shown in Table 9.10.

TABLE 9.8   Data Format Used in SPSS

S.N.	Playing_ Abl_X1	Accuracy_ X2	Dribbling_ X3	Dribble_ X4	Distance_ Throw_X5	Wall_ Bounce_X6
1	9	9	10.75	19	42	67
2	7	6	10.05	17	45	68
3	6	8	11.47	16	39	60
4	6	7	9.54	18	38	68
5	4	6	11.31	21	34	70
6	7	8	10.62	19	38	71
7	7	5	12.05	16	42	72
8	8	6	10.11	16	41	71
9	5	4	11.00	18	39	65
10	5	6	10.82	17	40	70
11	7	7	9.81	17	42	66
12	5	5	12.20	19	41	61
13	8	7	11.63	21	38	63
14	5	4	10.60	20	41	64
15	5	8	10.73	20	38	64
16	5	5	11.25	17	42	57
17	5	4	11.38	19	39	67
18	6	5	10.61	21	42	63
19	8	7	9.60	16	39	62
20	4	7	10.60	22	39	62
21	5	6	11.42	17	37	50
22	6	4	10.51	18	38	59
23	5	4	10.41	19	37	64
24	6	6	12.03	22	36	70
25	8	8	11.71	17	37	72
26	7	7	9.65	15	42	77
27	7	8	10.30	17	40	65
28	9	6	10.01	16	38	60
29	6	6	10.72	19	35	58
30	8	4	10.56	16	36	65

Playing_Abl: Playing ability (in score).
Accuracy: Accuracy in throws (in scores).
Dribbling: Dribbling speed (in sec).
Dribble: Dribble and Shoot test (in counts).
Distance_Throw: in mts.
Wall_Bounce: in sec.

TABLE 9.9   Regression Coefficients[a]

Model		Unstandardized Coefficients		Standardized Coefficients		
		B	Std. Error	Beta	t	Sig.
1	(Constant)	12.374	2.205		5.611	0.000
	Dribble-and-Shoot test	−0.334	0.121	−0.464	−2.770	0.010
2	(Constant)	10.038	2.280		4.403	0.000
	Dribble-and-Shoot test	−0.323	0.112	−0.449	−2.882	0.008
	Accuracy in throws	0.350	0.150	0.363	2.334	0.027

[a] Dependent variable: Playing ability.

TABLE 9.10   Model Summary

				Std. Error of	Change Statistics				
Model	R	R^2	Adjusted R^2	the Estimate	R Square Change	F Change	df1	df2	Sig. F Change
1	0.464[a]	0.215	0.187	1.27843	0.215	7.671	1	28	0.010
2	0.589[b]	0.347	0.298	1.18758	0.132	5.448	1	27	0.027

[a] Predictors: (constant), Dribble-and-Shoot test.
[b] Predictors: (constant), Dribble-and-Shoot test, accuracy in throws.

TABLE 9.11   ANOVA[a]

Model		Sum of Squares	df	Mean Square	F	Sig.
1	Regression	12.537	1	12.537	7.671	0.010[b]
	Residual	45.763	28	1.634		
	Total	58.300	29			
2	Regression	20.221	2	10.110	7.169	0.003[c]
	Residual	38.079	27	1.410		
	Total	58.300	29			

[a] Dependent variable: Playing ability.
[b] Predictors: (constant), Dribble-and-Shoot test.
[c] Predictors: (constant), Dribble-and-Shoot test, accuracy in throws.

Developing Regression Model

Table 9.9 shows the unstandardized (B) and standardized regression coefficients (Beta). By using the B coefficients, the following regression equation was developed:

Playing ability $= 10.038 - 0.323 \times$ (dribble-and-Shoot test) $+ 0.350 \times$ (Accuracy in throws)

It can be seen from the Table 9.9 that the regression coefficients for both the variables, that is, Dribble-and-Shoot ($p=0.008$) and Accuracy in throws ($p=0.027$) selected in the second model are significant. Thus, it may be concluded that these two variables contribute significantly to the developed model.

Testing Efficiency of the Model

Since '**Stepwise**' command was chosen in the analysis, two models were developed in the analysis. Since the value of R^2 for the second model is 0.589 which is higher than that of the first, that is, 0.464, the second model was chosen for developing the regression equation. Since adjusted R^2 for the model is 0.298, 29.8% variability of the Playing ability can be explained by the two independent variables selected in the model. F value for the regression of the second model in Table 9.11 is significant (0.003); therefore, it may be concluded that the developed model is significant. Further, the absolute value of beta coefficient for the Dribble-and-Shoot test (0.499) is higher than that of Accuracy in throws (0.363); hence, it is more useful in the model.

Reporting

- Only two independent variables Dribble and shoot and Accuracy in throws were found to be contributing to the model; hence, they were included in the model.
- The model is significant because F value for the model as shown in Table 9.11 is significant (p = 0.003)
- Since R^2 adjusted for the model is 0.298, only 29.8% variability of the Playing ability in basketball can be explained by this model.

Finally since the beta coefficient for the variable Dribble and shoot was higher, it was more useful in comparison to the Accuracy in throws in the model.

10

APPLICATION OF DISCRIMINANT FUNCTION ANALYSIS

LEARNING OBJECTIVES

After completing this chapter, you should be able to do the following:

- Learn the use of discriminant analysis (DA) in developing classification model in two groups
- Know the situation where DA can be used
- List the assumptions used in DA
- Understand different terms used in DA
- Learn the steps involved in using SPSS for DA
- Learn to apply discriminant analysis in explorative studies
- Understand to interpret the output obtained in DA
- Explain relative importance of variables in the model
- Know the procedure of developing discriminant function
- Explain the power of discriminant model in a study
- Learn to write the results of DA in standard format

Sports Research with Analytical Solution using SPSS®, First Edition. J. P. Verma.
© 2016 John Wiley & Sons, Inc. Published 2016 by John Wiley & Sons, Inc.
Companion website: www.wiley.com/go/Verma/Sportsresearch

10.1 INTRODUCTION

Discriminant function analysis, also known as discriminant analysis (DA), is used to classify a subject into one of the two groups on the basis of some independent traits. For instance, based on the maturity parameters, an individual may be classified in either junior or senior category. We often come across situations where classification strategy is required to be made. Many times, controversy arises during national and international tournaments regarding senior athletes playing in junior category on the basis of false testimony. Similarly, a coach may use his judgment to advice an athlete in opting for track or field event. During the match practice, one chooses a sport activity out of interest only and not because it suits them. In all these situations, DA can provide decision-making criteria.

DA is similar to the multiple regression analysis. The only difference is in the nature of dependent variable. In DA, the dependent variable is a dichotomous variable; whereas in multiple regression, it is a continuous variable.

In DA, only those independent variables that are found to have significant discriminating power in classifying a subject into any of the two groups are picked up. These identified independent variables are used to develop a discriminating function. On the basis of discriminant function so obtained, a criterion for classification is developed. The details of DA and the procedure of using SPSS in getting the solution have been discussed in the following sections.

10.2 BASICS OF DISCRIMINANT FUNCTION ANALYSIS

In discriminant analysis, a discriminant function is used to classify an individual or cases into two categories. If the function is effective for a set of data, the percentage of correct classification of cases in the classification table increases. Before discussing the procedure of this analysis we shall discuss the terminologies involved in it.

10.2.1 Discriminating Variables

These are the independent variables that construct a discriminant function. These variables are also known as predictors.

10.2.2 Dependent Variable

Dependent variable is also known as criterion variable. In SPSS, the dependent variable is known as grouping variable. It is the object of classification on the basis of independent variables. The dependent variable needs to be dichotomous.

10.2.3 Discriminant Function

A discriminant function is a latent variable, which is constructed as a linear combination of independent variables, such that

$$Z = a + b_1 X_1 + b_2 X_2 + \cdots + b_n X_n$$

where

b_1, b_2, …, b_n are discriminant coefficients,
X_1, X_2, …, X_n are discriminating variables, and
"a" is a constant.

The discriminant function is also known as canonical root.

10.2.4 Classification Matrix

A classification matrix is also known as confusion matrix, assignment matrix, or prediction matrix. It is used to assess the efficiency of DA. It tells us as to what percentage of the existing data points is correctly classified by the model developed in DA. This percentage is somewhat similar to R^2 (percentage of variation in the dependent variable explained by the model).

10.2.5 Stepwise Method of Discriminant Analysis

Discriminant function is developed either by using all independent variables or by identifying a few from a large set of independent variables. The choice of method depends upon whether the study is confirmatory or exploratory in nature. In exploratory study the independent variables are selected one by one in the model, depending upon its magnitude of contribution in the model. This method of identifying independent variables is known as stepwise method.

10.2.6 Power of Discriminating Variable

Power of discriminating variable (independent variable) refers to the capacity of the variable to discriminate cases into any of the two groups in the model. It can be determined by the coefficient of the discriminating variable in the model. SPSS provides these coefficients in the output and are named as standardized canonical discriminant function coefficients. The higher the value of coefficient, the better the discriminating power. Since these standardized coefficients are nothing but partial correlations that are free from units, a direct comparison of the coefficients can be made.

10.2.7 Canonical Correlation

The canonical correlation can be defined as the multiple correlation between the predictor variables and the discriminant function. In DA, it provides an index of overall model fit, which explains the proportion of variance explained (R^2).

10.2.8   Wilks' Lambda

The value of Wilks' lambda is the estimate of the variance of the dependent variable not explained by the independent variables in the model. Subtracting its value from 1 gives the value of eta square, which is the sign of robustness of the model. The value of Wilks' lambda lies in between 0 and 1, lesser its value, better is the model. If its value is less than 0.5, the discriminant model is considered to be good. Significance of Wilk's lambda is tested by the chi-square statistic.

10.3   ASSUMPTIONS IN DISCRIMINANT ANALYSIS

The following assumptions are made while using DA:

1. All variables have linear and homoscedastic relationships.
2. Dependent variable is a dichotomous variable.
3. The groups must be mutually exclusive, with every subject or case belonging to only one group.
4. All cases must be independent. One should not use correlated data like before–after, matched pairs data, etc.
5. Sample sizes of both the groups should not differ to a great extent. If the sample sizes are in the proportion 80 : 20, logistic regression may be preferred.
6. Sample size should be sufficient. As a guideline, there should be at least five to six times as many cases as independent variables.
7. No independent variable should have a zero variability in either of the groups formed by the dependent variable.

10.4   WHY TO USE DISCRIMINANT ANALYSIS

One may use DA for achieving one or more of the following objectives in a study:

1. Classifying subjects into groups
2. Testing a theory by observing whether cases are classified as predicted
3. Determining the percentage of variance in the dependent variable explained by the predictors
4. Assessing predictor's relative importance in discriminant model
5. Identifying and discarding those independent variables that do not have discriminating power in classification

10.5 STEPS IN DISCRIMINANT ANALYSIS

Applying DA requires the following steps:

1. The first step in the DA is to choose the independent variables having significant discriminant power. This is done either by taking all independent variables together or one by one in the analysis, and these can be done by choosing the option "Enter independents together" and "Use stepwise method," respectively in SPSS.

   In stepwise method, an independent variable is entered in the model if its corresponding regression coefficient is significant at 0.05 level. Thus, in developing discriminant function the model will enter only significant independent variables. The model so developed is required to be tested for its robustness.

2. In the second step, discriminant function model is developed by using the coefficients of independent variables and the value of constant in the "unstandardized canonical discriminant function coefficients" table generated in the SPSS output. This is similar to developing regression equation. This way the function so generated may be used to classify an individual into any of the two groups. The discriminant function shall look like as follows:

$$Z = a + b_1 X_1 + b_2 X_2 + \cdots + b_n X_n$$

   where

   "Z" is a discriminant function,

   X's are selected independent variables in the model,

   "a" is a constant, and

   b's are the discriminant coefficients.

3. The third step involves computing Wilks' lambda for testing the significance of discriminant function developed in the model. This acts as a sign of robustness of the discriminant model. The range of Wilk's lambda is from 0 and 1, and the lower value of it close to 0 indicates better discriminating power of the model. Further, significant value of chi-square indicates that the discrimination between two groups is highly significant.

   After selecting independent variables, the discriminant model is tested for its significance in classifying the subjects/cases correctly into groups. For this, SPSS generates a classification matrix. This is also known as confusion matrix. The matrix shows the number of correct and wrong classification of subjects in both the groups. High percentage of correct classification indicates the validity of the model. The level of accuracy shown in the classification matrix may not hold for all future classification of new subjects/cases.

4. In the fourth step, relative importance of independent variables selected in the model is reported. The SPSS generates the "standardized canonical

discriminant function coefficients". A variable having higher coefficient is more powerful in comparison to those having lesser value.

5. In fifth step, a criterion for classification is made by using the group centroids of both groups. The SPSS output provides the mean discriminant score (group centroid) in each group. The subject whose Z score is closer to the group centroid belongs to that group. In fact, a strategy can be developed for defining the group membership on the basis of the weighted means of the two group centroids. If equal number of cases is taken in both the groups of the dependent variable, then the weighted average of the group centroids will be just the average of the two. But in case the number of cases differs in both the groups, the weighted average can be computed using the following formula:

$$Z = \frac{n_1 \times \left(\text{Centroid}\_1\right) + n_2 \times \left(\text{Centroid}\_2\right)}{n_1 + n_2}$$

Here, n_1 and n_2 are the number of cases in the two groups, and Centroid_1 and Centroid_2 are the group centroids of the two groups.

10.6   APPLICATION OF DISCRIMINANT FUNCTION ANALYSIS

Consider an experiment in which a researcher is interested in identifying the discriminatory power of performance indicators between the players at guard and forward positions among national basketball players.

Sample consisting basketball players in the top performing teams during national championships may be drawn for the study. Further, only those players who play at guard and forward positions may be selected from the teams.

The data may be collected from each player by a trained group of observers on the parameters shown below:

Parameters of Study

1. Percent of success of three-point shots
2. Percent of success of free-throw shots
3. Percent of success of fast-break
4. Number of fouls made by
5. Number of fouls made on
6. Number of defensive rebounds
7. Number of offensive rebounds
8. Number of turn-over
9. Number of steals
10. Number of assists

11. Number of interceptions
12. Number of minutes played

Objectives

The objectives of this study may be described as follows:

- To identify independent variables having significant discriminating power in classifying a basketballer into guard or forward position specialist
- To develop a discriminant model for classifying a player into guard and forward position
- To test the validity of the model

Test

Discriminant function may be developed to solve the problem for discriminating players by game position.

Output in SPSS

The aforementioned objectives of the study can be achieved by using the five outputs generated in the SPSS as follows:

1. Box's M test
2. Standardized canonical discriminant function coefficients table
3. Unstandardized canonical discriminant function coefficients table
4. Functions at group centroids
5. Canonical correlation
6. Table of Wilks' lambda and chi-square test
7. Classification matrix.

The first output is used to test the assumption of variance–covariance matrix to be same in each group of the dependent variable. For this assumption to be true, Box's M test should not be significant. The second output provides the standardized coefficients of each variable. The variable having larger coefficient indicates more discriminating power. Thus, this output can be used to show the relative importance of variables in developing discriminant function.

The third output contains unstandardized coefficients of the variables selected in the model and are used to build the discriminant function for classifying subjects into groups.

The fourth output provides the group centroid of each group, which is used for developing criteria for defining the group membership.

The fifth output provides the canonical correlation which is an index of overall model fit. The value of Wilks' lambda in the sixth output explains the percentage variability of the dependent variable not explained by the predictor variables in the model, whereas its significance is tested by chi-square statistic. The seventh output provides the number of subjects classified correctly into groups by the model.

10.7   DISCRIMINANT ANALYSIS USING SPSS

Example 10.1

The data shown in Table 10.1 were obtained on 10 sub-junior and 10 junior male basketball players. Let us develop a discriminant function for classifying an individual into sub-junior or junior category. We shall test the significance of the model and discuss the efficiency of classification and relative importance of the independent variables retained in the model.

Solution: In this example, four things need to be done:

1. To develop a discriminant function for classifying an individual into sub-junior or junior category
2. To test the significance of the model
3. To find the efficiency of the model
4. To investigate the relative importance of the predictors retained in the model.

These issues shall be discussed using the outputs generated in the analysis. We shall first discuss the procedure of DA in SPSS.

10.7.1   Computation in Discriminant Analysis

10.7.1.1   Preparation of Data File   After starting the SPSS as discussed in Chapter 1, select the option 'Type in data.' The sequence of commands for starting SPSS on your computer is as follows:

Start → All Programs → SPSS Inc → SPSS 20.0 → Type in Data

Now you are ready for defining the variables row-wise.

10.7.1.2   Defining Variables   In this example, 12 variables need to be defined. Except *Category* that is nominal, all others variables are scale. Do the following:

1. Click **Variable View** in the left-hand bottom of the screen to define variables and their properties.
2. Write short name of these variables as *SBJ, Shut_run, Fifty_mt, Twelve_ min_R/W, Aner_cap, Wt, Ht, Leg_length, Calf_girth, Thigh_girth, Shl_width*, and *Category* under the column heading "Name."

TABLE 10.1 Data on Physical and Anthropometric Parameters on Junior and Senior College Male Basketballers

S.N.	SBJ (cm)	Shut_Run (s)	Fifty_Mt. (s)	Twelve_Min R/W (mt.)	Aner_Cap (s)	Wt (kg)	Ht (cm)	Leg_Len (cm)	Calf_Girth (cm)	Thigh_Girth (cm)	Shl_Width (cm)	Category
1	222	10.10	8.10	2810	57.55	39	137	72	26	36	41	Subjunior
2	210	10.20	7.92	2420	40.61	38	135	71	29	39	36	Subjunior
3	192	10.13	7.54	2755	45.30	32	143	70	28	36	36	Subjunior
4	199	11.01	8.26	2610	32.59	38	132	75	27	39	34	Subjunior
5	195	10.50	8.30	2205	36.74	32	130	72	25	33	36	Subjunior
6	210	10.22	7.41	2515	48.20	27	136	72	27	38	36	Subjunior
7	229	9.52	7.01	2702	51.30	31	145	76	28	40	37	Subjunior
8	215	10.45	7.15	2495	39.12	36	162	78	28	38	29	Subjunior
9	214	11.30	8.03	2535	31.09	32	144	77	26	38	33	Subjunior
10	223	10.12	8.40	2180	29.48	38	148	78	29	43	36	Subjunior
11	221	9.70	7.83	2418	52.40	38	145	76	31	45	38	Junior
12	212	9.88	6.95	2508	48.30	39	141	76	29	40	38	Junior
13	219	9.24	7.28	2416	45.30	42	158	74	29	42	39	Junior
14	208	9.14	7.48	2510	52.20	41	151	81	31	43	42	Junior
15	218	10.15	8.25	2520	44.53	45	156	76	27	42	36	Junior
16	211	9.35	7.45	2530	32.66	47	157	85	31	41	43	Junior
17	213	9.53	7.60	2405	25.22	49	158	74	31	45	44	Junior
18	213	10.08	7.20	2410	36.16	45	151	72	27	36	44	Junior
19	259	9.40	6.95	2730	59.23	49	157	81	32	45	45	Junior
20	222	9.12	7.30	2614	47.24	55	161	89	31	48	43	Junior

3. Under the column heading "Label," full name of these variables may be defined as *Standing broad jump, 4×10 Shuttle run, 50 Mt. timings, 12 min R/W, Anaerobic capacity, Weight, Height, Leg length, Calf girth, Thigh girth, Shoulder width*, and *Category of athlete*.

4. Under the column heading "Measure," select data type as 'Scale' for all the variables, except *Category* for which it is 'Nominal'.

5. For the variable *Category*, under the column heading "Values" enter 1 for sub-junior and 2 for junior by double clicking the cell, that is,

   1 = sub-junior

   2 = junior

6. Use default entries in rest of the columns.

After defining variables in the **Variable View**, the screen shall look like as shown in Figure 10.1.

10.7.1.3   Entering Data   After defining variables in the **Variable View**, click on **Data View** to open the data entry format. After entering the data column-wise, the screen will look like as shown in Figure 10.2. Save the data file in the desired location before further processing.

10.7.1.4   SPSS Commands   After entering data do the following steps:

1. *Initiating SPSS commands:* While being in the Data View, click the following commands in sequence:

$$\text{Analyze} \rightarrow \text{Classify} \rightarrow \text{Discriminant}$$

   The screen shall look like as shown in Figure 10.3.

2. *Selecting variables:* After clicking "Discriminant" option, the SPSS will ask you to select the variables for analysis.

   (a) Select *Category* variable from left panel and bring it to the "Grouping Variable" section in the right panel. Define minimum and maximum range of the grouping variable as "1" and "2."

   (b) Select all independent variables from the left panel and bring them into "Independents" section in the right panel.

   (c) Check "Use stepwise method" option. The screen will look like as shown in Figure 10.4.

3. *Selecting options for computation:* After selecting variables, different option needs to be defined for generating the output in DA. Do the following:

   (a) Click on the **Statistics** command on the screen shown in Figure 10.4.

   (b) Check 'Means' option in the "Descriptive" section.

   (c) Check 'Box's M' option.

	Name	Type	Width	Decimals	Label	Values	Missing	Columns	Align	Measure
1	SBJ	Numeric	8	2	Standing broa...	None	None	8	Right	Scale
2	Shut_run	Numeric	8	2	4x10 Shuttle r...	None	None	8	Right	Scale
3	Fifty_mt	Numeric	8	2	50 Mt. timings	None	None	8	Right	Scale
4	Twelve_mi...	Numeric	8	2	12 min R/W	None	None	8	Right	Scale
5	Aner_cap	Numeric	8	2	Anaerobic cap...	None	None	8	Right	Scale
6	Wt	Numeric	8	2	Weight	None	None	8	Right	Scale
7	Ht	Numeric	8	2	Height	None	None	8	Right	Scale
8	Leg_length	Numeric	8	2	Leg length	None	None	8	Right	Scale
9	Calf_girth	Numeric	8	2	Calf girth	None	None	8	Right	Scale
10	Thigh_girth	Numeric	8	2	Thigh girth	None	None	8	Right	Scale
11	Shl_width	Numeric	8	2	Shoulder width	None	None	8	Right	Scale
12	Category	Numeric	8	2	Category of at...	›-junior}...	None	8	Right	Nominal

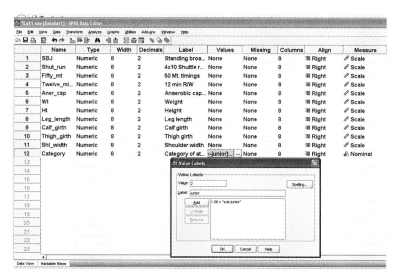

FIGURE 10.1 Defining variables in discriminant analysis.

	SBJ	Shut_run	Fifty_mt	Twelve_min_R_W	Aner_cap	Wt	Ht	Leg_length	Calf_girth	Thigh_girth	Shl_width	Category
1	222.00	10.10	8.10	2810.00	57.55	39.00	137.00	72.00	26.00	36.00	41.00	1.00
2	210.00	10.20	7.92	2420.00	40.61	38.00	135.00	71.00	29.00	39.00	36.00	1.00
3	192.00	10.13	7.54	2755.00	45.30	32.00	143.00	70.00	28.00	36.00	36.00	1.00
4	199.00	11.01	8.26	2610.00	32.59	38.00	132.00	75.00	27.00	39.00	34.00	1.00
5	195.00	10.50	8.30	2205.00	36.74	32.00	130.00	72.00	25.00	33.00	36.00	1.00
6	210.00	10.22	7.41	2515.00	48.20	27.00	136.00	72.00	27.00	38.00	36.00	1.00
7	229.00	9.52	7.01	2702.00	51.30	31.00	145.00	76.00	28.00	40.00	37.00	1.00
8	215.00	10.45	7.15	2495.00	39.12	36.00	162.00	78.00	28.00	38.00	29.00	1.00
9	214.00	11.30	8.03	2535.00	31.09	32.00	144.00	77.00	26.00	38.00	33.00	1.00
10	223.00	10.12	8.40	2180.00	29.48	38.00	148.00	78.00	29.00	43.00	36.00	1.00
11	221.00	9.70	7.83	2418.00	52.40	38.00	145.00	76.00	31.00	45.00	38.00	2.00
12	212.00	9.88	6.95	2508.00	48.30	39.00	141.00	76.00	29.00	40.00	38.00	2.00
13	219.00	9.24	7.28	2416.00	45.30	42.00	158.00	74.00	29.00	42.00	39.00	2.00
14	208.00	9.14	7.48	2510.00	52.20	41.00	151.00	81.00	31.00	43.00	42.00	2.00
15	218.00	10.15	8.25	2520.00	44.53	45.00	156.00	76.00	27.00	42.00	36.00	2.00
16	211.00	9.35	7.45	2530.00	32.66	47.00	157.00	85.00	31.00	41.00	43.00	2.00
17	213.00	9.53	7.60	2405.00	25.22	49.00	158.00	74.00	27.00	45.00	44.00	2.00
18	213.00	10.08	7.20	2410.00	36.16	45.00	151.00	72.00	27.00	36.00	44.00	2.00
19	259.00	9.40	6.95	2730.00	59.23	49.00	157.00	81.00	32.00	45.00	45.00	2.00
20	222.00	9.12	7.30	2614.00	47.24	55.00	161.00	89.00	31.00	48.00	43.00	2.00

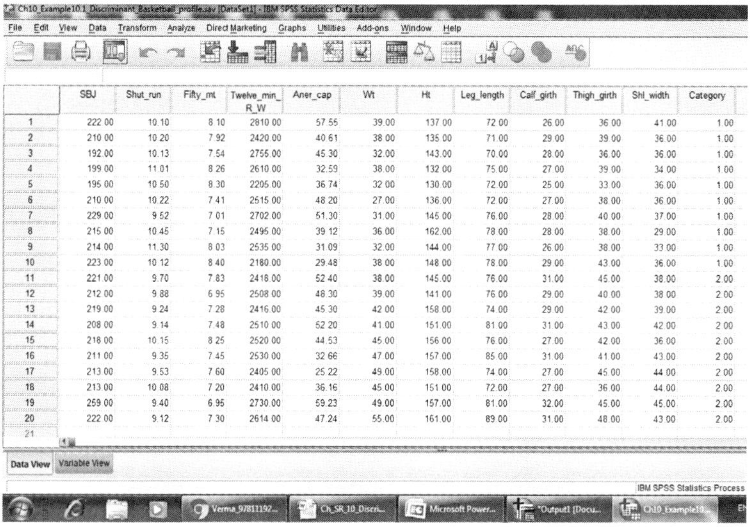

FIGURE 10.2 Screen showing data in the data view.

(d) Check 'Fisher's' and 'Unstandardized' options in the "Function Coefficients" section. The screen showing these options shall look like as shown in Figure 10.5.

(e) Click on **Continue**. This will take you back to the screen shown in Figure 10.4.

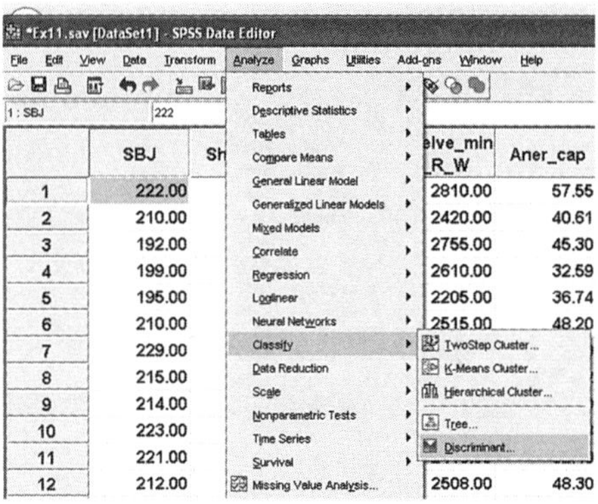

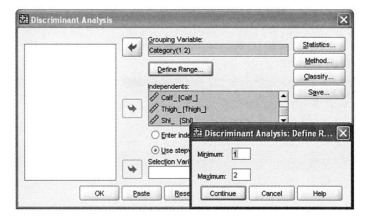

FIGURE 10.3   Screen showing SPSS commands for discriminant analysis.

FIGURE 10.4   Screen showing selection of variables for discriminant analysis.

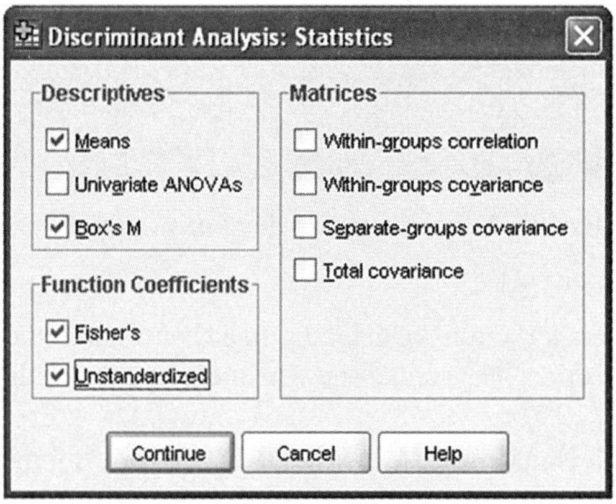

FIGURE 10.5   Screen showing the options for statistics and discriminant coefficients.

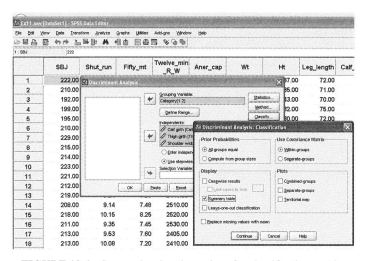

FIGURE 10.6 Screen showing the options for classification matrix.

(f) Click on **Classify** command and check the option 'Summary table' in the "Display" section. The screen for this option shall look like as shown in Figure 10.6.

(g) Click on the **Continue** and **OK** commands for generating outputs.

4. *Getting the output:* Select relevant outputs from the output window and copy them into word file for interpretation. We have selected the following outputs for discussion:

(a) Group statistics including mean and standard deviation

(b) Box's M test

(c) Unstandardized canonical discriminant function coefficients

(d) Canonical correlation

(e) Wilks' lambda and chi-square test

(f) Classification matrix

(g) Standardized canonical discriminant function coefficients

(h) Functions at group centroids.

10.7.2 Interpretation of Findings

The outputs picked up in DA are shown in Tables 10.2, 10.3, 10.4, 10.5, 10.6, 10.7, and 10.8.

1. Table 10.2 shows descriptive statistics containing mean and standard deviation for all the variables in sub-junior, junior, and overall categories. You may show this table in your analysis.

TABLE 10.2   Group Statistics: Mean and Standard Deviation of All Parameters in Different Groups

Category		Mean	Std. Deviation
Sub-junior	Standing broad jump	210.90	12.37
	4×10 Shuttle run	10.36	0.50
	50 Mt. timings	7.81	0.50
	12 min R/W	2522.70	212.44
	Anaerobic capacity	41.20	9.27
	Weight	34.30	4.03
	Height	141.20	9.41
	Leg length	74.10	3.03
	Calf girth	27.30	1.34
	Thigh girth	38.00	2.67
	Shoulder width	35.40	3.06
Junior	Standing broad jump	219.60	14.59
	4×10 Shuttle run	9.56	0.38
	50 Mt. timings	7.43	0.40
	12 min R/W	2506.10	104.29
	Anaerobic capacity	44.32	10.23
	Weight	45.00	5.23
	Height	153.50	6.40
	Leg length	78.40	5.44
	Calf girth	29.50	1.96
	Thigh girth	42.70	3.34
	Shoulder width	41.20	3.16
Total	Standing broad jump	215.25	13.90
	4×10 Shuttle run	9.96	0.59
	50 Mt. timings	7.62	0.48
	12 min R/W	2514.40	163.10
	Anaerobic capacity	42.76	9.64
	Weight	39.65	7.13
	Height	147.35	10.06
	Leg length	76.25	4.82
	Calf girth	28.40	1.98
	Thigh girth	40.35	3.80
	Shoulder width	38.30	4.24

2. In order to use DA, the variance–covariance matrix must be same in each categories of the dependent variable. This can be tested by Box's M test as shown in Table 10.3. Since Box's M test is not significant ($p = 0.586$), it may be concluded that the variance–covariance matrices in both categories of the dependent variable are same.

3. The unstandardized discriminant coefficients shown in Table 10.4 are used for constructing discriminant function. The stepwise method was used in this analysis, and only two variables, namely, 4×10 shuttle run and weight could be retained in the model due to its significant discriminating power. The remaining

TABLE 10.3   Box's M Test

Box's M		2.201
F	Approx.	0.645
	df1	3
	df2	5.832E4
	Sig.	0.586

Tests null hypothesis of equal population covariance matrices.

TABLE 10.4   Unstandardized Canonical Discriminant Function Coefficients

Variables Selected	Function 1
4×10 shuttle run	−1.269
Weight	0.164
(Constant)	6.125

TABLE 10.5   Eigenvalues Table

Function	Eigenvalue	% of Variance	Cumulative %	Canonical Correlation
1	2.126[a]	100.0	100.0	0.825

[a] First 1 canonical discriminant functions were used in the analysis.

TABLE 10.6   Wilks' Lambda and Chi-Square Test

Test of Function(s)	Wilks' Lambda	Chi-Square	df	Sig.
1	0.320	19.374	2	0.000

TABLE 10.7   Classification Matrix[a]

		Predicted Group Membership		
	Category of Athlete	Sub-Junior	Junior	Total
Original count	Sub-junior	10	0	10
	Junior	1	9	10
%	Sub-junior	100.0	0.0	100.0
	Junior	10.0	90.0	100.0

[a] 95.0% of original grouped cases correctly classified.

nine variables did not get selected in the model as they were not found to have sufficient discriminating power. Thus, discriminant function can be constructed by using the values of constant and coefficients of these two selected variables as shown below:

$$Z = 6.125 - 1.269 \times (4 \times 10 \text{ Shuttle run}) + 0.164 \times (\text{Weight})$$

TABLE 10.8   Standardized Canonical Discriminant Function Coefficients

Variables Selected	Function 1
4 × 10 shuttle run	−0.563
Weight	0.766

4. The canonical correlation provides an index of overall model fit. In Table 10.5, a canonical correlation of 0.825 suggests that the model explains 68.06% (square of canonical correlation) of the variation in the grouping variable by the predictor variables.

5. The value of Wilks' lambda shown in Table 10.6 is the estimate of variance of the dependent variable not explained by the predictor variables in the model. The eta square can be obtained by subtracting the value of Wilks' lambda from 1. This is a sign of robustness of the discriminant model. Since in this example the value of eta square is 0.68 (1.00 − 0.32), it can be interpreted that the model explains 68% variation in the grouping variable. The readers can note that this is same as what we have interpreted using the canonical correlation in Table 10.5.

   The significance of Wilks' lambda is tested by chi-square statistic. It can be seen from the Table 10.6 that the chi-square is significant as its p value is equal to 0.000, which is less than 0.05, hence it may be inferred that the discriminant model is significant as well.

6. Table 10.7 is a classification matrix that shows the summary of correct and wrong classification of subjects in both the groups on the basis of the developed discriminant model. It can be seen that out of 10 subjects belonging to subjunior category all were correctly classified in the same category, whereas out of 10 subjects in the junior category nine were classified in the same category. Thus, out of 20 cases 19 (95%) were correctly classified by the model, which is quite high, hence the model can be considered valid. Since this model is developed on the basis of a small sample, the level of accuracy shown in the classification matrix may not be true for all future classification of new cases.

7. Table 10.8 shows the discriminating power of the variables selected in the model. The variable having higher magnitude of the absolute function value is more powerful in discriminating the two groups. Since absolute function value of the weight is 0.766, which is higher than that of 4 × 10 shuttle run (0.563), weight is more powerful predictor in this model in comparison to 4 × 10 shuttle run in discriminating the two groups.

8. The purpose of using DA is to have a decision model for classifying a basketballer into any of the two categories: sub-junior and junior. Table 10.9 shows the means for the transformed group centroids. Thus, the new mean for group 1 (sub-junior basketballer) is −1.383, and for group 2 (junior basketballer) it is +1.383. This indicates that the midpoint of these two is 0.

   These two means can be plotted on a straight line by locating the midpoint as shown in Figure 10.7.

TABLE 10.9 Functions at Group Centroids

Category of Athlete	Function 1
Sub-junior	−1.383
Junior	1.383

Unstandardized canonical discriminant functions evaluated at group means.

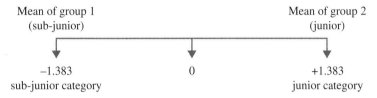

FIGURE 10.7 Means of the transformed group centroids.

The figure gives the decision rule for classifying any new subject into any of the two categories. If the discriminant score of any male basketballer falls to the right of the midpoint (Z>0), he is classified into the junior category, and if it falls to the left of the midpoint (Z<0), he is classified into sub-junior category.

The procedure of classification on the basis of discriminant score for a basketballer can be seen in the following example.

Example 10.2

Performance of the two basketballers on 4×10 meter shuttle run and their weights are given as follows:

Subjects	4×10 meter shuttle run (sec)	Weight (kg)
A	10.42	36
B	9.50	42

Using the discriminant model developed earlier, classify these two individuals into any of the two categories: sub-junior and junior.

Solution: The discriminant score for each subject on the basis of the developed regression equation can be computed as follows:

Since the discriminant model here is

$$Z = 6.125 - 1.269 \times (4 \times 10 \text{ shuttle run}) + 0.164 \times (\text{weight})$$

For subject A

$$Z = 6.125 - 1.269 \times 10.42 + 0.164 \times 36 = -1.19398$$

Since the value of Z is −1.19398, which is less than 0, the subject A is classified in the sub-junior category.

Similarly, for subject B

$$Z = 6.125 - 1.269 \times 9.50 + 0.164 \times 42 = 0.9575$$

Since the value of Z is 0.9575, which is greater than 0, the subject B may be classified in the junior category.

10.8   SUMMARY OF THE SPSS COMMANDS FOR DISCRIMINANT ANALYSIS

1. Start SPSS by using the following sequence of commands:

    Start → All Programs → SPSS Inc → SPSS 20.0

2. Click on **Variable View** and define *SBJ, Shut_run, Fifty_mt, Twelve_min_R_W, Aner_cap, Wt, Ht, Leg_length, Calf_girth, Thigh_girth, and Shl_width* as scale variables and *Category* as nominal.

3. For the dependent variable *Category* under the column heading "Values," define '1' for sub junior and '2' for junior.

4. After defining variables, type data column-wise for these variables by clicking on "Data View."

5. In the Data View, follow the command sequence as shown below:

    Analyze → Classify → Discriminant

6. Select *Category* from left panel, and bring it to the "Grouping Variables" section in the right panel and define its minimum and maximum range as '1' and '2.' Further, select all independent variables from the left panel and bring them to the "Independents" section of the right panel. Check "Use stepwise method" option.

7. Click on **Statistics** command and check 'Means', 'Fisher's,' and 'Unstandardized' options in it. Click on **Continue**.

8. Click on the **Classify** command and check 'Summary table' option.

9. Click on the **Continue** and **OK** for generating outputs.

10.9   EXERCISE

10.9.1   Short Answer Questions

Note: Write answers to each of the following questions in not more than 200 words.

Q.1   What do you mean by discriminating variable? What is its significance in discriminant analysis?

Q.2   In discriminant analysis what does dependent variable refers to? What is the data type of dependent variable in SPSS?

Q.3   What is discriminant function, and how is it developed? How is this function used in decision-making?

Q.4   What is the role of classification matrix in discriminant analysis? How is the percentage of correct classification similar to R^2?

Q.5   In SPSS what happens if stepwise method is selected for discriminant analysis? What criteria are adopted by SPSS in selecting and dropping variable in the model?

Q.6   What do you mean by discriminating power of a variable?

10.9.2   Multiple Choice Questions

Note: Questions 1–10 have four alternative answers for each question. Tick mark the one which is closest to the correct answer.

1   In discriminant analysis, dependent variables are defined as
   (a) Scale
   (b) Nominal
   (c) Ordinal
   (d) Ratio

2   Criterion for classifying discriminant analysis is as follows:
   Classify in group I if $Z < 0$
   Classify in group II if $Z > 0$
   The above criteria holds true
   (a) If size of the samples in both the groups is equal
   (b) If size of the samples in both the groups is nearly equal
   (c) If size of the samples in both the groups is in the proportion of $4:1$
   (d) In all the situations

3   Dependent variable in SPSS is denoted as
   (a) Scale variable
   (b) Grouping variable
   (c) Ordinal variable
   (d) Criterion variable

4   Discriminant function is also known as
   (a) Eigenvalue
   (b) Regression coefficient
   (c) Canonical root
   (d) Discriminant coefficient

5   Confusion matrix is used to denote
   (a) Correctly classified cases
   (b) Discriminant coefficients
   (c) F values
   (d) Robustness of different models

6 In stepwise method of discriminant analysis, a variable is included in the model
   if it is found significant at
   (a) 2% level
   (b) 1% level
   (c) 10% level
   (d) 5% level

7 Value of Wilks' lambda ranges from
   (a) −1 to +1
   (b) 0 to 1
   (c) −1 to 0
   (d) −2 to 2

8 Wilks' lambda is a measure of significance of
   (a) Discriminant function
   (b) Regression coefficient
   (c) Discriminant coefficient
   (d) Means of group

9 One of the assumptions in discriminant analysis is
   (a) All variables have curvilinear and homoscedastic relationships.
   (b) All variables have linear and non-homoscedastic relationships.
   (c) All variables have curvilinear and non-homoscedastic relationships.
   (d) All variables have linear and homoscedastic relationships.

10 Choose the correct statement about the assumption in discriminant analysis
   (a) Dependent variable is an ordinal variable.
   (b) The groups should not be mutually exclusive.
   (c) Sample sizes should differ to a great extent.
   (d) No independent variables should have a zero variability in either of the
       groups formed by the dependent variable.

11 Correct sequence of commands in SPSS for discriminant analysis is
   (a) Analyze → Discriminant → Classify
   (b) Analyze → Classify → Discriminant
   (c) Discriminant → Analyze → Classify
   (d) Discriminant → Classify → Analyze

12 Discriminant function is developed on the basis of the
   (a) Standardized coefficients
   (b) Unstandardized coefficients
   (c) Classification matrix
   (d) Functions at group centroids

10.9.3 Assignment

In a senior national volleyball championship for men, a group cohesion questionnaire
was administered on 48 high and low-performing players. The data on four parameters of a group cohesion questionnaire along with their performance category so
obtained is shown in Table 10.10.

TABLE 10.10 Data on the Group Cohesion Parameters Obtained on the High-Performer and Low-Performer Volleyballers

Performance category	Group Integration-Task	Group Integration-Social	Individual Attraction to the Group-Task	Individual Attraction to the Group-Social
1	20	14	24	13
1	20	14	24	13
1	20	14	24	13
1	20	14	19	13
2	18	26	29	15
1	13	19	13	16
2	18	26	29	19
2	18	26	29	19
1	20	14	13	12
1	20	14	23	15
2	11	26	29	19
2	26	26	22	14
2	12	15	28	23
1	8	11	21	20
1	10	12	19	13
1	12	13	19	16
1	15	13	20	16
1	12	14	22	18
1	13	18	16	13
1	12	12	22	14
1	12	22	13	14
1	9	14	20	16
2	16	16	26	22
1	7	11	23	18
2	22	27	24	17
2	23	22	32	25
2	17	21	32	14
2	20	25	20	23
1	14	16	26	20
2	16	33	27	25
2	22	25	18	17
2	19	28	27	25
2	23	21	24	18
1	18	20	16	18
2	16	33	27	24
2	19	24	18	18
2	15	16	22	25
1	16	20	18	14
1	11	24	15	23
1	15	21	28	11
2	17	27	30	13
2	17	30	17	17
1	18	19	21	17
2	17	22	17	26
1	19	16	20	19
2	26	27	27	16
2	21	23	32	32
2	18	16	19	26

Performance category: 1 - Low, 2 - High.

Apply discriminant analysis and
(a) Develop a discriminant function and the decision rule for classifying a volleyballer into high- and low-performer groups.
(b) Test the significance of discriminant model so developed.
(c) Comment on the efficiency of the model.
(d) Find the relative importance of independent variables in the model.

10.10   CASE STUDY ON DISCRIMINANT ANALYSIS

Objective

A badminton coach organized an experiment to develop a model for classifying badminton players into high- and low-performance groups on the basis of their physical and anthropometric variables. He selected 12 players randomly from the first six best teams in a tournament and 12 from the low-performing teams. Different physical and anthropometric measurements were obtained on them. The data so obtained is shown in Table 10.11.

Research Issues

The following research issues were investigated:

1. Can an efficient discriminant model be developed for classifying a badminton player into high- or low-performance categories?
2. Will the developed model be significant and efficient?

Data Format

The format used for preparing data file in SPSS is shown in Table 10.11.

Analyzing Data

In this study the dependent variable was categorical and independent variables were numerical, hence the discriminant model was developed for classifying the subjects into any one of the two categories on the basis of identified discriminating variables. This model was developed by using the discriminant coefficients generated by the SPSS in its output. SPSS identifies those independent variables that have significant discriminating power in classifying subjects into two categories.

The DA was carried out in SPSS by using the commands: **Analyze, Classify,** and **Discriminant** in sequence. Independent variables and group variables were placed in the appropriate locations in the dialog box. The option for 'Means', 'Box's M,' and 'Unstandardized' coefficient were checked by clicking on the **Statistics** command and 'Summary table' by clicking on the **Classify** command. Outputs in the analysis

TABLE 10.11 Data Format Used in SPSS for Discriminant Analysis

S.N.	Pla_Abl	Age (year)	Ht (cm)	Wt (kg)	Arm_Len (cm)	Leg_Len (cm)	Trunk_Len (cm)	Hand_Girth (cm)	Thigh_Girth (cm)	Calf_Girth (cm)	Shoul_Width (cm)	Hip_Width (cm)	50 Mt_Run (s)	Explo_Stren (kg)
1	Low	18	171	65.6	77	85	86	27	54	34	41	34	7.10	33
2	Low	18	163	61.5	76	84	79	27	54	36	42	32	7.18	33
3	Low	22	167	65.5	74	89	78	33	52	37	43	30	7.05	35
4	Low	21	163	74.5	70	85	78	28	58	38	42	36	7.29	33
5	Low	20	162	66.3	72	84	78	27	50	36	43	33	7.34	33
6	Low	22	167	59.7	76	84	83	27	50	35	43	32	7.08	33
7	Low	24	173	69.9	75	86	87	29	55	36	38	31	7.00	33
8	Low	28	172	78.5	72	92	80	31	53	36	42	35	7.00	43
9	Low	22	175	65.5	72	91	84	33	52	37	43	30	7.30	33
10	Low	23	165	67.3	70	87	78	27	50	35	43	35	7.33	30
11	Low	20	168	76.6	78	88	80	28	53	35	42	35	7.14	35
12	Low	24	173	69.9	80	86	87	29	55	36	38	31	7.00	33
13	High	33	176	68.3	73	92	84	30	52	35	44	35	7.17	40
14	High	30	184	64.3	76	94	90	26	54	36	43	31	6.90	50
15	High	26	180	66.7	79	95	85	31	51	35	44	31	6.98	53
16	High	23	177	76.7	80	90	87	30	57	40	45	33	6.75	53
17	High	36	181	98.8	79	89	92	36	54	40	48	35	6.92	56
18	High	23	178	67.3	84	88	90	25	51	35	46	35	6.95	59
19	High	19	180	67.8	86	88	92	27	50	35	43	35	6.90	55
20	High	31	188	78.8	82	95	92	28	54	36	49	36	6.80	45
21	High	24	176	72.8	82	88	88	28	51	34	44	36	6.75	57
22	High	24	187	73.5	84	94	93	28	50	33	43	35	6.90	55
23	High	23	181	68.8	85	97	84	26	52	33	41	34	7.20	60
24	High	24	174	67.3	77	88	86	27	53	34	45	33	7.05	58

Playing ability code: 1, Low; 2, High.

were obtained by selecting stepwise method. The outputs so obtained are shown in Tables 10.12, 10.13, 10.14, 10.15, 10.16, and 10.17 and in Figure 10.8.

Testing Assumption

One of the main assumptions in the discriminant analysis is that the variance–covariance matrix must be same in each categories of the dependent variable. This is tested by means of Box's M test as shown in Table 10.12. Since Box's M test is not significant

TABLE 10.12   Box's M Test

Box's M		9.710
F	Approx.	1.376
	df1	6
	df2	3.507E3
	Sig.	0.220

Tests null hypothesis of equal population covariance matrices.

TABLE 10.13   Canonical Discriminant Function Coefficients

	Function
	1
Ht	0.130
Shoul_width	0.231
Explo_stren	0.175
(Constant)	−40.201

Unstandardized coefficients.

TABLE 10.14   Standardized Canonical Discriminant Function Coefficients

	Function
	1
Ht	0.575
Shoul_width	0.471
Explo_stren	0.826

TABLE 10.15   Functions at Group Centroids

	Function
Pla_Abl	1
Low	−2.816
High	2.816

Unstandardized canonical discriminant functions evaluated at group means.

TABLE 10.16   Wilks' Lambda

Test of Function(s)	Wilks' Lambda	Chi-Square	df	Sig.
1	0.104	46.477	3	0.000

TABLE 10.17   Classification Results[a]

			Predicted Group Membership		
		Pla_Abl	Low	High	Total
Original	Count	Low	12	0	12
		High	1	11	12
	%	Low	100.0	0.0	100.0
		High	8.3	91.7	100.0

[a]95.8% of original grouped cases correctly classified.

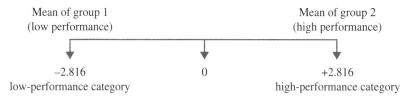

FIGURE 10.8   Means of the transformed group centroids.

($p > 0.05$); hence, it may be concluded that the variance–covariance matrices in both the categories of the dependent variable are same.

Developing Discriminant Model

The unstandardized discriminant coefficients shown in Table 10.13 were used for constructing discriminant function. The stepwise method used in this analysis identified only three variables, namely, height, shoulder width, and explosive strength that were retained in the model due to its significant discriminating power. Thus, discriminant function, Z, was constructed by using the values of constant and coefficients of these three selected variables.

$$Z = -40.201 + 0.130 \times (\text{height}) + 0.231 \times (\text{shoulder width}) + 0.175 \times (\text{explosive strength})$$

Table 10.14 shows discriminating power of the variables selected in the model. The higher the magnitude of the absolute function, the more powerful the variable in defining group membership. Since absolute function value of the explosive strength is 0.826, which is higher than the other two variables in the model, it is the most contributing predictor in the model.

A decision model was developed for classifying a badminton player into any of the two low- and high-performance categories. Table 10.15 shows the means for the transformed group centroids. Thus, the new mean for group 1 (low performance) is −2.816, and for group 2 (high performance) it is +2.816. This indicates that average of these two is 0. These two means were plotted on a straight line by locating this average value as shown in Figure 10.8.

Figure 10.8 shows the decision rule for classifying any new subject into any of the two categories. A badminton player is classified into high performance category if his discriminant score is more than zero ($Z > 0$) and in low performance if it is less than zero ($Z < 0$).

Testing Efficiency of the Model

Wilks' lambda in Table 10.16 is 0.104. This indicates the percentage variability in the dependent variable not explained by the independent variables in the model. Thus, only 10.4% of the variability in dependent variable was not explained by the developed model. Since the value of chi-square associated with the Wilks' lambda is significant, the model was significant.

Table 10.17 is a classification matrix, which shows the summary of correct and wrong classification of subjects in both the groups on the basis of the developed discriminant model. It can be seen from the table that out of 12 subjects belonging to the low-performance category, all were correctly classified; whereas out of 12 subjects in the high-performance category, only 11 were correctly classified. Thus, out of 24 cases, 95.8% cases were correctly classified.

Reporting

- The discriminant model was developed on the basis of only three independent variables: height, shoulder width, and explosive strength.
- Out of these three variables, explosive strength was found to have maximum discriminating power.
- Since chi-square was significant, the model was efficient. Wilks' lambda suggested that only 10.4% of the variability in dependent variable could not be explained by the developed model.
- In sampled data model, 95.8% cases were classified correctly.

11

LOGISTIC REGRESSION FOR DEVELOPING LOGIT MODEL IN SPORT

LEARNING OBJECTIVE

After completing this chapter, you should be able to do the following:

- Understand the situation where the logistic regression can be used
- Know the difference between the logistic regression and the ordinary least square regression
- Understand the procedure involved in developing logit model in sport
- Learn to apply SPSS for developing logit model
- Understand the assumptions used in logistic regression
- Learn to interpret the outputs generated by SPSS in logistic regression

---

11.1 INTRODUCTION

Sports scientists always aspire for researching those parameters that can help sportspersons to win their game. Parameters that can influence the performance may be identified by analyzing data using different statistical techniques. If player's performance can be measured quantitatively, the technique like regression analysis

---

Sports Research with Analytical Solution using SPSS®, First Edition. J. P. Verma.
© 2016 John Wiley & Sons, Inc. Published 2016 by John Wiley & Sons, Inc.
Companion website: www.wiley.com/go/Verma/Sportsresearch

discussed in Chapter 9 can be used to identify such parameters that are responsible for performance provided assumptions used in the analysis are satisfied. But if the measure of performance is categorical in nature say win/loss or success/failure, then the regression technique fails to provide solution. In such situations, discriminant analysis discussed in Chapter 10 may be used to identify parameters that can discriminate such performance parameters. Discriminant analysis provides efficient results only if the independent variables are measured either on interval or ratio scale. Further, independent variables need to be normally distributed, linearly related, and should have equal variance within each group of dependent variable (Tabachnick and Fidell, 2001). In a situation where independent variables are measured either on nominal, interval, ratio, or a mix of these scales, then the discriminant analysis cannot be used to predict group membership in dependent variable. In such situations, another statistical technique known as logistic regression is used to develop a model for predicting a group membership of a dichotomous dependent variable. Another advantage of using logistic regression is that it does not require independent variables to follow the assumptions of normality, linearity, and equal variance within each group of the dependent variable. Thus, the logistic regression is the most efficient technique of predicting group membership of a dichotomous dependent variable if the independent variables are metric, nominal, or a mix of both, and the assumptions about the distribution of independent variables are not satisfied. This chapter discusses the logistic regression in detail and its application in developing the model in sports research.

11.2 UNDERSTANDING LOGISTIC REGRESSION

Logistic regression is used to develop a predictive model when the dependent variable is dichotomous and independent variables are categorical. This analysis can also be used if the independent variables are a mix of both categorical and numerical. Here dependent variable takes value 1 or 0 where 1 represents occurrence of phenomenon and 0 indicates its nonoccurrence. For instance, dependent variable may be success/failure in field goal, winning/losing in a tennis match, injury/no injury in a football match, etc.

In logistic regression, we are interested in predicting the probability p that the dependent variable takes value 1 rather than 0 on the basis of the independent variables, rather than predicting precise value of the dependent variable as is done in case of least square regression analysis. We wish that we could use this probability as the dependent variable in an ordinary regression, that is, as a simple linear function of independent variables. But it is not possible because by including large number of independent variables the value of p may exceed 1, which is not permissible. Due to this reason in logistic regression, instead of predicting the probability p (that the dependent variable will take value 1 rather 0), log of odds that the dependent variable takes value 1 is estimated by the predictor variables in the model. The model in logistic regression looks like as follows:

$$\log(\text{Odds}) = \log\left(\frac{\hat{p}}{1-\hat{p}}\right) = b_0 + b_1 x_1 + b_2 x_2 + \cdots + b_n x_n$$

Thus in logistic regression instead of estimating the probability p (that $Y = 1$), log of odds is estimated. This log(Odds) is also known as logit, hence the name logistic regression.

Here b_0 is a constant and b_1, b_2, ..., b_n are the regression coefficients of x_1, x_2, ..., x_n, respectively.

Since in logistic regression log of Odds acts as a dependent variable which is regressed on the basis of the independent variables, the interpretation of regression coefficients is not straightforward as in the case of multiple regression. In simple regression, the regression coefficient b represents the amount of change in Y with 1 unit change in X, but this concept is not valid in case of logistic regression; instead, the regression coefficient b is converted into odds ratio to interpret the happening of outcome variable. If a logistic model has only one independent variable, then the model will look like as follows:

$$\log\left(\frac{\hat{p}}{1-\hat{p}}\right) = b_0 + b_1 x_1$$

$\Rightarrow$

$$\frac{\hat{p}}{1-\hat{p}} = e^{b_0 + b_1 x_1}$$

$\Rightarrow$

$$\hat{p} = \frac{e^{b_0 + b_1 x_1}}{1 + e^{b_0 + b_1 x_1}} = \frac{e^z}{1 + e^z}$$

Where $z = b_0 + b_1 x_1$. In case of more than one independent variables in the model, the z can be obtained by using the linear function of the independent variables as $z = b_0 + b_1 x_1 + b_2 x_2 + \cdots + b_n x_n$. Thus, the probability $p(y = 1)$ is a function of z and it can be represented as follows:

$$p = f(z) = \frac{e^z}{1 + e^z}$$

This function f is known as logistic function and the curve so obtained is known as logistic curve. The logistic curve is a sigmoid curve having shape just like letter "S" as shown in Figure 11.1. In logistic curve, the argument z is marked along the horizontal axis and value of the function f(z) along the vertical axis.

The advantage of using the logit function is that the variable z can assume any value from minus $-\infty$ to $+\infty$, but the outcome variable p will always have values in the range 0–1. This function is used to find the probability p that the target variable occurs for a given set of values of the independent variables in the logistic regression model.

11.3   APPLICATION OF LOGISTIC REGRESSION IN SPORTS RESEARCH

Logistic regression is useful in a situation where the researcher is interested in predicting the occurrence of any happening. In order to get the reliable findings, a minimum of 10 cases per independent variable need to be taken in the study. Several

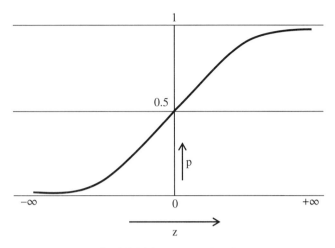

FIGURE 11.1   Logistic function.

situations may arise in sports research where this technique may be used. Some of these are mentioned in the following text:

1. In hockey, the success of penalty kick depends upon different factors say speed of the hit, height of the players, accuracy, arm strength, and eye–hand coordination. In this case, penalty kick is a dependent variable which is binary in nature. Converting penalty kick into goal is a success and missing is a failure. Here logistic model may be used to identify the significant variables that can be used to predict the success in the penalty kick. Here the likelihood of success may be determined by each of the independent variable in the model. The advantage of using this model is that independent variables can be categorical as well as quantitative. For instance, the subject's height may be classified as tall versus short, and eye–hand coordination may be classified into excellent, good, and average.

2. Since victory in football match depends upon the parameters like number of passes, number of turnovers, penalty yardage, number of fouls committed by the team. One may like to identify as to what independent parameters may be useful for winning in a football match. The obvious advantage in using this model is that the researcher is not required to ascertain the assumptions of normality, linearity, and equal variance within each group of the dependent variable.

3. In horse racing, a logistic regression model may be used to determine the likelihood of a particular horse finishing first in a specific race.

4. This technique can be used to classify field goal attempts as either makes or misses based upon the independent variables identified in the model.

11.4 ASSUMPTIONS IN LOGISTIC REGRESSION

The following assumptions are made in using logistic regression:

1. The dependent variable is binary. However, if it is continuous, one may decide criterion to convert it into binary.
2. The independent variables can either be categorical, numerical, or a mix of both. If categorical variable has more than two categories, a dummy variable may be defined to make it dichotomous.
3. Logit transformation of the dependent variable has a linear relationship with the independent variables.

11.5 STEPS IN DEVELOPING LOGISTIC MODEL

Following steps are involved in logistic regression:

1. Define coding of the dependent variable, 1 for the event to occur and 0 otherwise.
2. If independent variable is categorical having more than two categories, define the coding as 1, 2, 3, etc. The highest code needs to be given to the reference category.
3. Use SPSS to generate the following outputs:
   (a) Coding of dependent and independent variables
   (b) Omnibus tests of model coefficients
   (c) Model summary
   (d) Hosmer–Lemeshow test
   (e) Classification table
   (f) Variables in the equation
   (g) Variables not in the equation
4. Develop logistic regression equation by using regression coefficient of the variables selected in the model for predicting log of odds for the dependent variable to occur against its nonoccurrence.
5. Report the findings on the basis of Exp(B) for each variable.

11.6 LOGISTIC ANALYSIS USING SPSS

Example 11.1

A basketball coach wanted to investigate the factors that are responsible for winning a match. During a tournament, he collected the data on average height, number of pass, offensive rebound, free throws, and blocks for each team. In every match, performance (1 for winning and 0 for losing) of both the teams was noted. The score for each team on the "number of pass" was obtained as either 1 or 0 (If team's total number of pass was higher than that of the opponent, the score was noted as 0, otherwise 1). Similarly, scores on other independent variables such as offensive rebound, free throws, and blocks were obtained for each team as either 0 or 1. The data so obtained are shown in Table 11.1. Let us develop a logistic model for estimating the probability of winning in a basketball match on the basis of team statistics using SPSS. We shall also discuss the comparative importance of the independent variables in winning basketball match.

Solution
In this problem, it is required to develop a logistic model for estimating the likelihood of winning a basketball match on the basis of the identified independent variables. This shall be done by using the SPSS. Step-by-step procedure shall be shown for developing the logistic model. Once the outputs are generated, it will then be discussed to achieve the objectives. The SPSS provides findings of the logistic regression in two blocks: "Block 0" and "Block 1." In "Block 0," a logistic model is developed without using any of the explanatory variables. The model so obtained is based on only regression constant. In "Block 1," the regression model is developed using predictor variables. The model with constant only is used as a reference for

TABLE 11.1 Result of Different Basketball Matches in a Tournament Along with Selected Match Statistics

Match	Result	Number of Pass	Offensive Rebound	Free Throws	Blocks
1	1	0	0	1	0
2	0	1	1	1	1
3	1	0	0	1	1
4	1	1	1	1	0
5	0	1	0	1	1
6	0	0	1	0	0
7	1	1	0	0	1
8	0	0	1	1	0
9	1	1	0	0	0
10	0	1	1	1	1
11	1	0	0	0	1
12	0	1	1	0	0
13	1	1	0	1	1
14	0	0	1	0	0
15	1	1	0	1	0
16	0	0	0	0	0
17	0	1	1	1	1
18	1	0	0	0	0
19	0	1	1	1	1
20	1	0	0	0	1
21	0	1	1	1	0
22	1	0	0	0	0

Number of pass: 1=lower, 0=higher; *Offensive rebound:* 1=lower, 0=higher; *Free throws:* 1=lower, 0=higher; *Blocks:* 1=lower, 0=higher; *Result:* 0=loser, 1=winner.

checking improvement in the model having predictor variables. The entire procedure used in the logistic regression shall be discussed in a sequential manner in this example for easy understanding of readers.

11.6.1   Block 0

In this block, since logistic model is developed with no predictors and just the intercept, this is known as null model. Along with the model, its efficiency is also shown by means of classification table. The percentage of correct classification is then compared with the model developed by using the predictors in "Block 1." The relevant outputs of the first step are shown under the heading "Block 0" in SPSS output window.

11.6.2   Block 1

In "Block 1," a logistic model is developed by using the predictor variables along with the intercept. The SPSS provides different options for developing this model, which depends upon the nature of the research problem. If the study is exploratory in nature where it is desired to identify the predictor variables out of large number of independent variables, then the option "Forward:LR" is used. On the other hand, if the study is confirmatory type where all the predictors identified by the researcher are used to test the model, then 'Enter' method is used. In this study, we shall use 'Enter' method for the logistic regression model. The relevant outputs generated in the second step are shown under the heading "Block 1" in the SPSS output window.

These outputs include the knowledge about the variables that are included and excluded from the analysis and coding of the dependent and independent variables. The output generated in this section is used to test the significance of the model, regression coefficients, and odds ratios.

11.6.3   Computation in Logistic Regression with SPSS

11.6.3.1   Preparation of Data File   In order to generate the outputs in logistic regression, the first step is to prepare a data file. The readers who are using SPSS for the first time are advised to refer to Chapter 1 for detail procedure in preparing the data file. The data file will look like as shown in Figure 11.2.

11.6.3.2   SPSS Commands   After saving the data file, perform the following steps:

1. *Initiating SPSS commands*: While being in the **data view**, click on the following commands in sequence.

Analyze → Regression → Binary Logistic

The screen shall look like as shown in Figure 11.3.

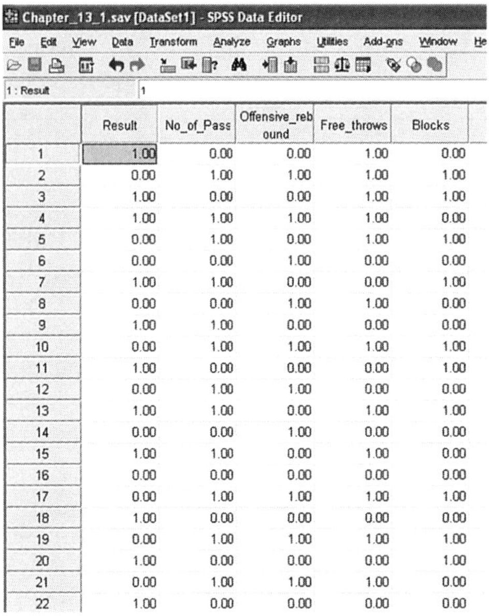

	Result	No_of_Pass	Offensive_rebound	Free_throws	Blocks
1	1.00	0.00	0.00	1.00	0.00
2	0.00	1.00	1.00	1.00	1.00
3	1.00	0.00	0.00	1.00	1.00
4	1.00	1.00	1.00	1.00	0.00
5	0.00	1.00	0.00	1.00	1.00
6	0.00	0.00	1.00	0.00	0.00
7	1.00	1.00	0.00	0.00	1.00
8	0.00	0.00	1.00	1.00	0.00
9	1.00	1.00	0.00	0.00	0.00
10	0.00	1.00	1.00	1.00	1.00
11	1.00	0.00	0.00	0.00	1.00
12	0.00	1.00	1.00	0.00	0.00
13	1.00	1.00	0.00	1.00	1.00
14	0.00	0.00	1.00	0.00	0.00
15	1.00	1.00	0.00	1.00	0.00
16	0.00	0.00	0.00	0.00	0.00
17	0.00	1.00	1.00	1.00	1.00
18	1.00	0.00	0.00	0.00	0.00
19	0.00	1.00	1.00	1.00	1.00
20	1.00	0.00	0.00	0.00	1.00
21	0.00	1.00	1.00	1.00	0.00
22	1.00	0.00	0.00	0.00	0.00

FIGURE 11.2 Data file of match statistics in basketball for logistic regression analysis.

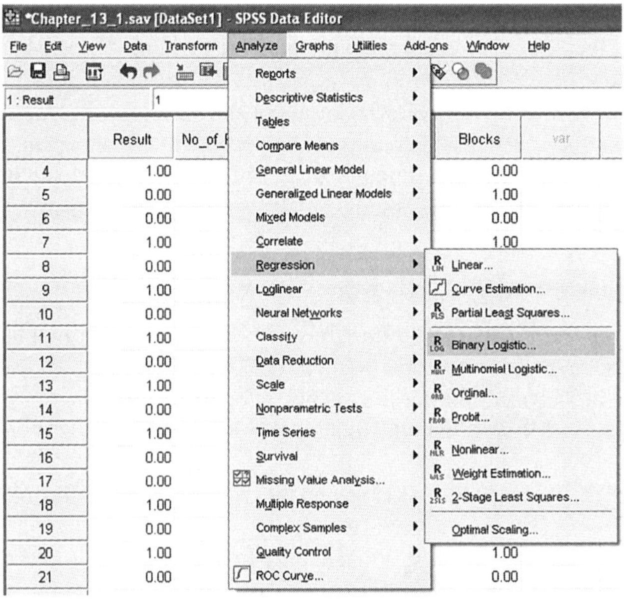

FIGURE 11.3 Command sequence for logistic regression.

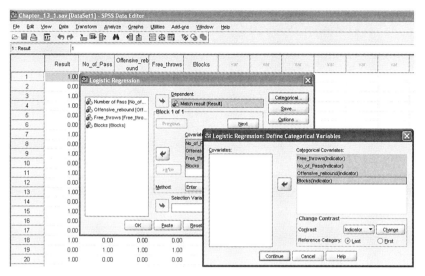

FIGURE 11.4   Selecting dependent and independent variables in logistic regression.

2. *Selecting variables:* After clicking the 'Binary Logistic' option, next screen shall be obtained for selecting dependent and independent variables. After selecting all the independent variables, you need to identify categorical independent variables included in it. Identify the variables by doing the following:

   (a) Select dependent variable from the left panel and bring it to the "Dependent" section in the right panel.

   (b) Select all independent variables from left panel and bring them to the "Covariates" section in the right panel.

   (c) Click on **Categorical** command and select the categorical variables from the "Covariates" section, and bring them to the "Categorical Covariates" section in the right panel. The screen will look like as shown in Figure 11.4.

   (d) Click on **Continue**.

3. *Selecting options for computation:* Once variables are selected, different options need to be defined for generating outputs. Do the following:

   (a) Click on **Options** command in the screen shown in Figure 11.4, which will take you to the screen shown in Figure 11.5 for generating the required outputs. Do the following:

      (i) Check 'Hosmer–Lemeshow goodness-of-fit' option.

      (ii) Let all other options be selected by default.

      (iii) Click on **Continue**.

4. *Selecting option for method to be used in the logistic regression*: Depending on whether the study is exploratory or confirmatory, option needs to be defined for the method to be used in SPSS. For confirmatory study, 'Enter' option has

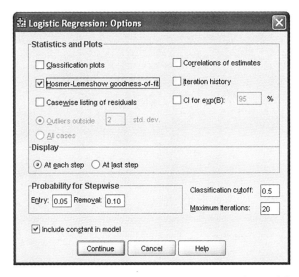

FIGURE 11.5   Option for generating Hosmer–Lemeshow goodness-of-fit and confidence intervals.

TABLE 11.2   Case Processing Summary

Unweighted Cases[a]		N	Percent
Selected cases	Included in analysis	22	100.0
	Missing cases	0	0.0
	Total	22	100.0
Unselected cases		0	0.0
Total		22	100.0

[a] If weight is in effect, see classification table for the total number of cases.

been provided by the SPSS; whereas for exploratory study one can choose any one of the option from the following: Forward: LR, Forward: Wald, Backward: LR, or Backward: Wald. The Forward: LR option is mostly used by the researchers in case the study is exploratory in nature. Since in this study all predictor variables shall be used in the model, the **Enter** method has been used in the screen shown in Figure 11.4. In fact, this option is selected by default. Click on **OK** to get the outputs.

11.6.3.3 SPSS Output   In SPSS, lots of outputs are generated in the output window. Relevant outputs selected from the output window are shown in Tables 11.2, 11.3, 11.4, 11.5, 11.6, 11.7, 11.8, and 11.9. Understanding the interpretation of these outputs shall facilitate you to report the findings of logistic regression in an appropriate manner. While reporting the findings in a research paper, it would be sufficient to mention the outputs shown in Tables 11.6, 11.7, 11.8, and 11.9 only.

TABLE 11.3   Dependent Variable Encoding

Original Value	Internal Value
Losing	0
Winning	1

TABLE 11.4   Categorical Variables Coding

		Parameter Coding	
		Frequency	(1)
Blocks	Lower	12	0.000
	Higher	10	1.000
Offensive_rebound	Lower	12	0.000
	Higher	10	1.000
Free_throws	Lower	10	0.000
	Higher	12	1.000
Number of pass	Lower	10	0.000
	Higher	12	1.000

TABLE 11.5   Classification Table[a,b] (Model without Predictors)

			Predicted		
			Match Result		
	Observed		Losing	Winning	Percentage Correct
Step 0	Match result	Losing	0	11	0.0
		Winning	0	11	100.0
	Overall percentage				50.0

[a] Constant is included in the model.
[b] The cut value is 0.500.

TABLE 11.6   Variables in the Equation

		B	S.E.	Wald	df	Sig.	Exp(B)
Step 0	Constant	0.000	0.426	0.000	1	1.000	1.000

TABLE 11.7   Variables Not in the Equation

			Score	df	Sig.
Step 0	Variables	No_of_Pass(1)	0.733	1	0.392
		Offensive_rebound(1)	11.733	1	0.001
		Free_throws(1)	0.733	1	0.392
		Blocks(1)	0.000	1	1.000
		Overall statistics	11.942	4	0.018

TABLE 11.8   Omnibus Tests of Model Coefficients

		Chi-Square	df	Sig.
Step 1	Step	13.604	4	0.009
	Block	13.604	4	0.009
	Model	13.604	4	0.009

TABLE 11.9   Model Summary

Step	−2 Log Likelihood	Cox and Snell R^2	Nagelkerke R^2
1	16.895[a]	0.461	0.615

[a] Estimation terminated at iteration number 5 because parameter estimates changed by less than 0.001.

11.7   INTERPRETATION OF FINDINGS

The following outputs have been selected from the output window of SPSS for interpretation:

- Case processing summary (Table 11.2)
- Dependent variable encoding (Table 11.3)
- Categorical variables coding (Table 11.4)
- Classification table (model without predictors) (Table 11.5)
- Variables in the equation (Table 11.6)
- Variables not in the equation (Table 11.7)
- Omnibus tests of model coefficients (Table 11.8)
- Model summary (Table 11.9)
- Hosmer–Lemeshow test (Table 11.10)
- Classification table (model with predictors) (Table 11.11)
- Variables in the equation (with predictors) (Table 11.12)

11.7.1   Case Processing and Coding Summary

Table 11.2 shows the number of cases (N) in each category (e.g., included in the analysis, missing, and total) and their percentage. SPSS does the list-wise deletion of missing data. Since there is no missing data, the number of missing cases is shown as 0. The coding of the dependent variable has been shown in Table 11.3.

In Table 11.4, coding of all the categorical independent variables and their frequencies has been shown. In coding categorical variable, highest number should be allotted to the reference category because by default SPSS considers the category with the highest coding as the reference category and gives the code as 0. For instance, if you define the coding of the variable "Block" as 1 for "Lower" and 0 for "Higher,"

TABLE 11.10   Hosmer–Lemeshow Test

Step	Chi-Square	df	Sig.
1	6.834	8	0.555

TABLE 11.11   Classification Table[a]

			Predicted		
			Match Result		
	Observed		Losing	Winning	Percentage Correct
Step 1	Match result	Losing	9	2	81.8
		Winning	1	10	90.9
	Overall percentage				86.4

[a] The cut value is 0.500.

TABLE 11.12   Variables in the Equation

		B	S.E.	Wald	df	Sig.	Exp(B)
Step 1[a]	No_of_pass(1)	−0.337	1.452	0.054	1	0.817	0.714
	Offensive_rebound(1)	4.190	1.556	7.249	1	0.007	65.990
	Free_throws(1)	−0.337	1.452	0.054	1	0.817	0.714
	Blocks(1)	0.834	1.390	0.360	1	0.548	2.303
	Constant	−2.539	1.416	3.213	1	0.073	0.079

[a] Variable(s) entered on step 1: No_of_Pass, Offensive_rebound, Free_throws, Blocks.

then the SPSS will consider Lower as the reference category and convert its code to 0 and the other category Higher as 1.

This fact can be easily verified by looking to the coding of the independent categorical variables in Table 11.1, that is, number of pass (1 : lower, 0 : higher), free throws (1 : lower, 0 : higher), offensive rebound (1 : lower, 0 : higher), and blocks (1 : lower, 0 : higher). These coding have been reversed by the SPSS as shown in Table 11.4. The SPSS also provides you the facility of changing the reference category as the lowest coding as shown in Figure 11.4.

11.7.2   Analyzing Logistic Models

Results of the logistic regression have been obtained in two blocks: Block 0 and Block 1. In Block 0, the logistic model has been developed using only intercept and no predictive variable; whereas in Block 1, the model with predictive variables has been developed.

11.7.2.1   Block 0: Logistic Model without Predictors   Results of the logistic regression with intercept only are shown in Tables 11.5, 11.6, and 11.7. This model developed in Block 0 is used to compare the efficiency of the model developed in

Block 1 with one or more predictors. Table 11.5 indicates that if nothing is known about the independent variables and one simply guesses that a particular team would win in the match, he would be correct 50% of the time. Table 11.6 shows that the Wald statistics is not significant as its significance value is 1.00, which is more than 0.05. Thus, it may be concluded that the model with constant is not worth and is equivalent to simply guessing about the winning of a particular team in the match without having the knowledge about any predictor variable.

Table 11.7 indicates whether each independent variable may improve the model or not. Here only offensive rebound variable is significant; hence it may improve the model if included. If none of the variables had been significant the analysis would have been terminated at this stage.

Since the model with intercept only has no practical utility, this may be ignored in reporting the findings.

11.7.2.2   Block 1: Logistic Model with Predictors   In Block 1, the logistic model is developed by the SPSS using all the four predictive variables: number of pass, free throws, offensive rebound, and blocks. This is the actual model in which we are interested. The results of this model are shown in Tables 11.8, 11.9, 11.10, 11.11, and 11.12.

11.7.2.2.1   Testing Significance of the Model   Omnibus tests for the model coefficients in Table 11.8 give us a chi-square of 13.604 with 4 df, which is significant beyond 0.01. This is the test of the null hypothesis that adding these four variables in the model will not be significant predictors if included.

The model summary in Table 11.9 shows that the −2 Log Likelihood statistic is 16.895. This statistic indicates how poorly the model predicts the decisions about winning a team. The smaller the value of −2 Log Likelihood statistic, the better the model. The SPSS does not give the value of this statistic for the model that has only the intercept, but we know that it is equal to 30.499. Adding all the four variables, that is, number of pass, free throws, offensive rebound, and blocks, the value of the −2 Log Likelihood statistic has reduced by 13.604(=30.499 − 16.895). This is equal to χ^2 statistic we just discussed in the previous paragraph. In Table 11.9, the Cox and Snell R Square and Nagelkerke R Square can be interpreted like R^2 in a multiple regression. The value of Cox and Snell R^2 cannot reach maximum value of 1, but the Nagelkerke R^2 can reach a maximum of 1. The reader should report the value of Nagelkerke R^2 as a measure of efficiency of the model. Thus, 61.5% variability of the dependent variable can be explained by all the four predictors together.

11.7.2.2.2   Testing Goodness of Fit of the Model   In order to know whether the developed logistic model is efficient in predicting the happening of the event (dependent variable taking value 1), a Hosmer–Lemeshow test is used. This test is used for assessing the goodness of fit of the logistic model. The Hosmer–Lemeshow test statistic follows a chi-square distribution. Since the value of chi-square is not significant as shown in Table 11.10, the logistic model is good in estimating the happening of the event (dependent variable taking value 1). In other words, the Hosmer–Lemeshow test (p=0.555) indicates that the numbers of winning are not significantly different from those predicted by the model, and that the overall model fit is good.

11.7.2.2.3 Model Accuracy   Table 11.11 is a classification table that shows the observed and predicted values of the dependent variable. Out of 22 matches, two teams have been wrongly predicted to be the winner and only one team has been wrongly classified as loser by the developed model. However, nine teams have been correctly predicted as loser and ten have been correctly predicted as winner. Thus, the model correctly classified 86.4% cases. In comparing results with that of Table 11.5, it can be seen that when no predictor was used the model correctly classified 50% cases; whereas by including four independent variables in the model, the percentage of correct classification has increased to 86.4%. Thus, it may be inferred that introducing these independent variables has definitely improved the model efficiency.

11.7.2.2.4 Developing Logistic Model   Table 11.12 is the main result in logistic regression. It includes regression coefficients (B) and odds ratios (Exp(B)). It also includes Wald chi-square statistic that tests the unique contribution of each predictor. You can notice that only offensive rebound predictor is significant (p<0.05). Since we are developing the logistic model by including all the four independent variables, by using the coefficients shown in the table, the following logistic model can be developed:

$$\log\frac{p}{1-p} = -2.539 + 0.834 \times \text{Blocks} - 0.337 \times \text{Free throws}$$
$$+ 4.190 \times \text{Offensive\_rebound} - 0.337 \times \text{No.\_of\_pass} \qquad (11.1)$$

where p is the probability of winning the match. The dependent variable in the logistic regression is known as logit (p) which is equal to $\log(p/(1-p))$.

Only those variables that are found to be significant should be included in the logistic model but for describing the results comprehensively, other variables have been included in this model.

The estimates of regression coefficients provided by the Equation 11.1 explain the relationship between the independent and dependent variables, where the dependent variable is on the logit scale. These estimates show the amount of increase (or decrease, if the sign of the coefficient is negative) in the estimated log odds ("Match result"=1) that would be predicted by a 1 unit increase (or decrease) in the independent variable, holding all other variables constant.

Since regression coefficients (B) are in log odds unit, they are often difficult to interpret, and thus they are converted into odds ratios that are equal to Exp(B). These odds ratios are shown in Table 11.12.

Significance of the Wald statistic indicates that the variable significantly predicts the winning of a team. The logistic regression should be used if the sample size is quite large, preferably more than 500 (or at least 10 cases per independent variable). In case of small sample due to inflating the level of significance, it does not give the correct picture.

11.7.2.2.5   Explanation of Odds Ratios and Logistic Model   In Table 11.12, the odds ratio Exp(B) for all the predictors has been shown. The larger the value of odds ratio, the more the predictive value of the independent variable. In this example, the offensive rebound has a larger odds ratio 65.99, and hence this is the most important predictor in predicting the win in the match. It may be interpreted that the odds for the team to win are increased by a factor 65.99 if the average offensive rebounds of a team are higher in comparison with the other team provided other independent variables are constants. Let us understand this fact.

$$\text{Since odds ratio} = \frac{p}{1-p} \Rightarrow p = \frac{\text{odds ratio}}{1 + \text{odds ratio}}$$

$$\text{For offensive rebound, } p = \frac{65.99}{1 + 65.99} = 0.985$$

This indicates that if a team's average offensive rebound is more than that of the opponent team, his probability of winning would be 0.985 provided other variables remain constant.

Since the odds ratio for the Blocks is 2.303, it indicates that if the average number of blocks of a team is more in comparison with that of the opponent, its odds for winning would increase by a factor 2.303 provided other variables remain constant.

$$\text{For Block, } p = \frac{2.303}{1 + 2.303} = 0.697$$

Thus, if a team's average number of blocks is more than that of the opponent, its probability of winning would be 0.697 provided other variables remain constant.

Similarly for the number of pass, the 0.714 odds ratio means that the odds of winning for a team are only 0.714 times in comparison with the team whose average number of pass is lower.

Let us now understand the interpretation of the logistic regression model that we developed in Equation 11.1. If two teams A and B are playing a basketball match and the value of all the independent variables for the team A is as follows:

Blocks = 1 (average number of block of the team A is higher than that of team B)

Free throws = 1 (average number of free throws of the team A is higher than that of team B)

Offensive rebound = 1 (average number of offensive rebound of the team A is higher than that of team B)

Number of pass = 0 (average number of pass of the team A is lower than that of team B)

Then by substituting these values in Equation 11.1, we obtain the following:

$$\log \frac{p}{1-p} = -2.539 + 0.834 \times 1 - 0.337 \times 1 + 4.190 \times 1 - 0.337 \times 0 = 2.148$$

$$\Rightarrow \qquad \text{Odds ratio} = \frac{p}{1-p} = e^{2.148} = 8.5677$$

$$\Rightarrow \qquad p = \frac{8.5677}{1+8.5677} = 0.8955$$

Thus, it may be inferred that the probability of the team A to win in the match would be 0.8955. One of the main features of the logistic regression equation is that no matter how many variables are included in the model, the probability of the dependent variable to occur cannot exceed 1.

Remark: You can compute the value of $e^{2.148}$ in Excel.

11.7.2.3 Reporting in Logistic Regression   Let us see how to report the findings in the logistic regression by means of the results obtained in this example.

- The logistic model developed using only intercept and without any predictor in Block 0 classifies only 50% cases correctly (Table 11.5) about the match results in a basketball tournament. However, if all the four predictors (number of pass, offensive rebound, free throws, and blocks) were included in the model shown in Block 1, the efficiency increased because the number of cases classified correctly by this model was 86.4% (Table 11.11).
- Since the value of chi-square in omnibus test (Table 11.8) is significant, it may be concluded that the model with all the four independent variables has significantly increased our ability to predict the match results.
- The Nagelkerke R^2 statistic is reported as 0.615 (Table 11.9); hence, 61.5% variability in predicting the match result can be explained by all the four predictors in the model.
- Since Hosmer–Lemeshow test is not significant (Table 11.10), it may be concluded that the fit is good and the developed logistic model is good in estimating the result.
- Among all the four independent variables only for offensive rebound, the Wald statistic is significant ($p=0.007$); hence, it may be concluded that the offensive rebound is the most important variable for estimating the result (Table 11.12). Further, odds ratio for the blocks is the second highest, that is, 2.303, and hence this is the second important variable in the model. It may be concluded that the probability of winning a team is 0.985 if its average offensive rebound is higher than that of the opponent team provided other variables are held constants.
- Finally, the logistic regression model developed in (Eq. 11.1) can be used to predict the match result if the values of all four independent variables are known.

11.8   SUMMARY OF THE SPSS COMMANDS FOR LOGISTIC REGRESSION

1. After preparing the data file, follow the command sequence as given in the text while being in the **data view** for logistic regression:

   Analyze → Regression → Binary Logistic

2. Select the dependent variables from the left panel, and bring them to the "Dependent" section in the right panel, and select all independent variables including categorical variables from left panel to the "Covariates" section in the right panel.

3. By clicking on the **Categorical** command, select the categorical variables from the "Covariates" section and bring them to the "Categorical Covariates" in the right panel and click on **Continue**.

4. Click on the **Options** command and check 'Hosmer–Lemeshow goodness-of-fit' option and click on **Continue**.

5. Ensure that the 'Enter' option is chosen by default and then click on **OK** for output.

11.9   EXERCISE

11.9.1   Short Answer Questions

Q.1 How would you interpret the logistic regression equation? Describe the procedure of computing probability of dependent variable to happen if log odds is known.

Q.2 Discuss the meaning of odds ratio and explain the logistic curve. Why the probability of dependent variable to happen cannot exceed 1.

Q.3 Discuss the assumptions used in logistic regression.

Q.4 Discuss two situations in sports where logistic regression can be used.

Q.5 Discuss the procedure in logistic regression. What outputs are generated in SPSS?

Q.6 What is the difference in outputs generated by the SPSS in Block 0 and Block 1? What is the utility of the model developed in Block 0?

Q.7 Explain the following terms:
(a) −2 Log Likelihood
(b) Hosmer–Lemeshow Test
(c) Nagelkerke R^2
(d) Classification table
(e) Logit

11.9.2   Multiple Choice Questions

Note: Questions 1–10 have four alternative answers for each question. Tick mark the one that you consider the closest to the correct answer.

1 With the help of logistic regression equation, the value of the
   (a) Dependent variable is estimated
   (b) Probability that the dependent variable $y = 1$ is estimated
   (c) Logit is estimated
   (d) Odds for the dependent variable Y to assume 1 is estimated

2 In binary logistic regression which of the following statement is true?
   (a) The dependent variable is categorical and independent variables should be numerical.
   (b) The dependent variable is dichotomous and independent variables should be ordinal.
   (c) The dependent variable is categorical and independent variables should be nonparametric.
   (d) The dependent variable is dichotomous and independent variables can be either numerical, categorical, or a mix of both.

3 If $Exp(4) = 54.6$, then $Log(54.6)$ is
   (a) 58.6
   (b) 4
   (c) 54.6
   (d) 218.4

4 If the probability of success is 0.4, then the odds ratio for the success is
   (a) 0.67
   (b) 0.6
   (c) 0.24
   (d) 0.20

5 If odds ratio for the happening of an event is 3, then the probability of the happening of the event is
   (a) 0.70
   (b) 0.43
   (c) 0.30
   (d) 0.75

6 In a logistic regression if the odds ratio for an independent variable is 4.6, then the true statement is:
   (a) The probability of the happening of the dependent variable is 0.46.
   (b) The odds for the happening of the dependent variable is increased by a factor of 4.6 against 1 unit increase in the independent variable provided other independent variables are held constant.
   (c) The odds against the happening of the dependent variable is 4.6.
   (d) The odds for the happening of the dependent variable is 4.6.

7   If p is the probability of the happening of a dependent variable, then logit is computed by

(a) $\ln \dfrac{1-p}{p}$

(b) $\ln \dfrac{1+p}{p}$

(c) $\log \dfrac{p}{1-p}$

(d) $\log \dfrac{p}{1+p}$

8   If log odds is represented by L, then the probability of the happening of a dependent variable is obtained by

(a) $p = \dfrac{L}{1-L}$

(b) $p = \dfrac{1+L}{L}$

(c) $\log \dfrac{1-L}{L}$

(d) $p = \dfrac{L}{1+L}$

9   In the output of logistic regression, Odds ratio is denoted by
(a) Log(B)
(b) Exp(B)
(c) B coefficient
(d) $\dfrac{p}{1-p}$

10   The Hosmer–Lemeshow test is used to test
(a) Whether the model fit is good or not
(b) Whether the model with predictors and without predictors gives the same results
(c) Whether the predictors included in the model are worth including
(d) Whether model with constant only and no predictors is significant

11.9.3   Assignment

1. An exercise scientist wanted to investigate the likelihood for the men cricketer to be obese on the basis of different lifestyle parameters. A cricketer was identified as obese if his fat% was 20 or more. The data so obtained are shown in Table 11.13. Develop logistic regression and explain your findings. Discuss the likelihood of cricketer being obese due to change of each independent variable separately in the model.

TABLE 11.13   Data of the National-Level Men Cricketers

SN	Obesity Status	Smoking Status	Alcohol Consumption	Fat Consumption	Sleep Hour
1	1	1	1	2	4
2	1	0	1	1	5
3	0	0	0	1	6
4	1	1	1	0	4
5	0	1	0	0	5
6	0	0	1	1	7
7	1	1	1	2	6
8	0	0	0	0	4
9	1	1	1	2	8
10	1	1	1	1	7
11	0	0	0	0	8
12	0	1	1	1	5
13	0	1	0	0	6
14	1	0	1	0	7
15	0	0	0	2	4
16	1	1	0	1	5
17	1	1	1	1	7
18	0	0	0	2	6

Coding: 0, nonobese; 1, nonsmoker; 1, nonalcoholic; 2, less fatty diet.
1, obese; 0, smoker; 0, alcoholic; 1, medium fatty diet.
0, high fatty diet.

11.10   CASE STUDY ON LOGISTIC REGRESSION

Objective

A sports scientist wanted to develop a strategy for winning in women soccer match. During a soccer championship, she obtained the data on height, dietary habit (veg/nonveg), VO_2 max, body fat%, and 40 yrd dash timings on the players of each team. For each team, average score of height, VO_2 max, Fat%, and 40 yrd timings was computed. A team's diet score was noted as 1 if more number of players were nonveg in comparison with that of the opponent team; whereas, the other team's score was noted as 0 (representing veg). The data so obtained for the teams in 12 matches are shown in Table 11.14.

Research Issues

The following research questions were investigated:

1. Whether an efficient logistic model be developed for finding the likelihood of winning in soccer match on the basis of some predictor variables.
2. Whether the developed model would be significant and efficient.
3. Whether few independent variables will have better contribution in the model over others.

TABLE 11.14 Data Format Used in SPSS for Logistic Regression

SN	Team_Result[a]	Height (centimeters)	VO$_2$ max (ml.kg^{-1}.min^{-1})	Diet[b]	Fat (%)	Forty_Yrd (sec)
1	1	165	45	1	22	5.63
2	1	162	43.5	1	21	5.62
3	0	168	44	0	24	5.9
4	1	172	40	1	20	5.4
5	0	170	46	0	25	6.1
6	0	174	44	0	24	5.8
7	1	165	42	0	19	5.4
8	1	160	45	1	18	5.5
9	1	176	43	1	24	5.3
10	0	178	40	0	20	6.0
11	1	179	45	0	21	5.1
12	0	165	44	1	26	5.9
13	0	167	46	0	27	5.7
14	0	164	42	0	21	5.8
15	0	161	40	1	27	5.9
16	1	176	44	1	22	5.4
17	1	180	40	1	21	5.3
18	0	168	41	0	25	5.0
19	1	172	46	0	21	5.6
20	1	175	43	1	22	5.7
21	0	168	46	1	22	5.1
22	1	173	45	1	24	5.7
23	0	168	38	0	26	5.9
24	1	176	42	1	22	6.2

[a] 0 = loser, 1 = winner.
[b] 0 = veg, 1 = nonveg.

Data Format

The format used for preparing data file in SPSS is shown in Table 11.14.

Analyzing Data

In this study, it was required to develop a model for estimating the likelihood of winning in women soccer match on the basis of the identified predictor variables. Since the dependent variable was categorical and independent variables were a mix of both categorical and numerical, the logistic regression was used. The analysis was carried out in SPSS by using the following commands: **Analyze, Regression,** and **Binary Logistic** in sequence. The dependent variable and covariates were placed in the appropriate locations in the dialog box by identifying the categorical variable. By choosing the option 'Hosmer–Lemeshow goodness-of-fit' and 'Enter,' the output was generated in two sections: Blocks 0 and Block 1. Since 'Enter' method was chosen, the model was developed by taking all the predictor variables in the model. The output in Block 0 shows a logistic model without using any of the explanatory variables. In Block 1, the logistic model was developed using all the explanatory variables in the study. The outputs generated by the SPSS are shown in Tables 11.15, 11.16, 11.17, 11.18, 11.19, 11.20, and 11.21. Findings of the logistic regression shall be discussed in two blocks.

TABLE 11.15 Classification Table[a,b]

			Predicted		
			Team_Result		Percentage Correct
Observed			Loser	Winner	
Step 0	Team_result	Loser	0	11	0.0
		Winner	0	13	100.0
	Overall percentage				54.2

[a] Constant is included in the model.
[b] The cut value is 0.500.

TABLE 11.16 Variables Not in the Equation

			Score	df	Sig.
Step 0	Variables	Height	2.018	1	0.155
		VO$_2$ max	0.321	1	0.571
		Diet(1)	5.916	1	0.015
		Fat	8.771	1	0.003
		Forty_Yrd	2.615	1	0.106
	Overall statistics		14.965	5	0.011

TABLE 11.17   Omnibus Tests of Model Coefficients

		Chi-Square	df	Sig.
Step 1	Step	20.243	5	0.001
	Block	20.243	5	0.001
	Model	20.243	5	0.001

TABLE 11.18   Model Summary

Step	−2 Log Likelihood	Cox and Snell R^2	Nagelkerke R^2
1	12.862[a]	0.570	0.761

[a] Estimation terminated at iteration number 7 because parameter estimates changed by less than 0.001.

TABLE 11.19   Hosmer–Lemeshow Test

Step	Chi-Square	df	Sig.
1	6.711	8	0.568

TABLE 11.20   Classification Table[a]

			Predicted		
			Team_Result		
	Observed		Loser	Winner	Percentage Correct
Step 1	Team_result	Loser	9	2	81.8
		Winner	0	13	100.0
	Overall percentage				91.7

[a] The cut value is 0.500.

TABLE 11.21   Variables in the Equation

		B	S.E.	Wald	df	Sig.	Exp(B)
Step 1[a]	Height	0.161	0.138	1.355	1	0.244	1.175
	VO$_2$ max	0.430	0.478	0.807	1	0.369	1.537
	Diet(1)	−3.663	1.889	3.762	1	0.052	0.026
	Fat	−1.076	0.589	3.333	1	0.068	0.341
	Forty_yrd	−0.275	2.772	0.010	1	0.921	0.759
	Constant	−18.660	37.766	0.244	1	0.621	0.000

[a] Variable(s) entered on step 1: Height, VO$_2$ max, Diet, Fat, Forty_Yrd.

Block 0: Logistic Model without Predictors

Table 11.15 indicates that if nothing is known about the independent variables and one simply guesses about the match result, he would be correct 54.2% of the time.

Table 11.16 indicates whether each independent variable may improve the model or not if included. Here only diet and fat% variables seem to be significant; hence they may improve the model if included.

Block 1: Logistic Model with Predictors

In Block 1, the logistic model was developed by the SPSS using all the five predictors. This is the actual model of interest.

Testing significance of the model: Omnibus test of model coefficients in Table 11.17 shows that a chi-square value 20.243 is significant (p=0.001). This indicates that after adding the predictor variables, the ability of predicting match result in a women soccer match would significantly improve.

In Table 11.18, the Nagelkerke R^2 is 0.761. This indicates that 76.1% variability of the dependent variable can be explained by all the five predictors together.

Testing goodness of fit of the model: The Hosmer–Lemeshow test was used to test whether the developed logistic model is efficient in predicting the happening of the dependent variable. Since the value of chi-square is not significant (p=0.568) as shown in Table 11.19, the developed model is good in estimating the match result (a dependent variable).

Model accuracy: Table 11.20 shows that the model correctly classified 91.7% cases. In comparing the result of Table 11.15, it can be seen that when no predictor was used, model correctly classified 54.2% cases; whereas by including five independent variables in the model, the percentage of correct classification has increased to 91.7%. It may therefore be concluded that introducing these independent variables has definitely improved the model efficiency.

Developing logistic model: Table 11.21 is the main result in logistic regression. It includes regression coefficients (B) and odds ratios (Exp(B)). It also includes Wald chi-square statistic that tests the unique contribution of each predictor. It can be seen that no variable is significant independently. Since the logistic model was developed by including all the five independent variables, hence using the coefficients shown in the table the following logistic model was developed.

$$\log \frac{p}{1-p} = -18.660 + 0.161 \times \text{Height} + 0.430 \times \text{VO}_2 \max - 3.663$$
$$\times \text{Diet} - 1.076 \times \text{Fat} - 0.275 \times \text{Forty\_yrd}$$

where p is the probability of winning the match. The dependent variable in the logistic regression is known as logit (p), which is equal to $\log(p/(1-p))$.

Explanation of odds ratios and logistic model: In Table 11.21, the odds ratio Exp(B) for all the predictors has been shown. The larger the value of odds ratio, the more the predictive value of the independent variable. In this study, the VO_2 max has a larger odds ratio 1.537; hence, this is the most important predictor in predicting the win in the match. It may be interpreted that the odds for the team to win are increased by a factor 1.537 if the average VO_2 max of a team is increased by 1 unit provided other independent variables are constants. This fact can be understood like this

$$\text{Since odds ratio} = \frac{p}{1-p} \quad \Rightarrow \quad p = \frac{\text{odds ratio}}{1+\text{odds ratio}}$$

$$\text{For } VO_2 \text{ max}, \quad p = \frac{1.537}{1+1.537} = 0.61$$

This indicates that if a team's average VO_2 max is increased by one unit the log odds of the team will increase by 1.537 and in that case probability of winning the match will become 0.61 in comparison to opponent, then the probability of winning would be 0.61 provided other variables remain constant.

Since the odds ratio for the height is 1.175, it indicates that if the average height of the team players is increased by 1 unit, its log odds of winning would increase by 1.175 times provided other variables remain constant.

$$\text{For Height}, \quad p = \frac{1.175}{1+1.175} = 0.54$$

Thus, if the average height of a team's player is increased by 1 unit, its probability of winning would be 0.54 provided other variables remain constant.

Reporting in Logistic Regression

- The logistic model developed using only intercept and without any predictor in Block 0 classified only 54.2% cases correctly about the team result in soccer tournament. But after including all the five predictors (height, VO_2 max, diet, fat, and 40 yrd) in the model, the efficiency has increased because the number of cases classified correctly by this model became 91.7%.
- Since the chi-square in omnibus test is significant, it may be concluded that the model with all the five independent variables has significantly increased our ability to predict the decision about the team result.
- The Nagelkerke R^2 statistic is reported as 0.761; hence, 76.1% variability in predicting the winning of a team can be explained by all the five predictors in the model.
- Since Hosmer–Lemeshow test was not significant, it may be concluded that the fit is good and the developed logistic model is good in estimating the happening of winning in a match.
- The Wald statistic was not significant for any of the variable; hence, no variable was found to be independently significant in the model.
- If the mean score of VO_2 max and height of a team are increased by 1 unit, then its chances of winning would be marginally higher than that of the opponent.

12

APPLICATION OF FACTOR ANALYSIS

LEARNING OBJECTIVES

After completing this chapter, you should be able to do the following:

- Know the use of factor analysis in developing test battery
- Interpret various terms involved in factor analysis
- Identify the situation where factor analysis can be used
- Explain the procedure of retaining factors and identifying variables in it
- Understand the steps involved in factor analysis
- Learn the steps involved in using SPSS for factor analysis
- Describe the output obtained in factor analysis
- Learn to write the results of factor analysis in standard format.

12.1 INTRODUCTION

Talent identification is one of the thrust areas of research in sports. Different approaches are used in developing criteria for talent identification. Coaches and sport scientists use their knowledge to identify parameters for developing such criteria. The factor analysis approach provides a solution in this regard by reducing a large number of variables, considered to be associated with performance, into a few latent factors that can be more easily studied. For example, in studying a group of badminton players, their measures on height, weight, arm length, leg length, agility, speed, upper body flexibility, lower body flexibility, and knee flexibility might be summarized using factor analysis as anthropometric (height, weight, arm length, and

Sports Research with Analytical Solution using SPSS®, First Edition. J. P. Verma.
© 2016 John Wiley & Sons, Inc. Published 2016 by John Wiley & Sons, Inc.
Companion website: www.wiley.com/go/Verma/Sportsresearch

leg length), flexibility (upper body flexibility, lower body flexibility, sit and reach), and speedo-agility (agility, speed) factors. In this way, nine variables can be grouped into three different latent factors.

Thus, in factor analysis, a few factors are extracted out of the large set of variables. Since variables in each factor are associated among themselves, they represent the same phenomenon. In this way, instead of studying all the parameters, a few extracted factors are studied. These factors so extracted explain much of the variations of the group characteristics.

The factor analysis may be used for developing a test battery. For example, to assess fitness status of an individual, several parameters may be tested. But using a large number of variables is neither feasible nor advisable. Thus, these variables may be reduced to a few significant factors that may be used for developing a test battery for assessing fitness. These factors so extracted by the factor analysis technique explain much of the variation of an individual's fitness.

Consider another situation where flexibility of an individual needs to be assessed. This can be done by obtaining 20 measures of different joints flexibility using flexometer and goniometer. Since many of these measures of the flexibility may be associated among themselves, by using factor analysis these variables may be reduced to few factors that can explain the total flexibility of an individual. In each factor, the most dominant variable may be selected for inclusion in the test battery. Thus, a battery of few variables may explain most of the subject's flexibility.

12.2 TERMINOLOGIES USED IN FACTOR ANALYSIS

We have seen that a factor analysis is a data reduction technique that aims at reducing a large number of variables into fewer factors to study the variability of a group. It can also be used to study the structure of factors present in a data set. Before discussing the procedure involved in factor analysis, let us first discuss the terminologies involved in it. It is assumed that the readers are familiar with the basic logic of statistical reasoning and the concepts of variance and correlation; if not, it is advised that they should read the basic statistics topic at this point from some other standard texts of statistics.

12.2.1 Principal Component Analysis

Principal component analysis is the most widely used method of factor analysis. In this method, the factor explaining the maximum variance is extracted first. After that, it removes the variance explained by the first factor and then starts extracting maximum variance for the second factor. This process goes on to the last factor.

12.2.2 Eigenvalue

The eigenvalue is the variance explained by a factor. It is also known as characteristics root. The sum of all the eigenvalues is equal to the number of variables. The decision about the number of factors to be retained in the factor analysis is taken on the basis of eigenvalue.

12.2.3   Kaiser Criterion

In factor analysis, one needs to decide the number of factors to be selected. As per the Kaiser's criteria, only those factors having eigenvalues greater than 1 should be retained. Initially, each variable is supposed to have its eigenvalue 1. Thus, it may be said that unless a factor extracts at least as much as the equivalent of one original variable, it is dropped. This criterion was proposed by Kaiser (1960) and is widely used by the researchers.

12.2.4   The Scree Test

It is a graphical method of identifying the point where important factors stop and unimportant ones start. The scree test was developed by Cattell. "Scree" is a term used in geology. The scree is the rubble at the bottom of a cliff. A correlation matrix can be decomposed into independent weighted combinations of the original variables. Each set will have some variance associated with it. In scree test if a factor is important, it will have a large variance. Here eigenvalues are plotted against the factors. Then the factors above the elbow in the plot are retained. These are the important factors that account for the bulk of the correlations in the matrix. The scree test graph may look like as shown in Figure 12.1.

12.2.5   Communality

The communality is the amount of variance each variable in the analysis shares with other variables. More specifically, it is the squared multiple correlation for the variable as dependent using the factors as predictors and is denoted by h^2. The value of communality may be considered as an indicator of the usefulness of a variable in the factor analysis.

If a variable has a low communality, the factor model is not working well for that variable, and possibly it should be removed from the model. Low communalities

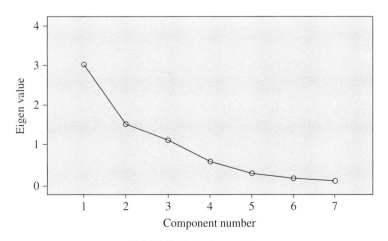

FIGURE 12.1   Scree plot.

across the set of variables indicate the variables are little related to each other. The communalities must be interpreted in relation to the interpretability of the factors. A communality of 0.80 may seem to be high but is meaningless unless the factor on which the variable is loaded is interpretable, though it usually will be. A communality of 0.30 may seem to be low but may be meaningful if the item is contributing to a well-defined factor.

Thus, it is not that only the value of communality coefficient is important, but the important consideration is the extent to which the item plays a role in the interpretation of the factor. Often the item would contribute more in explaining the factor if its communality is high.

12.2.6   Factor Loading

Factor loading can be defined as the correlation coefficient between the variable and the factor. It shows the variance explained by the variable on that particular factor. As a rule of thumb, 0.7 or higher factor loading represents that the factor extracts sufficient variance from that variable.

12.2.7   Varimax Rotation

In factor analysis, the factor loadings are plotted as a scatter plot. In the scatter plot, each variable is represented as a point. In this plot, one can rotate the axes in any direction without changing the relative locations of the points to each other. However, the actual coordinates of the points, that is, the factor loadings would of course change. Thus, if the axes are rotated by some degree, say $30°$ or $45°$, one might attain a clear pattern of loadings in each factor. Varimax rotation is the most widely used method of rotating the axes in the scatter plot. Other rotational strategies are Quartimax, Equamax, Direct oblimin, and Promax methods.

12.3   ASSUMPTIONS IN FACTOR ANALYSIS

The following assumptions are made in applying factor analysis:

1. Data used in the factor analysis is based on an interval scale or a ratio scale
2. Variables are normally distributed.
3. Relevant variables are included in the analysis. In other words, variables that theoretically go together have been included in the study.
4. Sufficient sample size has been taken for factor analysis. At least five cases per variable should be taken.
5. No outlier is present in the data.
6. Variables are linearly related with each other reasonably.
7. The spread about the line of best fit is homoscedastic.

12.4 STEPS IN FACTOR ANALYSIS

1. The first step in the factor analysis is to get unrotated factor solution by using the principal component method. This solution is obtained on the basis of the correlation matrix developed among the variables. This solution contains the factors extracted and loadings of all the variables on these factors. Factors are retained in the primary solution on the basis of their eigenvalues. Only those variables that have eigenvalues more than 1 are retained. The scree plot can be used to identify the factors to be retained.

2. The second phase of the analysis provides the final solution after rotating the factors. The researchers usually employ the varimax rotation. After the rotation, each variable can be exclusively classified in one or the other factors. Variables in each factor are identified on the basis of its factor loadings. As per the convention, in each factor only those variables that have factor loadings more than 0.7 are identified. After identifying variables in each factor, factors are named on the basis of the variable's characteristics identified in it.

3. Finally, one or two variables from each factor may be selected on the basis of highest loadings to develop a test battery. Usually, the first factor explains the maximum variance of the group and, therefore, two or three variables may be kept from it depending upon the nature of the variables and its explainability. From the rest of the factors, normally one variable per factor is selected as the sole purpose of the factor analysis is to reduce the variables so that the maximum variance in the group may be explained.

12.5 APPLICATION OF FACTOR ANALYSIS

Consider a situation where it is desired to develop an instrument in the form of questionnaire to assess the lifestyle of an individual. To do so, one must determine the parameters based on which the lifestyle can be assessed. On the basis of literature review, one may decide to identify 10 parameters. Now the two main issues of investigation are as follows: firstly, whether these parameters explain different dimensions of lifestyle and, secondly, if we could develop the lifestyle assessment instrument on less than 10 parameters. To address these two issues, factor analysis technique can be used. By using this technique, all these 10 parameters can be reduced to few factors. By selecting variables from these factors on the basis of their higher loadings, a questionnaire may be developed for assessing the lifestyle of an individual. This way, only relevant parameters would be used for assessment; and instead of 10 parameters, fewer numbers of variables may be required for developing the questionnaire.

Procedure Involved

After identifying the parameters responsible for the lifestyle as mentioned below, a questionnaire can be framed, where the respondent can get scores in between 1 and 5 depending upon the type of response selected for each question.

Parameters responsible for the lifestyle

1. Alcohol use
2. Tobacco use
3. Blood pressure
4. Body weight
5. Activity level
6. Stress level
7. Car safety
8. Relationships
9. Rest/sleep
10. Life satisfaction

After getting the scores on each of these 10 parameters, a data file can be prepared for using in the SPSS analysis. By using SPSS output, these parameters can be reduced to a few significant factors. From these factors, variables having higher loadings may be selected to form the final instrument for lifestyle assessment. Thus, the questionnaire so obtained shall be more reliable and will include less number of variables. The detailed procedure can be seen in the solved Example 12.1.

12.6   FACTOR ANALYSIS WITH SPSS

Example 12.1

In a study on swimmers, 11 physical and physiological parameters were measured and the data so obtained is shown in Table 12.1. Apply factor analysis technique to study the factor structure and suggest the test battery that can be used for screening the talents in swimming. Also apply the scree test for retaining factors graphically and Kaiser-Meyer-Olkin (KMO) test for testing the adequacy of data.

Solution: In this example, the following things are required to be done:

1. To decide the number of factors to be retained and the total variance explained by these factors
2. To identify the variables in each factor retained in the final solution on the basis of their factor loadings
3. To give a name to each factor on the basis of the nature of variables included in it
4. To suggest the test battery for screening talents in swimming
5. To test the adequacy of sample size used in factor analysis

TABLE 12.1   Data on Selected Physical and Physiological Parameters Obtained on Swimmers

S.N.	SBJ (cm)	Shut_Run (sec)	50_Mt (sec)	12Min_R/W (mt.)	Aner_Cap (sec)	Wt (kg)	Ht (cm)	Leg_Length (cm)	Calf_Girth (cm)	Thigh_Girth (cm)	Shoul_Width (cm)
1	218	10.20	7.90	2710	47.50	30	136	71	27	37	42
2	200	11.10	8.13	2410	20.60	27	136	70	28	39	35
3	195	10.43	7.99	2655	45.20	30	142	70	28	38	35
4	212	10.23	8.16	2510	32.67	41	157	76	28	38	33
5	185	10.91	8.50	2105	15.84	27	130	72	25	33	37
6	206	10.02	7.31	2615	50.20	27	135	72	27	38	35
7	235	09.60	6.88	2802	58.30	35	144	76	28	42	37
8	205	10.85	8.05	2395	29.00	42	161	78	29	38	28
9	213	10.30	8.13	2435	22.09	30	142	77	26	38	33
10	220	10.22	8.60	2080	30.48	40	149	78	29	43	37
11	208	09.70	7.73	2518	53.40	38	145	76	31	45	39
12	210	09.88	7.80	2608	49.30	34	141	76	29	40	38
13	201	09.84	7.98	2516	44.30	31	138	74	29	42	38
14	225	10.00	7.38	2610	50.20	41	154	82	30	43	41
15	200	11.15	8.15	2420	34.64	46	157	76	27	41	36
16	219	09.95	7.35	2630	34.55	42	158	86	31	41	43
17	215	09.73	7.50	2605	35.12	43	159	74	27	44	45
18	210	10.48	8.10	2310	34.16	43	153	71	27	36	44
19	260	09.50	6.85	2830	62.20	49	159	82	33	46	44
20	218	10.09	7.20	2514	52.10	52	164	90	32	47	44
21	205	11.10	8.88	1990	36.20	46	157	76	28	42	37

These objectives shall be achieved by generating the outputs in SPSS. Thus, the procedure of using SPSS for factor analysis in the given example shall be discussed first, and thereafter the output shall be explained in light of the objectives to be fulfilled in this study.

12.6.1 Computation in Factor Analysis Using SPSS

12.6.1.1 Preparation of Data File   To prepare data file, all the variables need to be defined first. This can be done by using the following sequence of commands:

Start → All Programs → SPSS Inc → SPSS 20.0 → Type in Data

This will open a window for defining variables row-wise.

12.6.1.2 Defining Variables   There are 11 variables in this example, which need to be defined along with their properties. All these variables are scale variables. The procedure of defining these variables and their characteristics is as follows:

1. Click on **Variable View** to define variables and their properties.
2. Write short name of the variables as *SBJ, Shut_Run, 50_Mt, 12_min_R/W, Aner_Cap, Wt, Ht, Leg_Length, Calf_Girth, Thigh_Girth, and Shl_Width* under the column heading "Name."
3. Under the column heading "Label," full name of these variables may be defined as *Standing Broad Jump, 4 × 10 Shuttle Run, 50 Mt. Timings, 12 min R/W, Anaerobic Capacity, Weight, Height, Leg Length, Calf Girth, Thigh Girth*, and *Shoulder Width*. Other names may be chosen for describing these variables.
4. Under the column heading "Measure," select 'Scale' option for all the variables.
5. Use default entries in rest of the columns.

After defining all the variables in **Variable View**, the screen shall look like as shown in Figure 12.2.

12.6.1.3 Entering Data   After defining the variables click on **Data View** on the screen shown in Figure 12.2 to open the format for entering the data column-wise.

After entering the data, the screen will look like as shown in Figure 12.3. Save the data file in the desired location before further processing.

12.6.1.4 SPSS Commands   While being in the **Data View**, do the following steps:

1. *Initiating SPSS commands:* Click the following commands in sequence:

Analyze → Data Reduction → Factor

The screen shall look like as shown in Figure 12.4.

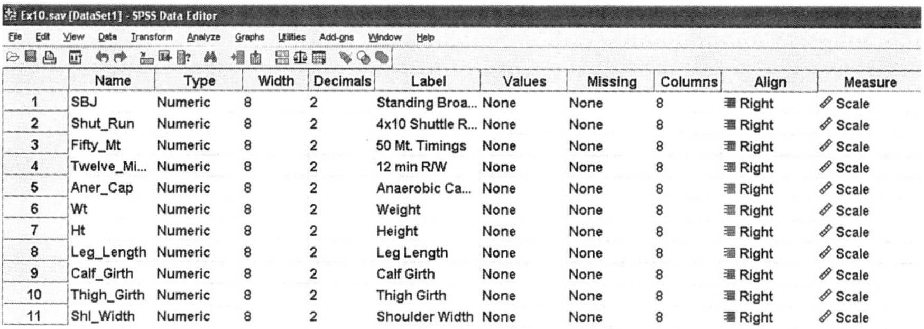

	Name	Type	Width	Decimals	Label	Values	Missing	Columns	Align	Measure
1	SBJ	Numeric	8	2	Standing Broa...	None	None	8	Right	Scale
2	Shut_Run	Numeric	8	2	4x10 Shuttle R...	None	None	8	Right	Scale
3	Fifty_Mt	Numeric	8	2	50 Mt. Timings	None	None	8	Right	Scale
4	Twelve_Mi...	Numeric	8	2	12 min R/W	None	None	8	Right	Scale
5	Aner_Cap	Numeric	8	2	Anaerobic Ca...	None	None	8	Right	Scale
6	Wt	Numeric	8	2	Weight	None	None	8	Right	Scale
7	Ht	Numeric	8	2	Height	None	None	8	Right	Scale
8	Leg_Length	Numeric	8	2	Leg Length	None	None	8	Right	Scale
9	Calf_Girth	Numeric	8	2	Calf Girth	None	None	8	Right	Scale
10	Thigh_Girth	Numeric	8	2	Thigh Girth	None	None	8	Right	Scale
11	Shl_Width	Numeric	8	2	Shoulder Width	None	None	8	Right	Scale

FIGURE 12.2 Defining variables along with their characteristics.

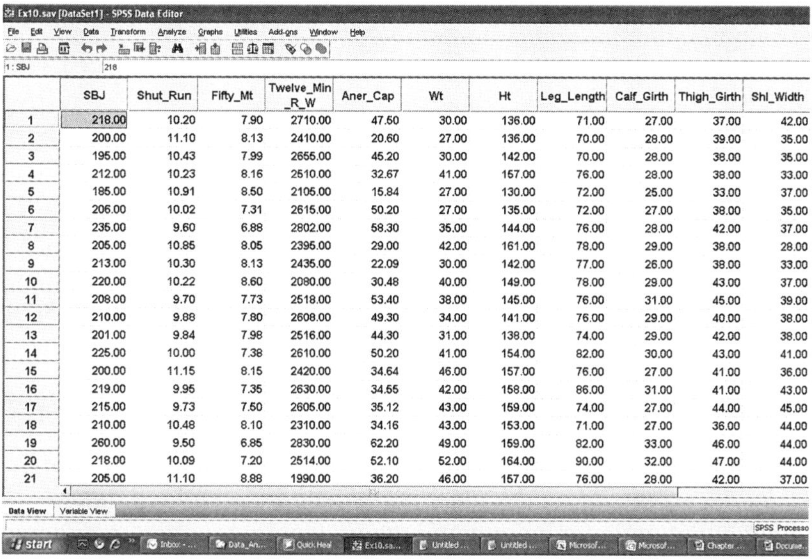

	SBJ	Shut_Run	Fifty_Mt	Twelve_Min_R_W	Aner_Cap	Wt	Ht	Leg_Length	Calf_Girth	Thigh_Girth	Shl_Width
1	218.00	10.20	7.90	2710.00	47.50	30.00	136.00	71.00	27.00	37.00	42.00
2	200.00	11.10	8.13	2410.00	20.60	27.00	136.00	70.00	28.00	39.00	35.00
3	195.00	10.43	7.99	2655.00	45.20	30.00	142.00	70.00	28.00	38.00	35.00
4	212.00	10.23	8.16	2510.00	32.67	41.00	157.00	76.00	28.00	38.00	33.00
5	185.00	10.91	8.50	2105.00	15.84	27.00	130.00	72.00	25.00	33.00	37.00
6	206.00	10.02	7.31	2615.00	50.20	27.00	135.00	72.00	27.00	38.00	35.00
7	235.00	9.60	6.88	2802.00	58.30	35.00	144.00	76.00	28.00	42.00	37.00
8	205.00	10.85	8.05	2395.00	29.00	42.00	161.00	78.00	29.00	38.00	28.00
9	213.00	10.30	8.13	2435.00	22.09	30.00	142.00	77.00	26.00	38.00	33.00
10	220.00	10.22	8.60	2080.00	30.48	40.00	149.00	78.00	29.00	43.00	37.00
11	208.00	9.70	7.73	2518.00	53.40	38.00	145.00	76.00	31.00	45.00	39.00
12	210.00	9.88	7.80	2608.00	49.30	34.00	141.00	76.00	29.00	40.00	38.00
13	201.00	9.84	7.98	2516.00	44.30	31.00	138.00	74.00	29.00	42.00	38.00
14	225.00	10.00	7.38	2610.00	50.20	41.00	154.00	82.00	30.00	43.00	41.00
15	200.00	11.15	8.15	2420.00	34.64	46.00	157.00	76.00	27.00	41.00	36.00
16	219.00	9.95	7.35	2630.00	34.55	42.00	158.00	86.00	31.00	41.00	43.00
17	215.00	9.73	7.50	2605.00	35.12	43.00	159.00	74.00	27.00	44.00	45.00
18	210.00	10.48	8.10	2310.00	34.16	43.00	153.00	71.00	27.00	36.00	44.00
19	260.00	9.50	6.85	2830.00	62.20	49.00	159.00	82.00	33.00	46.00	44.00
20	218.00	10.09	7.20	2514.00	52.10	52.00	164.00	90.00	32.00	47.00	44.00
21	205.00	11.10	8.88	1990.00	36.20	46.00	157.00	76.00	28.00	42.00	37.00

FIGURE 12.3 Data file of physical and physiological variables for factor analysis.

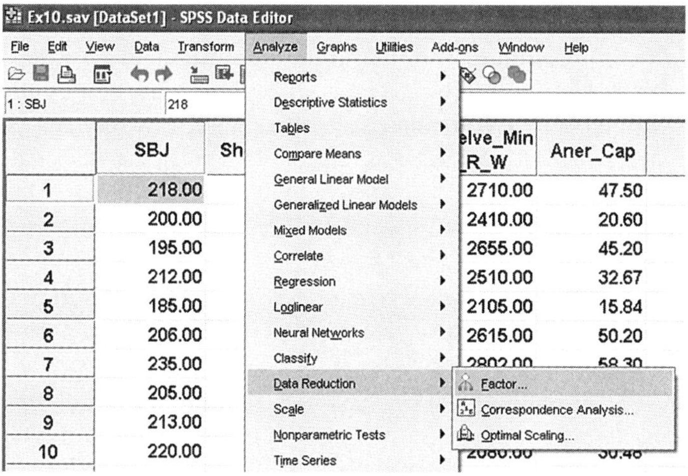

FIGURE 12.4 Command sequence for factor analysis.

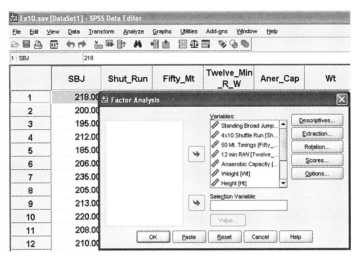

FIGURE 12.5   Selection of variables in factor analysis.

2. *Selecting variables for factor analysis:* Clicking the "Factor" option will take you to the next screen for selecting variables. Select all the variables from left panel and bring them to the "Variables" section in the right panel. The screen will look like as shown in Figure 12.5.

3. *Selecting option for computation:* After selecting the variables, various options need to be defined for generating the outputs in factor analysis. Do the following:

   (a) Click on **Descriptives** command on the screen shown in Figure 12.5.

   (b) Check 'Univariate descriptives' and 'Initial solution' options in "Statistics" section.

   (c) Check 'Coefficients,' 'Significance levels,' and 'KMO and Bartlett's test of sphericity' options in "Correlation Matrix" section. The screen will look like as shown in Figure 12.6.

   (d) Click on **Continue**. This will again take you back to the screen shown in Figure 12.5.

   (e) Now click on **Extraction** command and check 'Scree plot' option. Let other options remain as it is by default. The screen shall look like as shown in Figure 12.7.

   (f) Click on **Continue**. This will again take you back to the screen shown in Figure 12.5.

   (g) Now click on **Rotation** command and then check 'Varimax' rotation option. Let other options remain as it is by default. The screen shall look like as shown in Figure 12.8.

   (h) Click on **Continue** and **OK** to get the outputs.

4. *Getting the output:* After clicking on **OK** on in the screen shown in Figure 12.5, various outputs shall be generated in the output window. The SPSS shall

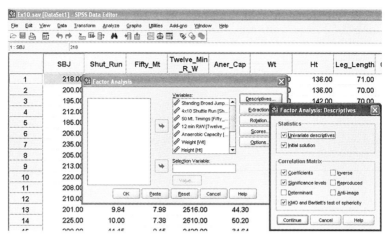

FIGURE 12.6 Selection of options for correlation matrix and initial factor solution.

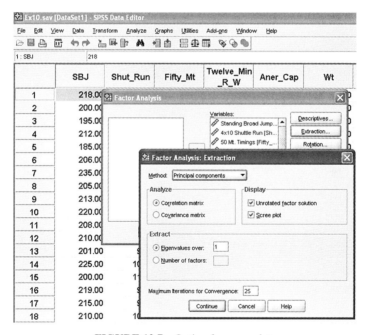

FIGURE 12.7 Option for scree plot.

generate many outputs, but the following relevant outputs have been picked up for the discussion:

(a) Descriptive statistics

(b) Correlation matrix

(c) KMO and Bartlett's test

(d) Total variance explained

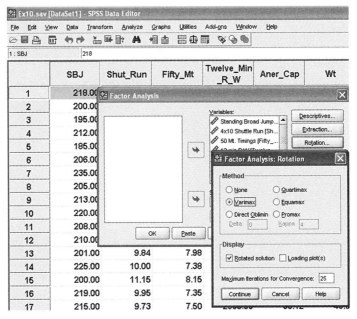

FIGURE 12.8   Option for factor rotation.

TABLE 12.2   Descriptive Statistics

	Mean	Std. Deviation	N
Standing broad jump	212.38	15.45793	21
4 × 10 shuttle run	10.2514	0.51167	21
50 mt. timings	7.8367	0.53814	21
12 min R/W	2489.0	222.46696	21
Anaerobic capacity	39.9071	12.70207	21
Weight	37.8095	7.67215	21
Height	148.43	10.23509	21
Leg length	76.3333	5.18009	21
Calf girth	28.5238	1.99045	21
Thigh girth	40.5238	3.51595	21
Shoulder width	38.1429	4.43041	21

(e) Scree plot

(f) Component matrix: unrotated factor solution

(g) Rotated component matrix: varimax rotated solution

12.6.1.5   Interpretation of Findings   The outputs generated in this example by the SPSS have been shown in Tables 12.2, 12.3, 12.4, 12.5, 12.6, and 12.7 and in Figure 12.9.

1. Table 12.2 shows the descriptive statistics that consists of mean and SD for all the variables. The researcher may select this table of descriptive statistics from

TABLE 12.3 Correlation Matrix for the Data on Selected Physical and Physiological Parameters of Swimmers

	SBJ	Shut_Run	50_Mt	12_Min_R/W	Aner_Cap	Wt	Ht	Leg_Length	Calf_Girth	Thigh_Girth	Shl_Width
	X1	X2	X3	X4	X5	X6	X7	X8	X9	X10	X11
X1	1	-0.651**	-0.672**	0.539*	0.608**	0.469*	0.415	0.513*	0.606**	0.584**	0.455*
X2	-0.651**	1	0.742**	-0.691**	-0.709**	-0.087	-0.052	-0.321	-0.495*	-0.515*	-0.483*
X3	-0.672**	0.742**	1	-0.858**	-0.723**	-0.194	-0.195	-0.442*	-0.534*	-0.479*	-0.446*
X4	0.539*	-0.691**	-0.858**	1	0.686**	-0.045	0.013	0.151	0.366	0.269	0.279
X5	0.608**	-0.709**	-0.723**	0.686**	1	0.255	0.139	0.292	0.602**	0.589*	0.41
X6	0.469*	-0.087	-0.194	-0.045	0.255	1	0.945**	0.687**	0.577**	0.632**	0.405
X7	0.415	-0.052	-0.195	0.013	0.139	0.945**	1	0.67**	0.516*	0.545*	0.25
X8	0.513*	-0.321	-0.442*	0.151	0.292	0.687**	0.67**	1	0.739**	0.646**	0.322
X9	0.606**	-0.495*	-0.534*	0.366	0.602**	0.577**	0.516*	0.739**	1	0.773**	0.377
X10	0.584**	-0.515*	-0.479*	0.269	0.589*	0.632**	0.545*	0.646**	0.773**	1	0.451*
X11	0.455*	-0.483*	-0.446*	0.279	0.41	0.405	0.25	0.322	0.377	0.451*	1

* Significant at 0.05 level. Value of "r" required for its significance at 0.05 level = 0.433. df = N − 2 = 19.
** Significant at 0.01 level. Value of "r" required for its significance at 0.01 level = 0.549. df = N − 2 = 19.

TABLE 12.4   KMO and Bartlett's Test

Kaiser-Meyer-Olkin (KMO) Measure of Sampling Adequacy		0.714
Bartlett's test of sphericity	Approx. chi-square	183.682
	df	55
	Sig.	0.000

the output. The readers may draw the conclusions as per their requirements from this table.

2. The first result in the factor analysis is the correlation matrix shown in Table 12.3. The SPSS provides significance value (p value) for each correlation coefficient. However, significant value of the correlation coefficients at 0.01 and at 0.05 level can be seen from any standard book of statistics. Meaningful conclusions can be drawn from this table about the relationships among the variables.

3. Table 12.4 is the output for KMO test. This test indicates whether the sample size is adequate or not for applying the exploratory factor analysis. The value of KMO should be at least 0.5 for adequacy of the sample.

   The Bartlett's test of sphericity is used to test whether the correlation matrix is an identity matrix, and if so in that case the factor model is inappropriate. Since chi-square associated with Bartlett's test is significant (p=0.000), correlation matrix is not an identity matrix; hence, the exploratory factor analysis can be applied.

4. Table 12.5 shows the factors that have been extracted and the variance explained by these factors. It can be seen that after rotating the factors, the first factor explains 39.091% of the total variance, whereas the second factor explains 35.337% of the total variance. Thus, both the factors together explain 74.428% of the total variance.

   The eigenvalues for each factor are given in Table 12.5. Only those factors have been retained whose eigenvalue is 1 or more than 1. Here you can see that the eigenvalue for the first factor is 5.820 and the second is 2.367, whereas all other factors have less than one eigenvalue. Thus, only two factors have been retained here.

5. Figure 12.9 shows the scree plot that is obtained by plotting the factors against their eigenvalues. This plot shows that only two factors have eigenvalues more than 1, whereas others have less than 1.

6. The first initial unrotated solution of the factor analysis is given in Table 12.6. Two factors have been extracted in this example. Factor loadings of all the variables on each of the two factors have been shown here. Since this is an unrotated factor solution, some of the variables may show their contribution in both the factors. In order to avoid this situation, the factors are rotated. Varimax rotation has been used in this example to rotate the factors as this is the most popular method used by the researchers due to its efficiency.

TABLE 12.5 Total Variance Explained

Component	Initial Eigenvalues			Extraction Sums of Squared Loadings			Rotation Sums of Squared Loadings		
	Total	% of Variance	Cumulative %	Total	% of Variance	Cumulative %	Total	% of Variance	Cumulative %
1	5.820	52.914	52.914	5.820	52.914	52.914	4.300	39.091	39.091
2	2.367	21.514	74.428	2.367	21.514	74.428	3.887	35.337	74.428
3	0.745	6.776	81.204						
4	0.582	5.290	86.494						
5	0.434	3.943	90.437						
6	0.367	3.335	93.772						
7	0.247	2.246	96.018						
8	0.184	1.677	97.695						
9	0.168	1.527	99.223						
10	0.072	0.653	99.876						
11	0.014	0.124	100.000						

Extraction method: principal component analysis.

TABLE 12.6   Component Matrix: Unrotated Factor Solution

	Component	
	1	2
Standing broad jump	0.826	−0.096
4 × 10 shuttle run	−0.735	0.506
50 mt. timings	−0.798	0.451
12 min R/W	0.612	−0.654
Anaerobic capacity	0.769	−0.398
Weight	0.635	0.714
Height	0.574	0.713
Leg length	0.725	0.452
Calf girth	0.837	0.185
Thigh girth	0.822	0.232
Shoulder width	0.600	−0.034

Extraction method: principal component analysis.
[a] Two components extracted.

TABLE 12.7   Rotated Component Matrix[a]: Varimax Rotated Solution

	Component[a]	
	1	2
Standing broad jump	0.681	0.476
4 × 10 shuttle run	−0.885	−0.109
50 mt. timings	−0.896	−0.192
12 min R/W	0.892	−0.084
Anaerobic capacity	0.839	0.213
Weight	0.001	0.956
Height	−0.044	0.914
Leg length	0.242	0.819
Calf girth	0.504	0.694
Thigh girth	0.461	0.719
Shoulder width	0.472	0.373

Extraction method: principal component analysis.
Rotation method: varimax with kaiser normalization.
[a] Rotation converged in three iterations.

The final solution of the factor analysis after the varimax rotation has been shown in Table 12.7. A clear picture emerges in this final solution about the variables, explaining the factors correctly as factors will have nonoverlapping variables in this final solution. If the variable has factor loadings more than 0.7, it indicates that the factor extracts sufficient variance from that variable. Thus, all those variables having loadings more than 0.7 or more on a particular factor are identified in that factor. However, a researcher may choose this threshold value anything more than 0.4. Owing to this criterion, the following variables have been grouped in each of the two factors shown in Tables 12.8 and 12.9.

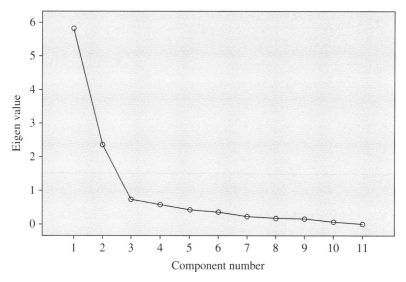

FIGURE 12.9 Scree plot for the data obtained on swimmers.

TABLE 12.8 Factor 1: Physical Factor

4 × 10 shuttle run	−0.885
50 mt. timings	−0.896
12 min R/W	0.892
Anaerobic capacity	0.839

TABLE 12.9 Factor 2: Growth Factor

Weight	0.956
Height	0.914
Leg length	0.819
Thigh girth	0.719

Factor 1 contains variables that define the physical performances of swimmers and, therefore, it may be termed *Physical Factor*. On the other hand, Factor 2 consists of those variables that define the growth dimension of the swimmers and, therefore, this factor may be termed *Growth Factor*. Thus, based on the data of Example 12.1, it may be concluded that the two factors, that is, "Physical" and "Growth" exist among the swimmers.

7. In order to develop the *test battery*, readers have a choice to select a few variables from each of the two factors retained. One such choice of the test battery for screening the swimmers may be like as shown in Table 12.10.

TABLE 12.10   Test Battery for Screening the Swimmers

50 mt. timings	−0.896
12 min R/W	0.892
Weight	0.956
Height	0.914

12.7   SUMMARY OF THE SPSS COMMANDS FOR FACTOR ANALYSIS

1. Start the SPSS by using the following sequence of commands:

   Start → All Programs → SPSS Inc → SPSS 20.0

2. Click on **Variable View** and define *SBJ, Shut_Run, 50_Mt, 12_min_R/W, Aner_Cap, Wt, Ht, Leg_Length, Calf_Girth, Thigh_Girth*, and *Shl_Width* as scale variables.

3. Once the variables are defined, type the data for these variables by clicking on **Data View**.

4. In the **Data View**, follow the command sequence for factor analysis as follows:

   Analyze → Data Reduction → Factor

5. Select all the variables from the left panel, and bring them into the "Variables" section in the right panel.

6. Click **Descriptives** command and check 'Univariate descriptives,' 'Initial Solution,' 'Coefficients,' 'Significance levels,' and 'KMO and Bartlett's test of sphericity' options. Click on **Continue.**

7. Click on **Extraction** command and then check 'Scree plot' option. Let other options remain by default. Click on **Continue.**

8. Click on **Rotation** command, and then check 'Varimax' rotation option. Let other options remain as they are by default. Click on **Continue** and **OK** commands for generating the outputs.

12.8   EXERCISE

12.8.1   Short Answer Questions

Note: Write answers to each of the following questions in not more than 200 words.

Q.1   How can the factor analysis be used in talent identification in sport? Discuss with a specific example.

Q.2   Can the factor analysis be used in developing a fitness index for assessing health status of an individual? If so, explain the procedure briefly.

Q.3   Why principal component analysis is mostly used in factor analysis?

Q.4 What do you mean by eigenvalue? How does the Kaiser's criterion work in retaining factors in the model?

Q.5 What do you mean by scree test? How is it useful in identifying the factors to be retained through graph?

Q.6 What is communality? How is it used to decide the reliability of variables in the factor model?

Q.7 What is the significance of factor loadings? How is it used to identify the variables to be retained in the factors?

Q.8 Why are the factors rotated to get the final solution in factor analysis? Which is the most popular rotation method and why?

12.8.2 Multiple Choice Questions

Note: Questions 1–10 have four alternative answers for each question. Tick mark the one that you consider the closest to the correct answer.

1 Choose the correct sequence of SPSS commands for factor analysis
  (a) Analyze → Data Reduction → Factor
  (b) Analyze → Factor → Data Reduction
  (c) Factor → Data Reduction → Analyze
  (d) Data Reduction → Factor → Analyze

2 Factor analysis is a technique for
  (a) Correlation analysis
  (b) Data reduction
  (c) Finding the most important variable
  (d) Comparing factors

3 Principal component analysis extracts the maximum variance in the
  (a) Last extracted factor
  (b) Second extracted factor
  (c) First extracted factor
  (d) Any extracted factor

4 Owing to Kaiser's criteria, the factor is retained if its eigenvalue is
  (a) Less than 1
  (b) Equal to 1
  (c) More than 2
  (d) More than 1

5 Scree test is the graph between
  (a) Eigenvalues and factors
  (b) Percentage variance explained and factors
  (c) Maximum factor loadings in the factors and factors
  (d) Communality and factor

6   Conventionally, a variable is retained in a factor if its loading is greater than or
    equal to
    (a) 0.4
    (b) 0.5
    (c) 0.7
    (d) 0.2

7   Varimax rotation is used to get the final solution. After rotation
    (a) Factor explaining maximum variance is extracted first.
    (b) All factors whose eigenvalues are more than 1 are extracted.
    (c) Three best factors are extracted.
    (d) Nonoverlapping of variables in the factors emerges.

8   Eigenvalue is also known as
    (a) Characteristics root
    (b) Factor loading
    (c) Communality
    (d) None of the above

9   KMO test in factor analysis is used to test whether
    (a) Factors extracted are valid or not?
    (b) Variables identified in each factor are valid or not?
    (c) Sample size taken for the factor analysis was adequate or not?
    (d) Multicollinearity among the variables exists or not?

10 While using factor analysis, certain assumptions need to be satisfied. Choose
    the most appropriate assumption.
    (a) Data used in the factor analysis is based on an interval scale or ratio scale
    (b) Multicollinearity among the variables exists.
    (c) Outlier is present in the data.
    (d) Size of the sample does not affect the analysis.

12.8.3   Assignment

Apply factor analysis on the data of physical characteristics obtained on the hockey
players as shown in Table 12.11. Use varimax rotation method for final solution.
Discuss your findings and answer the following questions:

1. Is data adequate for factor analysis?
2. Is sphericity significant?
3. How many factors have been extracted?
4. In your opinion what should be the name of the factors?
5. What factor loadings do you suggest for a variable to qualify in a factor?
6. Can you suggest the test battery for screening the hockey players on the basis
    of the data?

TABLE 12.11   Data on Physical Parameters of the College Hockey Players

S.N.	Height (cm) X_1	Weight (kg) X_2	Pulse Rate (beat/min) X_3	Explosive Power (kg.cm) X_4	9 Min. R/W (mt) X_5	Body Density (g/cc) X_6	Fat% X_7	LBW (kg) X_8
1	161	50	80	698.36	2800	1.05	21.23	47.26
2	174	60	80	937.83	3000	1.07	13.06	48.69
3	167	56	92	678.2	2000	1.05	21.76	43.81
4	165	55	96	697.7	2200	1.05	19.3	44.39
5	169	49	80	750.45	2400	1.07	11.66	43.28
6	154	48	88	754.61	2400	1.05	18.08	40.15
7	170	59	84	824.05	2400	1.06	19.3	49.65
8	163	49	80	726.5	1800	1.05	19.35	39.5
9	160	48	81	887.5	2400	1.06	12.58	41.95
10	158	50	84	924.85	2800	1.06	12.71	43.63
11	160	43	60	786.0	2000	1.07	11.92	37.84
12	157	57	100	678.0	3000	1.05	27.81	40.44
13	151	51	84	637.5	2600	1.06	17.46	42.6
14	161	57	92	744.45	2400	1.06	19.23	46.65
15	163	66	92	1220.85	2000	1.05	22.7	56.96

12.9   CASE STUDY ON FACTOR ANALYSIS

Objective

In a research study, yoga practitioners were studied for the latent profile characteristics possessed by them. Twenty-four practitioners of yoga were randomly selected in a college and were tested for their different physical and physiological parameters. The data so obtained are shown in Table 12.12.

Research Issues

The following research issues were investigated:

1. Whether any specific factor structure exists among yoga practitioners which explain the most of the variations about their physical and physiological profiles.
2. Whether the data was adequate to run the factor analysis.
3. How many factors would describe the characteristics of yoga practitioners?
4. How much variability would be measured by each factor?

TABLE 12.12 Data Format in SPSS with Physical and Physiological Parameters Obtained on Yoga Practitioners

S.N.	Flexi (cm) X_1	Max_End. (nos.) X_2	BP_Dia (Hg) X_3	BP_Sys (Hg) X_4	Res_Rate (nos.) X_5	Pulse_Rate (nos./min) X_6	BHT (sec) X_7	Vit_Cap (ml) X_8	Age (years) X_9	Wt (kg) X_{10}
1	20	35	80	120	15	68	36	2800	20	70
2	14	20	80	122	16	70	34	2300	22	74
3	12	27	82	124	17	72	30	2100	20	64
4	14	32	80	120	14	66	31	2750	23	74
5	22	28	80	120	16	74	32	1800	20	61
6	12	26	84	124	15	70	28	2150	22	54
7	12	28	80	120	16	69	38	2300	20	63
8	9	22	82	122	14	70	27	2350	25	62
9	14	31	86	126	15	68	34	2250	24	63
10	19	36	80	120	16	72	35	1900	22	54
11	12	24	82	120	16	77	29	2000	26	55
12	16	23	80	124	15	70	29	2250	25	69
13	18	22	80	122	13	69	30	2100	27	58
14	14	18	80	122	17	80	28	1750	22	48
15	13	28	80	118	14	68	31	2400	26	79
16	19	28	80	120	17	69	27	2150	22	59
17	17	31	82	120	15	72	30	1950	27	95
18	13	27	80	126	15	68	32	2150	21	49
19	13	21	80	120	16	70	28	2100	21	54
20	20	20	80	120	18	74	26	1750	26	67
21	9	25	80	123	16	74	30	2100	23	55
22	18	37	84	120	14	69	33	2000	23	86
23	17	21	80	120	17	72	27	2150	23	56
24	12	27	80	120	15	70	28	2400	21	66
25	17	26	80	120	14	70	28	2600	24	72

Data Format

The format used for preparing the data file in SPSS is shown in the Table 12.12.

Analyzing Data

In understanding the latent structure of the profile of yoga practitioners a factor analysis was carried out to classify the variables into meaningful factors. Before applying the factor analysis, adequacy of the data was tested by means of KMO test generated in the output by the SPSS. Factors were extracted by using the principal component analysis in the initial solution. The factors extracted in the initial solution were subjected to varimax rotation for getting the nonoverlapping factors. The variables having high factor loadings in each factor were identified, and the nomenclature of the factors was done on the basis of the nature of the variables retained in that factor.

The factor analysis was carried out in SPSS by using the commands: **Analyze, Data Reduction,** and **Factor** in sequence. All the variables were selected for the analysis and placed in the appropriate location in the dialog box. The option for 'Initial solution' and 'KMO and Bartlett's test of sphericity' was selected in Descriptive command, 'Scree plot' in extraction, and 'Varimax' in rotation. The outputs so generated in SPSS are shown in Tables 12.13, 12.14, 12.15, and 12.16 and in Figure 12.10.

Testing Assumptions

The KMO test is shown in Table 12.13. This test indicates the adequacy of the sample size for running the factor analysis. Since KMO is more than 0.5, the data was adequate for running the factor analysis. Further Bartlett's test is significant $(p = 0.000)$, hence the correlation matrix is not an identity matrix. And the factor analysis can be done.

Factors Extraction

Table 12.14 shows the factors that were extracted and the variance explained by these factors. In all, four factors were extracted, which together explained 78.461% of the total variability. The eigenvalues for each of the factors are given in Table 12.14. Only those factors were retained whose eigenvalues were 1 or more than 1. It can be seen from this table that the eigenvalues for the first four factors are 3.041, 1.798, 1.664, and 1.344, respectively; whereas for others, it is less than 1. Thus, only four factors were retained.

TABLE 12.13   KMO and Bartlett's Test

Kaiser-Meyer-Olkin Measure of Sampling Adequacy		0.581
Bartlett's test of sphericity	Approx. chi-square	85.427
	df	45
	Sig.	0.000

TABLE 12.14 Total Variance Explained

Component	Initial Eigenvalues			Extraction Sums of Squared Loadings			Rotation Sums of Squared Loadings		
	Total	% of Variance	Cumulative %	Total	% of Variance	Cumulative %	Total	% of Variance	Cumulative %
1	3.041	30.406	30.406	3.041	30.406	30.406	2.594	25.943	25.943
2	1.798	17.977	48.382	1.798	17.977	48.382	1.892	18.923	44.866
3	1.664	16.638	65.020	1.664	16.638	65.020	1.803	18.034	62.900
4	1.344	13.441	78.461	1.344	13.441	78.461	1.556	15.561	78.461
5	0.628	6.283	84.744						
6	0.505	5.052	89.797						
7	0.405	4.045	93.842						
8	0.220	2.201	96.043						
9	0.210	2.104	98.146						
10	0.185	1.854	100.000						

Extraction method: principal component analysis.

TABLE 12.15 Component Matrix[a]

	Component			
	1	2	3	4
Flex_X1	0.096	0.744	0.137	0.299
Max_end_X2	0.746	0.165	0.312	0.400
BP_dia_X3	0.230	−0.516	−0.183	0.714
BP_syS_X4	−0.123	−0.832	0.119	0.219
Res_rate_X5	−0.722	0.218	0.414	0.125
Pulse_Rate_X6	−0.823	0.178	−0.021	0.254
BHT_X7	0.567	0.007	0.590	0.210
Vit_cap_X8	0.703	−0.162	0.001	−0.586
Age_X9	−0.007	0.097	−0.906	0.165
WT_X10	0.626	0.378	−0.399	0.205

Extraction method: principal component analysis.
[a] Four components extracted.

TABLE 12.16 Rotated Component Matrix[a]

	Component			
	1	2	3	4
Flex_X1	−0.237	**0.758**	0.174	−0.104
Max_end_X2	0.349	0.499	0.576	0.373
BP_dia_X3	0.043	−0.087	−0.002	**0.924**
BP_syS_X4	−0.051	**−0.697**	0.120	0.517
Res_rate_X5	**−0.810**	−0.079	0.164	−0.256
Pulse_rate_X6	**−0.836**	−0.045	−0.261	−0.070
BHT_X7	0.244	0.196	**0.762**	0.192
Vit_cap_X8	**0.878**	−0.097	0.165	−0.238
Age_X9	0.125	0.264	***−0.836***	0.268
WT_X10	0.459	**0.670**	−0.159	0.224

Extraction method: principal component analysis.
Rotation method: varimax with Kaiser normalization.
Bold face indicates that the variable has been identified in that factor.
[a] Rotation converged in six iterations.

Figure 12.10 is a scree plot that is obtained by plotting the factors against their eigenvalues. This plot shows that only four factors have eigenvalues more than 1, whereas others have less than 1.

Identification of Factors

The factor loadings of all the variables on each of the four factors have been shown in the Table 12.15. Since this is an unrotated factor solution, some of the variables show their contribution in more than one factor. In order to avoid this situation, the factors were rotated by using the varimax rotation. The final solution has been shown in the Table 12.16.

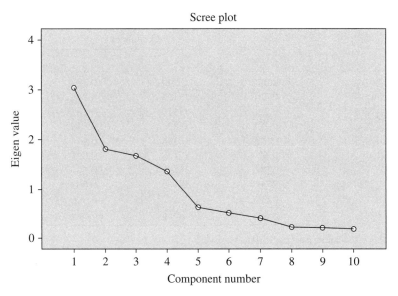

FIGURE 12.10 Scree plot for the data obtained on yoga practitioners.

TABLE 12.17 Factor 1

Cardio Health	
Variables	Loading
Respiratory rate	−0.810
Pulse rate	−0.836
Vital capacity	0.878

TABLE 12.18 Factor 2

Flexibility	
Variables	Loading
Flexibility	0.758
BP systolic	−0.697
Weight	0.670

A clear picture emerged in this final solution about the variables, explaining the factors correctly as shown in Table 12.16. Variables were retained in the factor if the factor loading was 0.6 or more. Owing to this criterion, the variables have been grouped in each of the four factors as shown in Tables 12.17, 12.18, 12.19, and 12.20. On the basis of the variable's characteristics identified in the factors, all the four factors were named as cardio health, flexibility, lungs health, and blood pressure, which explained 30.406, 17.977, 16.638, and 13.441% of the total variability, respectively.

TABLE 12.19   Factor 3

Lungs Health	
Variables	Loading
Breath holding time	0.762
Age	−0.836

TABLE 12.20   Factor 4

Blood Pressure	
Variables	Loading
BP diastolic	0.924

Reporting

- Since KMO value is 0.581, which is more than 0.5, the data was adequate to run the factor analysis.
- The four factors were extracted that together explained 78.461% of the total variability.
- Identified factors were named as cardio, health, flexibility, lungs health, and blood pressure, which explained 30.406, 17.977, 16.638, and 13.441% of the total variability, respectively.

APPENDIX

TABLE A.1 The Normal Curve Area Between the Mean and a Given z Value

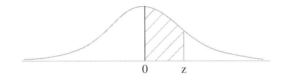

Z	0.00	0.01	0.02	0.03	0.04	0.05	0.06	0.07	0.08	0.09
0.0	0.0000	0.0040	0.0080	0.0120	0.0160	0.0199	0.0239	0.0279	0.0319	0.0359
0.1	0.0398	0.0438	0.0478	0.0517	0.0557	0.0596	0.0636	0.0675	0.0714	0.0753
0.2	0.0793	0.0832	0.0871	0.0910	0.0948	0.0987	0.1026	0.1064	0.1103	0.1141
0.3	0.1179	0.1217	0.1255	0.1293	0.1331	0.1368	0.1406	0.1443	0.1480	0.1517
0.4	0.1554	0.1591	0.1628	0.1664	0.1700	0.1736	0.1772	0.1808	0.1844	0.1879
0.5	0.1915	0.1950	0.1985	0.2019	0.2054	0.2088	0.2123	0.2157	0.2190	0.2224
0.6	0.2257	0.2291	0.2324	0.2357	0.2389	0.2422	0.2454	0.2486	0.2517	0.2549
0.7	0.2580	0.2611	0.2642	0.2673	0.2704	0.2734	0.2764	0.2794	0.2823	0.2852
0.8	0.2881	0.2910	0.2939	0.2967	0.2995	0.3023	0.3051	0.3078	0.3106	0.3133
0.9	0.3159	0.3186	0.3212	0.3238	0.3264	0.3289	0.3315	0.3340	0.3365	0.3389
1.0	0.3413	0.3438	0.3461	0.3485	0.3508	0.3531	0.3554	0.3577	0.3599	0.3621
1.1	0.3643	0.3665	0.3686	0.3708	0.3729	0.3749	0.3770	0.3790	0.3810	0.3830
1.2	0.3849	0.3869	0.3888	0.3907	0.3925	0.3944	0.3962	0.3980	0.3997	0.4015
1.3	0.4032	0.4049	0.4066	0.4082	0.4099	0.4115	0.4131	0.4147	0.4162	0.4177
1.4	0.4192	0.4207	0.4222	0.4236	0.4251	0.4265	0.4279	0.4292	0.4306	0.4319
1.5	0.4332	0.4345	0.4357	0.4370	0.4382	0.4394	0.4406	0.4418	0.4429	0.4441
1.6	0.4452	0.4463	0.4474	0.4484	0.4495	0.4505	0.4515	0.4525	0.4535	0.4545
1.7	0.4554	0.4564	0.4573	0.4582	0.4591	0.4599	0.4608	0.4616	0.4625	0.4633
1.8	0.4641	0.4649	0.4656	0.4664	0.4671	0.4678	0.4686	0.4693	0.4699	0.4706
1.9	0.4713	0.4719	0.4726	0.4732	0.4738	0.4744	0.4750	0.4756	0.4761	0.4767
2.0	0.4772	0.4778	0.4783	0.4788	0.4793	0.4798	0.4803	0.4808	0.4812	0.4817
2.1	0.4821	0.4826	0.4830	0.4834	0.4838	0.4842	0.4846	0.4850	0.4854	0.4857
2.2	0.4861	0.4864	0.4868	0.4871	0.4875	0.4878	0.4881	0.4884	0.4887	0.4890
2.3	0.4893	0.4896	0.4898	0.4901	0.4904	0.4906	0.4909	0.4911	0.4913	0.4916
2.4	0.4918	0.4920	0.4922	0.4925	0.4927	0.4929	0.4931	0.4932	0.4934	0.4936
2.5	0.4938	0.4940	0.4941	0.4943	0.4945	0.4946	0.4948	0.4949	0.4951	0.4952
2.6	0.4953	0.4955	0.4956	0.4957	0.4959	0.4960	0.4961	0.4962	0.4963	0.4964
2.7	0.4965	0.4966	0.4967	0.4968	0.4969	0.4970	0.4971	0.4972	0.4973	0.4974
2.8	0.4974	0.4975	0.4976	0.4977	0.4977	0.4978	0.4979	0.4979	0.4980	0.4981
2.9	0.4981	0.4982	0.4982	0.4983	0.4984	0.4984	0.4985	0.4985	0.4986	0.4986
3.0	0.4987	0.4987	0.4987	0.4988	0.4988	0.4989	0.4989	0.4989	0.4990	0.4990

Sports Research with Analytical Solution using SPSS®, First Edition. J. P. Verma.
© 2016 John Wiley & Sons, Inc. Published 2016 by John Wiley & Sons, Inc.
Companion website: www.wiley.com/go/Verma/Sportsresearch

TABLE A.2   Critical Values of "t"

					Level of Significance for Two-Tailed Test					
df	1.00	0.50	0.40	0.30	0.20	0.10	0.05	0.02	0.01	0.002	0.001
1	0.000	1.000	1.376	1.963	3.078	6.314	12.71	31.82	63.66	318.31	636.62
2	0.000	0.816	1.061	1.386	1.886	2.920	4.303	6.965	9.925	22.327	31.599
3	0.000	0.765	0.978	1.250	1.638	2.353	3.182	4.541	5.841	10.215	12.924
4	0.000	0.741	0.941	1.190	1.533	2.132	2.776	3.747	4.604	7.173	8.610
5	0.000	0.727	0.920	1.156	1.476	2.015	2.571	3.365	4.032	5.893	6.869
6	0.000	0.718	0.906	1.134	1.440	1.943	2.447	3.143	3.707	5.208	5.959
7	0.000	0.711	0.896	1.119	1.415	1.895	2.365	2.998	3.499	4.785	5.408
8	0.000	0.706	0.889	1.108	1.397	1.860	2.306	2.896	3.355	4.501	5.041
9	0.000	0.703	0.883	1.100	1.383	1.833	2.262	2.821	3.250	4.297	4.781
10	0.000	0.700	0.879	1.093	1.372	1.812	2.228	2.764	3.169	4.144	4.587
11	0.000	0.697	0.876	1.088	1.363	1.796	2.201	2.718	3.106	4.025	4.437
12	0.000	0.695	0.873	1.083	1.356	1.782	2.179	2.681	3.055	3.930	4.318
13	0.000	0.694	0.870	1.079	1.350	1.771	2.160	2.650	3.012	3.852	4.221
14	0.000	0.692	0.868	1.076	1.345	1.761	2.145	2.624	2.977	3.787	4.140
15	0.000	0.691	0.866	1.074	1.341	1.753	2.131	2.602	2.947	3.733	4.073
16	0.000	0.690	0.865	1.071	1.337	1.746	2.120	2.583	2.921	3.686	4.015
17	0.000	0.689	0.863	1.069	1.333	1.740	2.110	2.567	2.898	3.646	3.965
18	0.000	0.688	0.862	1.067	1.330	1.734	2.101	2.552	2.878	3.610	3.922
19	0.000	0.688	0.861	1.066	1.328	1.729	2.093	2.539	2.861	3.579	3.883
20	0.000	0.687	0.860	1.064	1.325	1.725	2.086	2.528	2.845	3.552	3.850
21	0.000	0.686	0.859	1.063	1.323	1.721	2.080	2.518	2.831	3.527	3.819
22	0.000	0.686	0.858	1.061	1.321	1.717	2.074	2.508	2.819	3.505	3.792
23	0.000	0.685	0.858	1.060	1.319	1.714	2.069	2.500	2.807	3.485	3.768
24	0.000	0.685	0.857	1.059	1.318	1.711	2.064	2.492	2.797	3.467	3.745
25	0.000	0.684	0.856	1.058	1.316	1.708	2.060	2.485	2.787	3.450	3.725
26	0.000	0.684	0.856	1.058	1.315	1.706	2.056	2.479	2.779	3.435	3.707
27	0.000	0.684	0.855	1.057	1.314	1.703	2.052	2.473	2.771	3.421	3.690
28	0.000	0.683	0.855	1.056	1.313	1.701	2.048	2.467	2.763	3.408	3.674
29	0.000	0.683	0.854	1.055	1.311	1.699	2.045	2.462	2.756	3.396	3.659
30	0.000	0.683	0.854	1.055	1.310	1.697	2.042	2.457	2.750	3.385	3.646
40	0.000	0.681	0.851	1.050	1.303	1.684	2.021	2.423	2.704	3.307	3.551
60	0.000	0.679	0.848	1.045	1.296	1.671	2.000	2.390	2.660	3.232	3.460
80	0.000	0.678	0.846	1.043	1.292	1.664	1.990	2.374	2.639	3.195	3.416
100	0.000	0.677	0.845	1.042	1.290	1.660	1.984	2.364	2.626	3.174	3.390
1000	0.000	0.675	0.842	1.037	1.282	1.646	1.962	2.330	2.581	3.098	3.300
	0.000	0.674	0.842	1.036	1.282	1.645	1.960	2.326	2.576	3.090	3.291
	0.50	0.25	0.20	0.15	0.10	0.05	0.025	0.01	0.005	0.001	0.0005

Level of significance for one-tailed test

TABLE A.3   F-Table: Critical Values at 0.05 Level of Significance

n_1/n_2	1	2	3	4	5	6	7	8	9	10	11	12	n_1/n_2
3	10.13	9.55	9.28	9.12	9.01	8.94	8.89	8.85	8.81	8.79	8.76	8.74	3
4	7.71	6.94	6.59	6.39	6.26	6.16	6.09	6.04	6.00	5.96	5.94	5.91	4
5	6.61	5.79	5.41	5.19	5.05	4.95	4.88	4.82	4.77	4.74	4.70	4.68	5
6	5.99	5.14	4.76	4.53	4.39	4.28	4.21	4.15	4.10	4.06	4.03	4.00	6
7	5.59	4.74	4.35	4.12	3.97	3.87	3.79	3.73	3.68	3.64	3.60	3.57	7
8	5.32	4.46	4.07	3.84	3.69	3.58	3.50	3.44	3.39	3.35	3.31	3.28	8
9	5.12	4.26	3.86	3.63	3.48	3.37	3.29	3.23	3.18	3.14	3.10	3.07	9
10	4.96	4.10	3.71	3.48	3.33	3.22	3.14	3.07	3.02	2.98	2.94	2.91	10
11	4.84	3.98	3.59	3.36	3.20	3.09	3.01	2.95	2.90	2.85	2.82	2.79	11
12	4.75	3.89	3.49	3.26	3.11	3.00	2.91	2.85	2.80	2.75	2.72	2.69	12
13	4.67	3.81	3.41	3.18	3.03	2.92	2.83	2.77	2.71	2.67	2.63	2.60	13
14	4.60	3.74	3.34	3.11	2.96	2.85	2.76	2.70	2.65	2.60	2.57	2.53	14
15	4.54	3.68	3.29	3.06	2.90	2.79	2.71	2.64	2.59	2.54	2.51	2.48	15
16	4.49	3.63	3.24	3.01	2.85	2.74	2.66	2.59	2.54	2.49	2.46	2.42	16
17	4.45	3.59	3.20	2.96	2.81	2.70	2.61	2.55	2.49	2.45	2.41	2.38	17
18	4.41	3.55	3.16	2.93	2.77	2.66	2.58	2.51	2.46	2.41	2.37	2.34	18
19	4.38	3.52	3.13	2.90	2.74	2.63	2.54	2.48	2.42	2.38	2.34	2.31	19
20	4.35	3.49	3.10	2.87	2.71	2.60	2.51	2.45	2.39	2.35	2.31	2.28	20
22	4.30	3.44	3.05	2.82	2.66	2.55	2.46	2.40	2.34	2.30	2.26	2.23	22
24	4.26	3.40	3.01	2.78	2.62	2.51	2.42	2.36	2.30	2.25	2.22	2.18	24
26	4.23	3.37	2.98	2.74	2.59	2.47	2.39	2.32	2.27	2.22	2.18	2.15	26
28	4.20	3.34	2.95	2.71	2.56	2.45	2.36	2.29	2.24	2.19	2.15	2.12	28
30	4.17	3.32	2.92	2.69	2.53	2.42	2.33	2.27	2.21	2.16	2.13	2.09	30
35	4.12	3.27	2.87	2.64	2.49	2.37	2.29	2.22	2.16	2.11	2.08	2.04	35
40	4.08	3.23	2.84	2.61	2.45	2.34	2.25	2.18	2.12	2.08	2.04	2.00	40
45	4.06	3.20	2.81	2.58	2.42	2.31	2.22	2.15	2.10	2.05	2.01	1.97	45
50	4.03	3.18	2.79	2.56	2.40	2.29	2.20	2.13	2.07	2.03	1.99	1.95	50
60	4.00	3.15	2.76	2.53	2.37	2.25	2.17	2.10	2.04	1.99	1.95	1.92	60
70	3.98	3.13	2.74	2.50	2.35	2.23	2.14	2.07	2.02	1.97	1.93	1.89	70
80	3.96	3.11	2.72	2.49	2.33	2.21	2.13	2.06	2.00	1.95	1.91	1.88	80
100	3.94	3.09	2.70	2.46	2.31	2.19	2.10	2.03	1.97	1.93	1.89	1.85	100
200	3.89	3.04	2.65	2.42	2.26	2.14	2.06	1.98	1.93	1.88	1.84	1.80	200
500	3.86	3.01	2.62	2.39	2.23	2.12	2.03	1.96	1.90	1.85	1.81	1.77	500
1000	3.85	3.00	2.61	2.38	2.22	2.11	2.02	1.95	1.89	1.84	1.80	1.76	1000
>1000	1.04	3.00	2.61	2.37	2.21	2.10	2.01	1.94	1.88	1.83	1.79	1.75	>1000
n_1/n_2	1	2	3	4	5	6	7	8	9	10	11	12	n_1/n_2

n_1/n_2	13	14	15	16	17	18	19	20	22	24	26	28	n_1/n_2
3	8.73	8.71	8.70	8.69	8.68	8.67	8.67	8.66	8.65	8.64	8.63	8.62	3
4	5.89	5.87	5.86	5.84	5.83	5.82	5.81	5.80	5.79	5.77	5.76	5.75	4
5	4.66	4.64	4.62	4.60	4.59	4.58	4.57	4.56	4.54	4.53	4.52	4.50	5
6	3.98	3.96	3.94	3.92	3.91	3.90	3.88	3.87	3.86	3.84	3.83	3.82	6
7	3.55	3.53	3.51	3.49	3.48	3.47	3.46	3.44	3.43	3.41	3.40	3.39	7
8	3.26	3.24	3.22	3.20	3.19	3.17	3.16	3.15	3.13	3.12	3.10	3.09	8
9	3.05	3.03	3.01	2.99	2.97	2.96	2.95	2.94	2.92	2.90	2.89	2.87	9
10	2.89	2.86	2.85	2.83	2.81	2.80	2.79	2.77	2.75	2.74	2.72	2.71	10
11	2.76	2.74	2.72	2.70	2.69	2.67	2.66	2.65	2.63	2.61	2.59	2.58	11
12	2.66	2.64	2.62	2.60	2.58	2.57	2.56	2.54	2.52	2.51	2.49	2.48	12
13	2.58	2.55	2.53	2.51	2.50	2.48	2.47	2.46	2.44	2.42	2.41	2.39	13
14	2.51	2.48	2.46	2.44	2.43	2.41	2.40	2.39	2.37	2.35	2.33	2.32	14
15	2.45	2.42	2.40	2.38	2.37	2.35	2.34	2.33	2.31	2.29	2.27	2.26	15
16	2.40	2.37	2.35	2.33	2.32	2.30	2.29	2.28	2.25	2.24	2.22	2.21	16
17	2.35	2.33	2.31	2.29	2.27	2.26	2.24	2.23	2.21	2.19	2.17	2.16	17
18	2.31	2.29	2.27	2.25	2.23	2.22	2.20	2.19	2.17	2.15	2.13	2.12	18
19	2.28	2.26	2.23	2.21	2.20	2.18	2.17	2.16	2.13	2.11	2.10	2.08	19
20	2.25	2.23	2.20	2.18	2.17	2.15	2.14	2.12	2.10	2.08	2.07	2.05	20
22	2.20	2.17	2.15	2.13	2.11	2.10	2.08	2.07	2.05	2.03	2.01	2.00	22
24	2.15	2.13	2.11	2.09	2.07	2.05	2.04	2.03	2.00	1.98	1.97	1.95	24
26	2.12	2.09	2.07	2.05	2.03	2.02	2.00	1.99	1.97	1.95	1.93	1.91	26
28	2.09	2.06	2.04	2.02	2.00	1.99	1.97	1.96	1.93	1.91	1.90	1.88	28
30	2.06	2.04	2.01	1.99	1.98	1.96	1.95	1.93	1.91	1.89	1.87	1.85	30
35	2.01	1.99	1.96	1.94	1.92	1.91	1.89	1.88	1.85	1.83	1.82	1.80	35
40	1.97	1.95	1.92	1.90	1.89	1.87	1.85	1.84	1.81	1.79	1.77	1.76	40
45	1.94	1.92	1.89	1.87	1.86	1.84	1.82	1.81	1.78	1.76	1.74	1.73	45
50	1.92	1.89	1.87	1.85	1.83	1.81	1.80	1.78	1.76	1.74	1.72	1.70	50
60	1.89	1.86	1.84	1.82	1.80	1.78	1.76	1.75	1.72	1.70	1.68	1.66	60
70	1.86	1.84	1.81	1.79	1.77	1.75	1.74	1.72	1.70	1.67	1.65	1.64	70
80	1.84	1.82	1.79	1.77	1.75	1.73	1.72	1.70	1.68	1.65	1.63	1.62	80
100	1.82	1.79	1.77	1.75	1.73	1.71	1.69	1.68	1.65	1.63	1.61	1.59	100
200	1.77	1.74	1.72	1.69	1.67	1.66	1.64	1.62	1.60	1.57	1.55	1.53	200
500	1.74	1.71	1.69	1.66	1.64	1.62	1.61	1.59	1.56	1.54	1.52	1.50	500
1000	1.73	1.70	1.68	1.65	1.63	1.61	1.60	1.58	1.55	1.53	1.51	1.49	1000
>1000	1.72	1.69	1.67	1.64	1.62	1.61	1.59	1.57	1.54	1.52	1.50	1.48	>1000
n_1/n_2	13	14	15	16	17	18	19	20	22	24	26	28	n_1/n_2

(*Continued*)

TABLE A.3   (continued)

n_1/n_2	30	35	40	45	50	60	70	80	100	200	500	1000	>1000	n_1/n_2
3	8.62	8.60	8.59	8.59	8.58	8.57	8.57	8.56	8.55	8.54	8.53	8.53	8.54	3
4	5.75	5.73	5.72	5.71	5.70	5.69	5.68	5.67	5.66	5.65	5.64	5.63	5.63	4
5	4.50	4.48	4.46	4.45	4.44	4.43	4.42	4.42	4.41	4.39	4.37	4.37	4.36	5
6	3.81	3.79	3.77	3.76	3.75	3.74	3.73	3.72	3.71	3.69	3.68	3.67	3.67	6
7	3.38	3.36	3.34	3.33	3.32	3.30	3.29	3.29	3.27	3.25	3.24	3.23	3.23	7
8	3.08	3.06	3.04	3.03	3.02	3.01	2.99	2.99	2.97	2.95	2.94	2.93	2.93	8
9	2.86	2.84	2.83	2.81	2.80	2.79	2.78	2.77	2.76	2.73	2.72	2.71	2.71	9
10	2.70	2.68	2.66	2.65	2.64	2.62	2.61	2.60	2.59	2.56	2.55	2.54	2.54	10
11	2.57	2.55	2.53	2.52	2.51	2.49	2.48	2.47	2.46	2.43	2.42	2.41	2.41	11
12	2.47	2.44	2.43	2.41	2.40	2.38	2.37	2.36	2.35	2.32	2.31	2.30	2.30	12
13	2.38	2.36	2.34	2.33	2.31	2.30	2.28	2.27	2.26	2.23	2.22	2.21	2.21	13
14	2.31	2.28	2.27	2.25	2.24	2.22	2.21	2.20	2.19	2.16	2.14	2.14	2.13	14
15	2.25	2.22	2.20	2.19	2.18	2.16	2.15	2.14	2.12	2.10	2.08	2.07	2.07	15
16	2.19	2.17	2.15	2.14	2.12	2.11	2.09	2.08	2.07	2.04	2.02	2.02	2.01	16
17	2.15	2.12	2.10	2.09	2.08	2.06	2.05	2.03	2.02	1.99	1.97	1.97	1.96	17
18	2.11	2.08	2.06	2.05	2.04	2.02	2.00	1.99	1.98	1.95	1.93	1.92	1.92	18
19	2.07	2.05	2.03	2.01	2.00	1.98	1.97	1.96	1.94	1.91	1.89	1.88	1.88	19
20	2.04	2.01	1.99	1.98	1.97	1.95	1.93	1.92	1.91	1.88	1.86	1.85	1.84	20
22	1.98	1.96	1.94	1.92	1.91	1.89	1.88	1.86	1.85	1.82	1.80	1.79	1.78	22
24	1.94	1.91	1.89	1.88	1.86	1.84	1.83	1.82	1.80	1.77	1.75	1.74	1.73	24
26	1.90	1.87	1.85	1.84	1.82	1.80	1.79	1.78	1.76	1.73	1.71	1.70	1.69	26
28	1.87	1.84	1.82	1.80	1.79	1.77	1.75	1.74	1.73	1.69	1.67	1.66	1.66	28
30	1.84	1.81	1.79	1.77	1.76	1.74	1.72	1.71	1.70	1.66	1.64	1.63	1.62	30
35	1.79	1.76	1.74	1.72	1.70	1.68	1.66	1.65	1.63	1.60	1.57	1.57	1.56	35
40	1.74	1.72	1.69	1.67	1.66	1.64	1.62	1.61	1.59	1.55	1.53	1.52	1.51	40
45	1.71	1.68	1.66	1.64	1.63	1.60	1.59	1.57	1.55	1.51	1.49	1.48	1.47	45
50	1.69	1.66	1.63	1.61	1.60	1.58	1.56	1.54	1.52	1.48	1.46	1.45	1.44	50
60	1.65	1.62	1.59	1.57	1.56	1.53	1.52	1.50	1.48	1.44	1.41	1.40	1.39	60
70	1.62	1.59	1.57	1.55	1.53	1.50	1.49	1.47	1.45	1.40	1.37	1.36	1.35	70
80	1.60	1.57	1.54	1.52	1.51	1.48	1.46	1.45	1.43	1.38	1.35	1.34	1.33	80
100	1.57	1.54	1.52	1.49	1.48	1.45	1.43	1.41	1.39	1.34	1.31	1.30	1.28	100
200	1.52	1.48	1.46	1.43	1.41	1.39	1.36	1.35	1.32	1.26	1.22	1.21	1.19	200
500	1.48	1.45	1.42	1.40	1.38	1.35	1.32	1.30	1.28	1.21	1.16	1.14	1.12	500
1000	1.47	1.43	1.41	1.38	1.36	1.33	1.31	1.29	1.26	1.19	1.13	1.11	1.08	1000
>1000	1.46	1.42	1.40	1.37	1.35	1.32	1.30	1.28	1.25	1.17	1.11	1.08	1.03	>1000
n_1/n_2	30	35	40	45	50	60	70	80	100	200	500	1000	>1000	n_1/n_2

TABLE A.4 F-Table: Critical Values at 0.01 Level of Significance

n_1/n_2	1	2	3	4	5	6	7	8	9	10	11	12	n_1/n_2
3	34.12	30.82	29.46	28.71	28.24	27.91	27.67	27.49	27.35	27.23	27.13	27.05	3
4	21.20	18.00	16.69	15.98	15.52	15.21	14.98	14.80	14.66	14.55	14.45	14.37	4
5	16.26	13.27	12.06	11.39	10.97	10.67	10.46	10.29	10.16	10.05	9.96	9.89	5
6	13.75	10.92	9.78	9.15	8.75	8.47	8.26	8.10	7.98	7.87	7.79	7.72	6
7	12.25	9.55	8.45	7.85	7.46	7.19	6.99	6.84	6.72	6.62	6.54	6.47	7
8	11.26	8.65	7.59	7.01	6.63	6.37	6.18	6.03	5.91	5.81	5.73	5.67	8
9	10.56	8.02	6.99	6.42	6.06	5.80	5.61	5.47	5.35	5.26	5.18	5.11	9
10	10.04	7.56	6.55	5.99	5.64	5.39	5.20	5.06	4.94	4.85	4.77	4.71	10
11	9.65	7.21	6.22	5.67	5.32	5.07	4.89	4.74	4.63	4.54	4.46	4.40	11
12	9.33	6.93	5.95	5.41	5.06	4.82	4.64	4.50	4.39	4.30	4.22	4.16	12
13	9.07	6.70	5.74	5.21	4.86	4.62	4.44	4.30	4.19	4.10	4.02	3.96	13
14	8.86	6.51	5.56	5.04	4.70	4.46	4.28	4.14	4.03	3.94	3.86	3.80	14
15	8.68	6.36	5.42	4.89	4.56	4.32	4.14	4.00	3.89	3.80	3.73	3.67	15
16	8.53	6.23	5.29	4.77	4.44	4.20	4.03	3.89	3.78	3.69	3.62	3.55	16
17	8.40	6.11	5.19	4.67	4.34	4.10	3.93	3.79	3.68	3.59	3.52	3.46	17
18	8.29	6.01	5.09	4.58	4.25	4.01	3.84	3.71	3.60	3.51	3.43	3.37	18
19	8.19	5.93	5.01	4.50	4.17	3.94	3.77	3.63	3.52	3.43	3.36	3.30	19
20	8.10	5.85	4.94	4.43	4.10	3.87	3.70	3.56	3.46	3.37	3.29	3.23	20
22	7.95	5.72	4.82	4.31	3.99	3.76	3.59	3.45	3.35	3.26	3.18	3.12	22
24	7.82	5.61	4.72	4.22	3.90	3.67	3.50	3.36	3.26	3.17	3.09	3.03	24
26	7.72	5.53	4.64	4.14	3.82	3.59	3.42	3.29	3.18	3.09	3.02	2.96	26
28	7.64	5.45	4.57	4.07	3.75	3.53	3.36	3.23	3.12	3.03	2.96	2.90	28
30	7.56	5.39	4.51	4.02	3.70	3.47	3.30	3.17	3.07	2.98	2.91	2.84	30
35	7.42	5.27	4.40	3.91	3.59	3.37	3.20	3.07	2.96	2.88	2.80	2.74	35
40	7.31	5.18	4.31	3.83	3.51	3.29	3.12	2.99	2.89	2.80	2.73	2.66	40
45	7.23	5.11	4.25	3.77	3.45	3.23	3.07	2.94	2.83	2.74	2.67	2.61	45
50	7.17	5.06	4.20	3.72	3.41	3.19	3.02	2.89	2.79	2.70	2.63	2.56	50
60	7.08	4.98	4.13	3.65	3.34	3.12	2.95	2.82	2.72	2.63	2.56	2.50	60
70	7.01	4.92	4.07	3.60	3.29	3.07	2.91	2.78	2.67	2.59	2.51	2.45	70
80	6.96	4.88	4.04	3.56	3.26	3.04	2.87	2.74	2.64	2.55	2.48	2.42	80
100	6.90	4.82	3.98	3.51	3.21	2.99	2.82	2.69	2.59	2.50	2.43	2.37	100
200	6.76	4.71	3.88	3.41	3.11	2.89	2.73	2.60	2.50	2.41	2.34	2.27	200
500	6.69	4.65	3.82	3.36	3.05	2.84	2.68	2.55	2.44	2.36	2.28	2.22	500
1000	6.66	4.63	3.80	3.34	3.04	2.82	2.66	2.53	2.43	2.34	2.27	2.20	1000
>1000	1.04	4.61	3.78	3.32	3.02	2.80	2.64	2.51	2.41	2.32	2.25	2.19	>1000
n_1/n_2	1	2	3	4	5	6	7	8	9	10	11	12	n_1/n_2

(*Continued*)

TABLE A.4   (continued)

n_1/n_2	13	14	15	16	17	18	19	20	22	24	26	28	30	n_1/n_2
3	26.98	26.92	26.87	26.83	26.79	26.75	26.72	26.69	26.64	26.60	26.56	26.53	26.50	3
4	14.31	14.25	14.20	14.15	14.11	14.08	14.05	14.02	13.97	13.93	13.89	13.86	13.84	4
5	9.82	9.77	9.72	9.68	9.64	9.61	9.58	9.55	9.51	9.47	9.43	9.40	9.38	5
6	7.66	7.61	7.56	7.52	7.48	7.45	7.42	7.40	7.35	7.31	7.28	7.25	7.23	6
7	6.41	6.36	6.31	6.28	6.24	6.21	6.18	6.16	6.11	6.07	6.04	6.02	5.99	7
8	5.61	5.56	5.52	5.48	5.44	5.41	5.38	5.36	5.32	5.28	5.25	5.22	5.20	8
9	5.05	5.01	4.96	4.92	4.89	4.86	4.83	4.81	4.77	4.73	4.70	4.67	4.65	9
10	4.65	4.60	4.56	4.52	4.49	4.46	4.43	4.41	4.36	4.33	4.30	4.27	4.25	10
11	4.34	4.29	4.25	4.21	4.18	4.15	4.12	4.10	4.06	4.02	3.99	3.96	3.94	11
12	4.10	4.05	4.01	3.97	3.94	3.91	3.88	3.86	3.82	3.78	3.75	3.72	3.70	12
13	3.91	3.86	3.82	3.78	3.75	3.72	3.69	3.66	3.62	3.59	3.56	3.53	3.51	13
14	3.75	3.70	3.66	3.62	3.59	3.56	3.53	3.51	3.46	3.43	3.40	3.37	3.35	14
15	3.61	3.56	3.52	3.49	3.45	3.42	3.40	3.37	3.33	3.29	3.26	3.24	3.21	15
16	3.50	3.45	3.41	3.37	3.34	3.31	3.28	3.26	3.22	3.18	3.15	3.12	3.10	16
17	3.40	3.35	3.31	3.27	3.24	3.21	3.19	3.16	3.12	3.08	3.05	3.03	3.00	17
18	3.32	3.27	3.23	3.19	3.16	3.13	3.10	3.08	3.03	3.00	2.97	2.94	2.92	18
19	3.24	3.19	3.15	3.12	3.08	3.05	3.03	3.00	2.96	2.92	2.89	2.87	2.84	19
20	3.18	3.13	3.09	3.05	3.02	2.99	2.96	2.94	2.90	2.86	2.83	2.80	2.78	20
22	3.07	3.02	2.98	2.94	2.91	2.88	2.85	2.83	2.78	2.75	2.72	2.69	2.67	22
24	2.98	2.93	2.89	2.85	2.82	2.79	2.76	2.74	2.70	2.66	2.63	2.60	2.58	24
26	2.90	2.86	2.82	2.78	2.75	2.72	2.69	2.66	2.62	2.58	2.55	2.53	2.50	26
28	2.84	2.79	2.75	2.72	2.68	2.65	2.63	2.60	2.56	2.52	2.49	2.46	2.44	28
30	2.79	2.74	2.70	2.66	2.63	2.60	2.57	2.55	2.51	2.47	2.44	2.41	2.39	30
35	2.69	2.64	2.60	2.56	2.53	2.50	2.47	2.44	2.40	2.36	2.33	2.31	2.28	35
40	2.61	2.56	2.52	2.48	2.45	2.42	2.39	2.37	2.33	2.29	2.26	2.23	2.20	40
45	2.55	2.51	2.46	2.43	2.39	2.36	2.34	2.31	2.27	2.23	2.20	2.17	2.14	45
50	2.51	2.46	2.42	2.38	2.35	2.32	2.29	2.27	2.22	2.18	2.15	2.12	2.10	50
60	2.44	2.39	2.35	2.31	2.28	2.25	2.22	2.20	2.15	2.12	2.08	2.05	2.03	60
70	2.40	2.35	2.31	2.27	2.23	2.20	2.18	2.15	2.11	2.07	2.03	2.01	1.98	70
80	2.36	2.31	2.27	2.23	2.20	2.17	2.14	2.12	2.07	2.03	2.00	1.97	1.94	80
100	2.31	2.27	2.22	2.19	2.15	2.12	2.09	2.07	2.02	1.98	1.95	1.92	1.89	100
200	2.22	2.17	2.13	2.09	2.06	2.03	2.00	1.97	1.93	1.89	1.85	1.82	1.79	200
500	2.17	2.12	2.07	2.04	2.00	1.97	1.94	1.92	1.87	1.83	1.79	1.76	1.74	500
1000	2.15	2.10	2.06	2.02	1.98	1.95	1.92	1.90	1.85	1.81	1.77	1.74	1.72	1000
>1000	2.13	2.08	2.04	2.00	1.97	1.94	1.91	1.88	1.83	1.79	1.76	1.73	1.70	>1000
n_1/n_2	13	14	15	16	17	18	19	20	22	24	26	28	30	n_1/n_2

n_1/n_2	35	40	45	50	60	70	80	100	200	500	1000	>1000	n_1/n_2
3	26.45	26.41	26.38	26.35	26.32	26.29	26.27	26.24	26.18	26.15	26.13	26.15	3
4	13.79	13.75	13.71	13.69	13.65	13.63	13.61	13.58	13.52	13.49	13.47	13.47	4
5	9.33	9.29	9.26	9.24	9.20	9.18	9.16	9.13	9.08	9.04	9.03	9.02	5
6	7.18	7.14	7.11	7.09	7.06	7.03	7.01	6.99	6.93	6.90	6.89	6.89	6
7	5.94	5.91	5.88	5.86	5.82	5.80	5.78	5.75	5.70	5.67	5.66	5.65	7
8	5.15	5.12	5.09	5.07	5.03	5.01	4.99	4.96	4.91	4.88	4.87	4.86	8
9	4.60	4.57	4.54	4.52	4.48	4.46	4.44	4.42	4.36	4.33	4.32	4.32	9
10	4.20	4.17	4.14	4.12	4.08	4.06	4.04	4.01	3.96	3.93	3.92	3.91	10
11	3.89	3.86	3.83	3.81	3.78	3.75	3.73	3.71	3.66	3.62	3.61	3.60	11
12	3.65	3.62	3.59	3.57	3.54	3.51	3.49	3.47	3.41	3.38	3.37	3.36	12
13	3.46	3.43	3.40	3.38	3.34	3.32	3.30	3.27	3.22	3.19	3.18	3.17	13
14	3.30	3.27	3.24	3.22	3.18	3.16	3.14	3.11	3.06	3.03	3.01	3.01	14
15	3.17	3.13	3.10	3.08	3.05	3.02	3.00	2.98	2.92	2.89	2.88	2.87	15
16	3.05	3.02	2.99	2.97	2.93	2.91	2.89	2.86	2.81	2.78	2.76	2.75	16
17	2.96	2.92	2.89	2.87	2.83	2.81	2.79	2.76	2.71	2.68	2.66	2.65	17
18	2.87	2.84	2.81	2.78	2.75	2.72	2.71	2.68	2.62	2.59	2.58	2.57	18
19	2.80	2.76	2.73	2.71	2.67	2.65	2.63	2.60	2.55	2.51	2.50	2.49	19
20	2.73	2.69	2.67	2.64	2.61	2.58	2.56	2.54	2.48	2.44	2.43	2.42	20
22	2.62	2.58	2.55	2.53	2.50	2.47	2.45	2.42	2.36	2.33	2.32	2.31	22
24	2.53	2.49	2.46	2.44	2.40	2.38	2.36	2.33	2.27	2.24	2.22	2.21	24
26	2.45	2.42	2.39	2.36	2.33	2.30	2.28	2.25	2.19	2.16	2.14	2.13	26
28	2.39	2.35	2.32	2.30	2.26	2.24	2.22	2.19	2.13	2.09	2.08	2.07	28
30	2.34	2.30	2.27	2.25	2.21	2.18	2.16	2.13	2.07	2.03	2.02	2.01	30
35	2.23	2.19	2.16	2.14	2.10	2.07	2.05	2.02	1.96	1.92	1.90	1.89	35
40	2.15	2.11	2.08	2.06	2.02	1.99	1.97	1.94	1.87	1.83	1.82	1.81	40
45	2.09	2.05	2.02	2.00	1.96	1.93	1.91	1.88	1.81	1.77	1.75	1.74	45
50	2.05	2.01	1.97	1.95	1.91	1.88	1.86	1.82	1.76	1.71	1.70	1.69	50
60	1.98	1.94	1.90	1.88	1.84	1.81	1.78	1.75	1.68	1.63	1.62	1.60	60
70	1.93	1.89	1.85	1.83	1.78	1.75	1.73	1.70	1.62	1.57	1.56	1.54	70
80	1.89	1.85	1.82	1.79	1.75	1.71	1.69	1.65	1.58	1.53	1.51	1.50	80
100	1.84	1.80	1.76	1.74	1.69	1.66	1.63	1.60	1.52	1.47	1.45	1.43	100
200	1.74	1.69	1.66	1.63	1.58	1.55	1.52	1.48	1.39	1.33	1.30	1.28	200
500	1.68	1.63	1.60	1.57	1.52	1.48	1.45	1.41	1.31	1.23	1.20	1.17	500
1000	1.66	1.61	1.58	1.54	1.50	1.46	1.43	1.38	1.28	1.19	1.16	1.12	1000
>1000	1.64	1.59	1.56	1.53	1.48	1.44	1.41	1.36	1.25	1.16	1.11	1.05	>1000
n_1/n_2	35	40	45	50	60	70	80	100	200	500	1000	>1000	n_1/n_2

TABLE A.5 Critical Values of Chi-Square

Level of significance

df	0.995	0.99	0.975	0.95	0.90	0.10	0.05	0.025	0.01	0.005
1	—	—	0.001	0.004	0.016	2.706	3.841	5.024	6.635	7.879
2	0.010	0.020	0.051	0.103	0.211	4.605	5.991	7.378	9.210	10.597
3	0.072	0.115	0.216	0.352	0.584	6.251	7.815	9.348	11.345	12.838
4	0.207	0.297	0.484	0.711	1.064	7.779	9.488	11.143	13.277	14.860
5	0.412	0.554	0.831	1.145	1.610	9.236	11.070	12.833	15.086	16.750
6	0.676	0.872	1.237	1.635	2.204	10.645	12.592	14.449	16.812	18.548
7	0.989	1.239	1.690	2.167	2.833	12.017	14.067	16.013	18.475	20.278
8	1.344	1.646	2.180	2.733	3.490	13.362	15.507	17.535	20.090	21.955
9	1.735	2.088	2.700	3.325	4.168	14.684	16.919	19.023	21.666	23.589
10	2.156	2.558	3.247	3.940	4.865	15.987	18.307	20.483	23.209	25.188
11	2.603	3.053	3.816	4.575	5.578	17.275	19.675	21.920	24.725	26.757
12	3.074	3.571	4.404	5.226	6.304	18.549	21.026	23.337	26.217	28.300
13	3.565	4.107	5.009	5.892	7.042	19.812	22.362	24.736	27.688	29.819
14	4.075	4.660	5.629	6.571	7.790	21.064	23.685	26.119	29.141	31.319
15	4.601	5.229	6.262	7.261	8.547	22.307	24.996	27.488	30.578	32.801
16	5.142	5.812	6.908	7.962	9.312	23.542	26.296	28.845	32.000	34.267
17	5.697	6.408	7.564	8.672	10.085	24.769	27.587	30.191	33.409	35.718
18	6.265	7.015	8.231	9.390	10.865	25.989	28.869	31.526	34.805	37.156
19	6.844	7.633	8.907	10.117	11.651	27.204	30.144	32.852	36.191	38.582
20	7.434	8.260	9.591	10.851	12.443	28.412	31.410	34.170	37.566	39.997
21	8.034	8.897	10.283	11.591	13.240	29.615	32.671	35.479	38.932	41.401
22	8.643	9.542	10.982	12.338	14.041	30.813	33.924	36.781	40.289	42.796
23	9.260	10.196	11.689	13.091	14.848	32.007	35.172	38.076	41.638	44.181
24	9.886	10.856	12.401	13.848	15.659	33.196	36.415	39.364	42.980	45.559
25	10.520	11.524	13.120	14.611	16.473	34.382	37.652	40.646	44.314	46.928
26	11.160	12.198	13.844	15.379	17.292	35.563	38.885	41.923	45.642	48.290
27	11.808	12.879	14.573	16.151	18.114	36.741	40.113	43.195	46.963	49.645

28	12.461	13.565	15.308	16.928	18.939	37.916	41.337	44.461	48.278	50.993
29	13.121	14.256	16.047	17.708	19.768	39.087	42.557	45.722	49.588	52.336
30	13.787	14.953	16.791	18.493	20.599	40.256	43.773	46.979	50.892	53.672
40	20.707	22.164	24.433	26.509	29.051	51.805	55.758	59.342	63.691	66.766
50	27.991	29.707	32.357	34.764	37.689	63.167	67.505	71.420	76.154	79.490
60	35.534	37.485	40.482	43.188	46.459	74.397	79.082	83.298	88.379	91.952
70	43.275	45.442	48.758	51.739	55.329	85.527	90.531	95.023	100.425	104.215
80	51.172	53.540	57.153	60.391	64.278	96.578	101.879	106.629	112.329	116.321
90	59.196	61.754	65.647	69.126	73.291	107.565	113.145	118.136	124.116	128.299
100	67.328	70.065	74.222	77.929	82.358	118.498	124.342	129.561	135.807	140.169

Probability under H_0 that $\chi^2 \geq \chi_\alpha^2$.

TABLE A.6   Critical Values of the Correlation Coefficient

	Level of Significance for Two-Tailed Test			
df $(n-2)$	0.10	0.05	0.02	0.01
1	0.988	0.997	0.9995	0.9999
2	0.900	0.950	0.980	0.990
3	0.805	0.878	0.934	0.959
4	0.729	0.811	0.882	0.917
5	0.669	0.754	0.833	0.874
6	0.622	0.707	0.789	0.834
7	0.582	0.666	0.750	0.798
8	0.549	0.632	0.716	0.765
9	0.521	0.602	0.685	0.735
10	0.497	0.576	0.658	0.708
11	0.476	0.553	0.634	0.684
12	0.458	0.532	0.612	0.661
13	0.441	0.514	0.592	0.641
14	0.426	0.497	0.574	0.623
15	0.412	0.482	0.558	0.606
16	0.400	0.468	0.542	0.590
17	0.389	0.456	0.528	0.575
18	0.378	0.444	0.516	0.561
19	0.369	0.433	0.503	0.549
20	0.36	0.423	0.492	0.537
21	0.352	0.413	0.482	0.526
22	0.344	0.404	0.472	0.515
23	0.337	0.396	0.462	0.505
24	0.33	0.388	0.453	0.496
25	0.323	0.381	0.445	0.487
26	0.317	0.374	0.437	0.479
27	0.311	0.367	0.430	0.471
28	0.306	0.361	0.423	0.463
29	0.301	0.355	0.416	0.456
30	0.296	0.349	0.409	0.449
35	0.275	0.325	0.381	0.418
40	0.257	0.304	0.358	0.393
45	0.243	0.288	0.338	0.372
50	0.231	0.273	0.322	0.354
60	0.211	0.25	0.295	0.325
70	0.195	0.232	0.274	0.303
80	0.183	0.217	0.256	0.283
90	0.173	0.205	0.242	0.267
100	0.164	0.195	0.230	0.254
df $(n-2)$	0.050	0.250	0.010	0.005
	Level of significance for one-tailed test			

TABLE A.7 Critical Values of Studentized Range Distribution (q) for Family-wise ALPHA = 0.05

Denominator DF	Number of Groups (Treatments)							
	3	4	5	6	7	8	9	10
1	26.98	32.82	37.08	40.41	43.12	45.40	47.36	49.07
2	8.33	9.80	10.88	11.73	12.43	13.03	13.54	13.99
3	5.91	6.83	7.50	8.04	8.48	8.85	9.18	9.46
4	5.04	5.76	6.29	6.71	7.05	7.35	7.60	7.83
5	4.60	5.22	5.67	6.03	6.33	6.58	6.80	7.00
6	4.34	4.90	5.31	5.63	5.90	6.12	6.32	6.49
7	4.17	4.68	0.06	5.36	5.61	5.82	6.00	6.16
8	4.04	4.53	4.89	5.17	5.40	5.60	5.77	5.92
9	3.95	4.42	4.76	5.02	5.24	5.43	5.60	5.74
10	3.88	4.33	4.65	4.91	5.12	5.30	5.46	5.60
11	3.82	4.26	4.57	4.82	5.03	5.20	5.35	5.49
12	3.77	4.20	4.51	4.75	4.95	5.12	5.26	5.40
13	3.73	4.15	4.45	4.69	4.88	5.05	5.19	5.32
14	3.70	4.11	4.41	4.64	4.83	4.99	5.13	5.25
15	3.67	4.08	4.37	4.60	4.78	4.94	5.08	5.20
16	3.65	4.05	4.33	4.56	4.74	4.90	5.03	5.15
17	3.63	4.02	4.30	4.52	4.71	4.86	4.99	5.11
18	3.61	4.00	4.28	4.49	4.67	4.82	4.96	5.07
19	3.59	3.98	4.25	4.47	4.65	4.79	4.92	5.04
20	3.58	3.96	4.23	4.45	4.62	4.77	4.90	5.01
21	3.57	3.94	4.21	4.42	4.60	4.74	4.87	4.98
22	3.55	3.93	4.20	4.41	4.58	4.72	4.85	4.96
23	3.54	3.91	4.18	4.39	4.56	4.70	4.83	4.94
24	3.53	3.90	4.17	4.37	4.54	4.68	4.81	4.92
25	3.52	3.89	4.15	4.36	4.53	4.67	4.79	4.90
26	3.51	3.88	4.14	4.35	4.51	4.65	4.77	4.88
27	3.51	3.87	4.13	4.33	4.50	4.64	4.76	4.86
28	3.50	3.86	4.12	4.32	4.49	4.63	4.75	4.85
29	3.49	3.85	4.11	4.31	4.48	4.61	4.73	4.84
30	3.49	3.85	4.10	4.30	4.46	4.60	4.72	4.82
31	3.48	3.84	4.09	4.29	4.45	4.59	4.71	4.81
32	3.48	3.83	4.09	4.28	4.45	4.58	4.70	4.80
33	3.47	3.83	4.08	4.28	4.44	4.57	4.69	4.79
34	3.47	3.82	4.07	4.27	4.43	4.56	4.68	4.78
35	3.46	3.81	4.07	4.26	4.42	4.56	4.67	4.77
36	3.46	3.81	4.06	4.26	4.41	4.55	4.66	4.76
37	3.45	3.80	4.05	4.25	4.41	4.54	4.66	4.76
38	3.45	3.80	4.05	4.24	4.40	4.53	4.65	4.75
39	3.45	3.80	4.04	4.24	4.39	4.53	4.64	4.74
40	3.44	3.79	4.04	4.23	4.39	4.52	4.63	4.74
41	3.44	3.79	4.04	4.23	4.38	4.52	4.63	4.73
42	3.44	3.78	4.03	4.22	4.38	4.51	4.62	4.72

(*Continued*)

TABLE A.7   (continued)

Denominator DF	Number of Groups (Treatments)							
	3	4	5	6	7	8	9	10
43	3.43	3.78	4.03	4.22	4.37	4.50	4.62	4.72
44	3.43	3.78	4.02	4.21	4.37	4.50	4.61	4.71
45	3.43	3.77	4.02	4.21	4.36	4.49	4.61	4.71
46	3.43	3.77	4.02	4.21	4.36	4.49	4.60	4.70
47	3.42	3.77	4.01	4.20	4.36	4.49	4.60	4.70
48	3.42	3.76	4.01	4.20	4.35	4.48	4.59	4.69
49	3.42	3.76	4.01	4.19	4.35	4.48	4.59	4.69
50	3.42	3.76	4.00	4.19	4.34	4.47	4.58	4.68
51	3.41	3.76	4.00	4.19	4.34	4.47	4.58	4.68
52	3.41	3.75	4.00	4.18	4.34	4.47	4.58	4.67
53	3.41	3.75	3.99	4.18	4.33	4.46	4.57	4.67
54	3.41	3.75	3.99	4.18	4.33	4.46	4.57	4.67
55	3.41	3.75	3.99	4.18	4.33	4.46	4.57	4.66
56	3.41	3.75	3.99	4.17	4.33	4.45	4.56	4.66
57	3.40	3.74	3.98	4.17	4.32	4.45	4.56	4.66
58	3.40	3.74	3.98	4.17	4.32	4.45	4.56	4.65
59	3.40	3.74	3.98	4.17	4.32	4.44	4.55	4.65
60	3.40	3.74	3.98	4.16	4.31	4.44	4.55	4.65
61	3.40	3.74	3.98	4.16	4.31	4.44	4.55	4.64
62	3.40	3.73	3.97	4.16	4.31	4.44	4.55	4.64
63	3.40	3.73	3.97	4.16	4.31	4.43	4.54	4.64
64	3.39	3.73	3.97	4.16	4.31	4.43	4.54	4.64
65	3.39	3.73	3.97	4.15	4.30	4.43	4.54	4.63
66	3.39	3.73	3.97	4.15	4.30	4.43	4.54	4.63
67	3.39	3.73	3.97	4.15	4.30	4.43	4.53	4.63
68	3.39	3.73	3.96	4.15	4.30	4.42	4.53	4.63
69	3.39	3.72	3.96	4.15	4.30	4.42	4.53	4.62
70	3.39	3.72	3.96	4.14	4.29	4.42	4.53	4.62
71	3.39	3.72	3.96	4.14	4.29	4.42	4.53	4.62
72	3.38	3.72	3.96	4.14	4.29	4.42	4.52	4.62
73	3.38	3.72	3.96	4.14	4.29	4.41	4.52	4.62
74	3.38	3.72	3.95	4.14	4.29	4.41	4.52	4.61
75	3.38	3.72	3.95	4.14	4.29	4.41	4.52	4.61
76	3.38	3.72	3.95	4.14	4.28	4.41	4.52	4.61
77	3.38	3.71	3.95	4.13	4.28	4.41	4.51	4.61
78	3.38	3.71	3.95	4.13	4.28	4.41	4.51	4.61
79	3.38	3.71	3.95	4.13	4.28	4.40	4.51	4.60
80	3.38	3.71	3.95	4.13	4.28	4.40	4.51	4.60
81	3.38	3.71	3.95	4.13	4.28	4.40	4.51	4.60
82	3.38	3.71	3.95	4.13	4.28	4.40	4.51	4.60
83	3.38	3.71	3.94	4.13	4.27	4.40	4.50	4.60
84	3.37	3.71	3.94	4.13	4.27	4.40	4.50	4.60
85	3.37	3.71	3.94	4.12	4.27	4.40	4.50	4.60
86	3.37	3.71	3.94	4.12	4.27	4.39	4.50	4.59

TABLE A.7   (continued)

Denominator DF	Number of Groups (Treatments)							
	3	4	5	6	7	8	9	10
87	3.37	3.70	3.94	4.12	4.27	4.39	4.50	4.59
88	3.37	3.70	3.94	4.12	4.27	4.39	4.50	4.59
89	3.37	3.70	3.94	4.12	4.27	4.39	4.50	4.59
90	3.37	3.70	3.94	4.12	4.27	4.39	4.50	4.59
91	3.37	3.70	3.94	4.12	4.26	4.39	4.49	4.59
92	3.37	3.70	3.94	4.12	4.26	4.39	4.49	4.59
93	3.37	3.70	3.93	4.12	4.26	4.39	4.49	4.59
94	3.37	3.70	3.93	4.11	4.26	4.38	4.49	4.58
95	3.37	3.70	3.93	4.11	4.26	4.38	4.49	4.58
96	3.37	3.70	3.93	4.11	4.26	4.38	4.49	4.58
97	3.37	3.70	3.93	4.11	4.26	4.38	4.49	4.58
98	3.37	3.70	3.93	4.11	4.26	4.38	4.49	4.58
99	3.37	3.70	3.93	4.11	4.26	4.38	4.49	4.58
100	3.37	3.70	3.93	4.11	4.26	4.38	4.48	4.58

BIBLIOGRAPHY

Agresti, A. (2002). *Categorical data analysis*, 2nd ed. New York: John Wiley & Sons, Inc.

Agresti, A. (2007). *An introduction to categorical data analysis*, 2nd ed. Hoboken, NJ: John Wiley & Sons, Inc.

Allison, P. D. (2001). *Missing data*. Thousand Oaks, CA: SAGE.

Anderson, T. W. (2003). *Introduction to multivariate statistical analysis*, 3rd ed. Hoboken, NJ: John Wiley & Sons, Inc.

Anderson, J. C., Gebing, D. W., and Hunter, J. E. (1987). "On the assessment of unidimensional measurement: Internal and external consistency and overall consistency criteria." *Journal of Marketing Research* 24 (November): 432–437.

Armstrong, J. S. (2012). "Illusions in regression analysis." *International Journal of Forecasting (forthcoming)* 28 (3): 689. doi:10.1016/j.ijforecast.2012.02.001.

Babbie, E. (2007). *The practice of social research*, 11th ed. Belmont, CA: Thompson Wadsworth. pp. 87–89.

Bagdonavicius, V., Kruopis, J., and Nikulin, M. S. (2011). *Non-parametric tests for complete data*. London: ISTE & Wiley. ISBN 978-1-84821-269-5.

Baguley, T. (2012). *Serious stats: A guide to advanced statistics for the behavioral sciences*. Basingstoke: Palgrave Macmillan. p. 281. ISBN 9780230363557.

Bailey, R. A. (2008). *Design of comparative experiments*. Cambridge, UK: Cambridge University Press. ISBN 978-0-521-68357-9. Pre-publication chapters are available on-line.

Bakeman, R. (2005). "Recommended effect size statistics for repeated measures designs." *Behavior Research Methods* 37 (3): 379–384. doi:10.3758/bf03192707.

Sports Research with Analytical Solution using SPSS®, First Edition. J. P. Verma.
© 2016 John Wiley & Sons, Inc. Published 2016 by John Wiley & Sons, Inc.
Companion website: www.wiley.com/go/Verma/Sportsresearch

Bandalos, D. L. and Boehm-Kaufman, M. R. (2008). "Four common misconceptions in exploratory factor analysis." In Lance, C. E. and Vandenberg, R. J. (eds.), *Statistical and methodological myths and urban legends: Doctrine, verity and fable in the organizational and social sciences*. New York: Taylor & Francis. pp. 61–87. ISBN 978-0-8058-6237-9.

Bartholomew, D. J., Steele, F., Galbraith, J., and Moustaki, I. (2008). *Analysis of multivariate social science data*, 2nd ed. Boca Raton, FL: Taylor & Francis. Statistics in the Social and Behavioral Sciences Series. ISBN 1584889608.

Beebee, H., Hitchcock, C., and Menzies, P. (2009). *The Oxford handbook of causation*. Oxford: Oxford University Press. ISBN 978-0-19-162946-4.

Blair, R. C. and Higgins, J. J. (1980). "A comparison of the power of Wilcoxon's rank-sum statistic to that of Student's t statistic under various nonnormal distributions." *Journal of Educational Statistics* 5 (4): 309–335. doi:10.2307/1164905. JSTOR 1164905.

Bobko, P. (2001). *Correlation and regression*, 2nd ed. Thousand Oaks, CA: SAGE. Introductory text which includes coverage of range restriction, trivariate correlation.

Bock, R. D. (1975). *Multivariate statistical methods in behavioral research*. New York: McGraw Hill.

Borgatta, E. F., Kercher, K., and Stull, D. E. (1986). "A cautionary note on the use of principal components analysis." *Sociological Methods and Research* 15: 160–168.

Bryant, F. B. and Yarnold, P. R. (1995). Principal components analysis and exploratory and confirmatory factor analysis. In Grimm, L. G. and Yarnold, P. R. (eds.), *Reading and understanding multivariate analysis*. Washington, DC: American Psychological Association.

Carroll, J. D., Green, P. E., and Chaturvedi, A. (1997). *Mathematical tools for applied multivariate analysis*, 2nd ed. New York: Academic Press.

Chen, P. Y. and Popovich, P. M. (2002). *Correlation: Parametric and nonparametric measures*. Thousand Oaks, CA: SAGE. Covers tests of difference between two dependent correlations, and the difference between more than two independent correlations.

Cliff, N. (1987). *Analyzing multivariate data*. San Diego, CA: Harcourt Brace Jovanovich.

Cohen, J., West, S. G., Aiken, L., and Cohen, P. (2002). *Applied multiple regression/correlation analysis for the behavioral sciences*, 3rd ed. Hillsdale, NJ: Lawrence Erlbaum Associates.

Conover, W. J. (1980). *Practical nonparametric statistics*, 2nd ed. New York: John Wiley & Sons, Inc.

Cooley, W. W. and Lohnes, P. R. (1971). *Multivariate data analysis*. New York: John Wiley & Sons, Inc.

Corder, G. W. and Foreman, D. I. (2014). *Nonparametric statistics: A step-by-step approach*. Hoboken, NJ: John Wiley & Sons, Inc. ISBN 978-1118840313.

Cox, D. R. (1958). "The regression analysis of binary sequences (with discussion)." *Journal of the Royal Statistical Society. Series B* 20: 215–242.

Cox, D. R. (2006). *Principles of statistical inference*. Cambridge, UK: Cambridge University Press. ISBN 978-0-521-68567-2.

Darlington, R. B., Weinberg, S., and Walberg, H. (1973). "Canonical variate analysis and related techniques." *Review of Educational Research* 43 (4): 453–454.

David, H. A. and Gunnink, J. L. (1997). "The paired t test under artificial pairing." *The American Statistician* 51 (1): 9–12. doi:10.2307/2684684. JSTOR 2684684.

Dillon, W. R. and Goldstein, M. (1984). *Multivariate analysis: Methods and applications.* New York: John Wiley & Sons, Inc.

Duncan, T. E., Omen, R., and Duncan, S. C. (1994). "Modeling incomplete data in exercise behavior using structural equation methodology." *Journal of Sport and Exercise Psychology* 16: 187–205.

Dunteman, G. H. (1984). *Introduction to multivariate analysis.* Thousand Oaks, CA: SAGE. Chapter 5 covers classification procedures and discriminant analysis.

Dunteman, G. H. (1989). *Principal components analysis.* Thousand Oaks, CA: SAGE. Quantitative Applications in the Social Sciences Series, No. 69.

Fabrigar, L. R., Wegener, D. T., MacCallum, R. C., and Strahan, E. J. (1999). "Evaluating the use of exploratory factor analysis in psychological research." *Psychological Methods* 4 (3): 272–299.

Fagerland, M. W. (2012). "t-Tests, non-parametric tests, and large studies—a paradox of statistical practice?" *BioMed Central Medical Research Methodology* 12: 78. doi:10.1186/1471-2288-12-78.

Fay, M. P. and Proschan, M. A. (2010). "Wilcoxon–Mann–Whitney or t-test? On assumptions for hypothesis tests and multiple interpretations of decision rules." *Statistics Surveys* 4: 1–39. doi:10.1214/09-SS051. PMC 2857732. PMID 20414472.

Flury, B. (1997). *A first course in multivariate statistics.* New York: Springer.

Freedman, D. A. (2005). *Statistical models: Theory and practice.* Cambridge, UK: Cambridge University Press. ISBN 978-0-521-67105-7.

Freedman, D. A. (2009). *Statistical models: Theory and practice.* Cambridge, UK: Cambridge University Press. p. 128.

Glantz, S. A. and Slinker, B. K. (2001). *Primer of applied regression & analysis of variance,* 2nd ed. New York: McGraw-Hill.

Gnanedesikan, R. (1977). *Methods for statistical analysis of multivariate distributions.* New York: John Wiley & Sons, Inc.

Good, P. I. and Hardin, J. W. (2009). *Common errors in statistics (and how to avoid them),* 3rd ed. Hoboken, NJ: John Wiley & Sons, Inc. p. 211. ISBN 978-0-470-45798-6.

Gorsuch, R. L. (1983). *Factor analysis.* Hillsdale, NJ: Lawrence Erlbaum. Original ed. 1974.

Green, P. E. (1978). *Analyzing multivariate data.* Hinsdale, IL: Holt, Rinehart and Winston.

Green, P. E. and Carroll, J. D. (1978). *Mathematical tools for applied multivariate analysis.* New York: Academic Press.

Green, S. B. and Salkind, N. J. (2008). *Using SPSS for Windows and Macintosh: Analyzing and understanding data,* 6th ed. Boston, MA: Prentice Hall. ISBN 978-0-205-02040-9.

Gueorguieva, R. and Krystal, J. H. (2004). "Move over ANOVA: Progress in analyzing repeated-measures data and its reflection in papers published in the Archives of General Psychiatry." *Archives of General Psychiatry* 61: 310–317. doi:10.1001/archpsyc.61.3.310.

Hair, J. F., Jr., Anderson, R. E., Tatham, R. L., and Black, W. C. (1998). *Multivariate data analysis with readings,* 5th ed. Englewood Cliffs, NJ: Prentice-Hall.

Hand, D. J. and Taylor, C. C. (1987). *Multivariate analysis of variance and repeated measures.* London: Chapman & Hall.

Harrell, F. E. (2001). *Regression modeling strategies.* New York: Springer-Verlag. ISBN 0-387-95232-2.

Hellevik, O. (1988). *Introduction to causal analysis: Exploring survey data by cross-tabulation*, 2nd ed. New York: Oxford University Press. Contemporary Social Research Series, No. 9.

Hinkelmann, K. and Kempthorne, O. (2008). *Design and analysis of experiments*, Vols. I and II, 2nd ed. Hoboken, NJ: John Wiley & Sons, Inc. ISBN 978-0-470-38551-7.

Hollander, M., Wolfe, D. A., and Chicken, E. (2014). *Nonparametric statistical methods*. Hoboken, NJ: John Wiley & Sons, Inc.

Hopkins, W. G. (2000). "Quantitative research design." *Sportscience* (1). http://sportsci.org/jour/0001/wghdesign.html (accessed September 24, 2015).

Hopkins, W. G. (2008). "Research designs: Choosing and fine-tuning a design for your study." *Sportscience* 12: 12–21.

Howell, D. C. (2002). *Statistical methods for psychology*, 5th ed. Pacific Grove, CA: Duxbury/Thomson Learning. ISBN 0-534-37770-X.

http://evolutionarymedia.com/cgi-bin/wiki.cgi?StatisticalMethods (accessed September 24, 2015).

http://people.richland.edu/james/lecture/m170/tbl-chi.html (accessed September 24, 2015).

http://www.ma.utexas.edu/users/davis/375/popecol/tables/f005.html (accessed September 24, 2015).

http://www.sjsu.edu/faculty/gerstman/StatPrimer/t-table.pdf (accessed September 24, 2015).

http://www.statisticssolutions.com/methods-chapter/statistical-tests/factor-analysis/ (accessed September 24, 2015).

Hubert, C. J. and Morris, J. D. (1989). Multivariate analysis versus multiple univariate analyses. *Psychological Bulletin* 105 (2): 302–308.

Huberty, C. J. (1984). Issues in the use and interpretation of discriminant analysis. *Psychological Bulletin* 95 (1): 156–171.

Huberty, C. J. (1994). *Applied discriminant analysis*. New York: Wiley-Interscience. Wiley Series in Probability and Statistics.

Huitema, B. (1980). *The analysis of covariance and alternatives*. New York: John Wiley & Sons, Inc.

Hutcheson, G., & Sofroniou, N. (1999). *The multivariate social scientist: Introductory statistics using generalized linear models*. Thousand Oaks, CA: SAGE.

Jaccard, J. and Wan, C. K. (1996). *LISREL approaches to interaction effects in multiple regression*. Thousand Oaks, CA: SAGE.

Johnson, R. A. and Wichern, D. W. (2002). *Applied multivariate statistical analysis*, 5th ed. Upper Saddle River, NJ: Prentice Hall.

Kaiser, H. F. (1960). "The application of electronic computers to factor analysis". *Educational and Psychological Measurement* 20: 141–151. doi:10.1177/001316446002000116.

Kempthorne, O. (1979). *The design and analysis of experiments (corrected reprint of (1952) Wiley ed.)*. Huntington, NY: Robert E. Krieger. ISBN 0-88275-105-0.

Kendall, M. G. (1980). *Multivariate analysis*, 2nd ed. London: Griffin.

Kim, J.-O. (1975). "Multivariate analysis of ordinal variables." *American Journal of Sociology* 81: 261–298.

Kim, J.-O. and Curry, J. (1977). "The treatment of missing data in multivariate analysis." *Sociological Methods and Research* 6: 215–241.

Kim, J.-O. and Mueller, C. W. (1978a). *Factor analysis: Statistical methods and practical issues*. Newbury Park, CA: SAGE. SAGE University Paper Series on Quantitative Applications in the Social Sciences Series, No. 07-014.

Kim, J.-O. and Mueller, C. W. (1978b). *Introduction to factor analysis: What it is and how to do it*. Newbury Park, CA: SAGE.

Kirk, R. E. (1994). *Experimental design: Procedures for the behavioral sciences*, 3rd ed. Belmont, CA: Wadsworth Publishing.

Klecka, W. R. (1980). *Discriminant analysis*. Thousand Oaks, CA: SAGE. Quantitative Applications in the Social Sciences Series, No. 19.

Kreuger, C. and Tian, L. (2004). "A comparison of the general linear mixed model and repeated measures ANOVA using a dataset with multiple missing data points." *Biological Research for Nursing* 6: 151–157. doi:10.1177/1099800404267682.

Kruskal, W. H. and Wallis, W. A. (1952). "Use of ranks in one-criterion variance analysis." *Journal of the American Statistical Association* 47 (260): 583–621. doi:10.1080/01621459.1952.10483441.

Labovitz, S. (1970). "The assignment of numbers to rank order categories." *American Sociological Review* 35: 515–524.

Lachenbruch, P. A. (1975). *Discriminant analysis*. New York: Hafner. For detailed notes on computations.

Lance, C. E., Butts, M. M., and Michels, L. C. (2006). "The sources of four commonly reported cutoff criteria: What did they really say?" *Organizational Research Methods* 9 (2): 202–220. Discusses Kaiser and other criteria for selecting number of factors.

Lawley, D. N. and Maxwell, A. E. (1962). "Factor analysis as a statistical method." *The Statistician* 12 (3): 209–229.

Lawley, D. N. and Maxwell, A. E. (1971). *Factor analysis as a statistical method*. London: Butterworth and Co.

Lebart, L., Morineau, A. and Warwick, K. M. (1984). *Multivariate descriptive statistical analysis*. New York: John Wiley & Sons, Inc.

Lee, J. (1994). "Odds ratio or relative risk for cross-sectional data?" *International Journal of Epidemiology* 23 (1): 201–203. doi:10.1093/ije/23.1.201. PMID 8194918.

Lehmann, E. L. and Romano, J. P. (2005). *Testing statistical hypotheses*, 3rd ed. New York: Springer. ISBN 0-387-98864-5.

Levine, M. S. (1977). *Canonical analysis and factor comparison*. Newbury Park, CA: SAGE.

Liebetrau, A. M. (1983). *Measures of association*. Newbury Park, CA: SAGE. Quantitative Applications in the Social Sciences Series, No. 32.

Little, R. J. A. and Rubin, D. B. (1987). *Statistical analysis with missing data*. New York: John Wiley & Sons, Inc.

Liu, I. and Agresti, A. (2005). "The analysis of ordered categorical data: An overview and a survey of recent developments." *TEST* 14: 1–73.

Mason, C. H. and Perreailt, W. D., Jr. (1991). "Collinearity, power, and interpretation of multiple regression analysis." *Journal of Marketing Research* 28 (August): 268–280.

Matthews, G., Deary, I. J., and Whiteman, M. C. (2003). *Personality traits*, 2nd ed. Cambridge: Cambridge University Press.

Menard, S. W. (2002). *Applied logistic regression*, 2nd ed. Thousand Oaks, CA: SAGE. pp. 7–106. ISBN 978-0-7619-2208-7.

Meyers, J. L. (1979). *Fundamentals of experimental design*. Boston, MA: Allyn & Bacon.

Montgomery, D. (2009). *Design and analysis of experiments*. Hoboken, NJ: John Wiley & Sons, Inc. ISBN 978-0-470-12866-4.

Moore, D. S. (1995). *The basic practice of statistics*. New York: W. H. Freeman

Morrison, D. F. (2002). *Multivariate statistical methods*, 4th ed. Belmont, CA: Duxbury Press.

Moses, L. E. (1952). "A two-sample test." *Psychometrika* 17: 239–247.

Mosteller, F. and Tukey, J. W. (1977). *Data analysis and regression*. Reading, MA: Addison-Wesley.

Muller, K. E. and Barton, C. N. (1989). "Approximate power for repeated-measures ANOVA lacking sphericity." *Journal of the American Statistical Association* 84 (406): 549–555. doi: 10.1080/01621459.1989.10478802.

Neter, J., Kutner, M. H., Nachtsheim, C. J., and Wasserman, W. (1996). *Applied linear statistical models*, 4th ed. Boston, MA: McGraw-Hill.

Norman, G. R. and Streiner, D. L. (1994). *Biostatistics: The bare essentials*. St. Louis, MO: Mosby.

Norušis, M. J. (2005). *SPSS 13.0 statistical procedures companion*. Chicago, IL: SPSS, Inc.

Olejnik, S. and Algina, J. (2003). "Generalized eta and omega squared statistics: Measures of effect size for some common research designs." *Psychological Methods* 8: 434–447. doi:10.1037/1082-989x.8.4.434.

Overall, J. E. and Klett, C. J. (1972). *Applied multivariate analysis*. New York: McGraw-Hill.

Park, T. (1993). "A comparison of the generalized estimating equation approach with the maximum likelihood approach for repeated measurements." *Statistics in Medicine* 12: 1723–1732. doi:10.1002/sim.4780121807.

Rice, J. A. (2006). *Mathematical statistics and data analysis*, 3rd ed. Belmont, CA: Duxbury Advanced.

Rohlf, F. J. and Sokal, R. R. (1995). *Statistical tables*, 3rd ed. New York: W. H. Freeman.

Roy, S. N. (1957). *Some aspects of multivariate analysis*. New York: John Wiley & Sons, Inc.

Rubin, D. B. (1987). *Multiple imputation for nonresponse in surveys*. New York: John Wiley & Sons, Inc.

Ruscio, J. and Roche, B. (2012). "Determining the number of factors to retain in an exploratory factor analysis using comparison data of known factorial structure." *Psychological Assessment* 24: 282–292. doi:10.1037/a0025697.

Russell, D. W. (2002). "In search of underlying dimensions: The use (and abuse) of factor analysis in Personality and Social Psychology Bulletin." *Personality and Social Psychology Bulletin* 28 (12): 1629–1646. doi:10.1177/014616702237645.

Ruxton, G. D. (2006). "The unequal variance t-test is an underused alternative to Student's t-test and the Mann–Whitney U test." *Behavioral Ecology* 17: 688–690. doi:10.1093/beheco/ark016.

Sawilowsky, S. S. (2005). "Misconceptions leading to choosing the t test over the Wilcoxon Mann–Whitney test for shift in location parameter." *Journal of Modern Applied Statistical Methods* 4 (2): 598–600.

Schafer, J. L. (1997). *Analysis of incomplete multivariate data*. London: Chapman & Hall. Chapman & Hall Series Monographs on Statistics and Applied Probability, Book No. 72.

Schmidt, C. O. and Kohlmann, T. (2008). "When to use the odds ratio or the relative risk?" *International Journal of Public Health* 53 (3): 165–167. doi:10.1007/s000-00-7068-3. PMID 19127890.

Shields, P. and Rangarjan, N. (2013). *A playbook for research methods: Integrating conceptual frameworks and project management*. Stillwater, OK: New Forums Press. See Chapter 4 for an extensive discussion of descriptive research.

Shuttleworth, M. (2009). "Repeated measures design". Experiment-resources.com. Retrieved September 2, 2013.

Siegel, S. and Castellan, N. J. (1988). *Nonparametric statistics for the behavioral sciences*, 2nd ed. New York: McGraw-Hill. Social Sciences Series, No. 19.

Srtevens, J. P. (1980). "Power of the multivariate analysis of variance tests." *Psychological Bulletin* 88:728–737.

Tabachnick, B. G. and Fidell, L. S. (2001). *Using multivariate statistics*, 4th ed. Boston, MA: Allyn & Bacon. Chapter 11 covers discriminant analysis.

Tatsuoka, M. M. (1988). *Multivariate analysis*, 2nd ed. New York: John Wiley & Sons, Inc.

Truett, J., Cornfield, J., and Kannel, W. (1967). "A multivariate analysis of the risk of coronary heart disease in Framingham." *Journal of Chronic Diseases* 20 (7): 511–524. PMID 6028270.

Van de Geer, J. P. (1971). *Introduction to multivariate analysis for the social sciences*. San Francisco, CA: W. H. Freeman.

Verma, J. P. (2014). *Statistics for exercise science and health with Microsoft Office Excel*. New York: John Wiley & Sons, Inc.

Verma, J. P. (2015). *Repeated measures design for empirical researchers*. New York: John Wiley & Sons, Inc.

Verma, J. P. (2013). *Data Analysis in Management with SPSS Software*. India: Springer.

Verma, J. P. (2012). *Statistics for Psychology*. India: Tata McGraw Hills.

Verma J. P. (2011). *Statistical Methods for Sports and Physical Education*. India: Tata McGraw Hill Higher Education.

Walker, S. H. and Duncan, D. B. (1967). "Estimation of the probability of an event as a function of several independent variables." *Biometrika* 54: 167–178.

Welch, B. L. (1947). "The generalization of 'Student's' problem when several different population variances are involved." *Biometrika* 34 (1–2): 28–35. doi:10.1093/biomet/34.1-2.28. MR 19277.

Widaman, K. F. (1993). "Common factor analysis versus principal component analysis: Differential bias in representing model parameters?" *Multivariate Behavioral Research* 28: 263–311. Cited with regard to preference for common factor analysis over PCA in confirmatory factor analysis in SEM.

Wildt, A. R. and Ahtola, O. T. (1978). *Analysis of covariance*. Thousand Oaks, CA: SAGE.

Wilkinson, L. (1975). "Tests of significance in stepwise regression." *Psychological Bulletin* 86: 168–174.

Wilson, T. (1971). "Critique of ordinal variables." In Blalock, H. M. (ed.), *Causal models in the social sciences*. Chicago, IL: Aldine. Ch. 24.

Yates, F. (1934). "Contingency table involving small numbers and the χ2 test." *Supplement to the Journal of the Royal Statistical Society* 1 (2): 217–235. JSTOR 2983604.

Zimmerman, D. W. (1997). "A note on interpretation of the paired-samples t test." *Journal of Educational and Behavioral Statistics* 22 (3): 349–360. doi:10.3102/10769986022003349. JSTOR 1165289.

Zumbo, B. D. and Zimmerman, D. W. (1993). "Is the selection of statistical methods governed by level of measurement?" *Canadian Psychology* 34: 390–399. Defends robustness of parametric techniques even when using ordinal data.

INDEX

Sports Research with Analytical Solution using SPSS®, First Edition. J. P. Verma.
© 2016 John Wiley & Sons, Inc. Published 2016 by John Wiley & Sons, Inc.
Companion website: www.wiley.com/go/Verma/Sportsresearch